Sue,
Never forget how
much we need you.

Springer Series on Social Work

Albert R. Roberts, PhD., Series Editor

Advisory Board: Gloria Bonilla-Santiago, PhD, Barbara Berkman, PhD, Elaine P. Congress, DSW, Gilbert J. Greene, PhD, Jesse Harris, DSW, C. Aaron McNeece, DSW

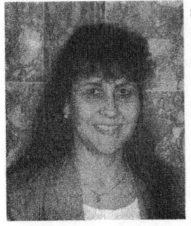

Sophia F. Dziegielewski, PhD, LCSW, is Professor in the School of Social Work, University of Cincinnati, Ohio. Prior to this appointment Dr. Dziegielewski was professor and co-chair of the Institutional Review Board, University of Central Florida, and in The University of Alabama, Tuscaloosa, AL; the Departments of Family and Preventive Medicine and Psychiatry at Meharry Medical College, Nashville, TN; The School of Social Work at the University of TN; and in the U.S. Army Military College stationed at Fort Benning, GA. Throughout her social work career she has been active in part-time clinical practice.

Educational qualifications include her MSW and PhD in Social Work from Florida State University, Tallahassee, FL. Among other numerous professional awards, in 1995 Dr. Dziegielewski was named Social Worker of the Year for the State of Tennessee by the National Association of Social Workers (NASW).

Her professional social work interests focus primarily on two major areas: time-limited empirically based practice and research. As a Licensed Clinical Social Worker she is firm on the importance of joining practice and research and applying measurement to establish treatment effectiveness in the short-term therapy setting. Her practice interest centers on the establishment of outcome-based treatments in the health care setting. Relying on experience in practice and research, she has served as the methodologist on numerous research and grant-writing projects. In addition, she has also conducted over 300 professional workshops and community presentations on implementing medical, and mental health-related counseling practices and strategies in today's managed care environment.

The Changing Face of Health Care Social Work

Professional Practice in Managed Behavioral Health Care

Second Edition

Sophia F. Dziegielewski, PhD, LCSW

with Contributors

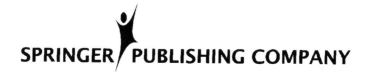

SPRINGER PUBLISHING COMPANY

SPRINGER/PUBLISHING COMPANY
11 West 42nd Street
New York, NY 10036-8002
www.springerpub.com

Acquisitions Editor: Sheri W. Sussman
Production Editor: Pamela Lankas
Cover design by Joanne Honigman

10 11 12 / 9 8 7

Library of Congress Cataloging-in-Publication Data

Dziegielewski, Sophia F.
    The changing face of health care social work : professional practice in managed behavioral health care / Sophia F. Dziegielewski. — 2nd ed.
        p. ; cm. – (Springer series on social work)
    Includes bibliographical references and index.
    ISBN 0-8261-8145-7   ISBN 13:   978-0-8261-8145-9
    1. Medical social work—United States—Methodology.   2. Managed care plans (Medical care)—United States.   3. Hospitals—Case management services—United States.   4. Hospitals—United States—Administration.   5. Social work administration—United States.   6. Medical care—Computer network resources.   I. Title.   II. Springer series on social work (Unnumbered).
    HV687.5.U5D95 2004
    362.1'0425—dc22

                                                                                            2003057356

Printed in the United States of America by Yurchak Printing, Inc.

In my life I have come to believe that intelligence consists of the knowledge that one acquires over a lifetime, wisdom, however, is far greater. Wisdom requires having intelligence but realizing that it means nothing if it is not shared. In wisdom there is a natural giving of the self to others, where there is no fear of loss. It means realizing that the knowledge we have is measured purely by what we can teach.

This book is dedicated to the memory of my earliest and wisest teachers, my mother and father, Mary and Joseph Dziegielewski, and my "other" parents, Winston and Esther Mooney.

This page intentionally left blank

Contents

**Part III   Fields of Clinical Social Work Practice
in Health Care Settings**

**Chapter 9   Practice of Social Work in Acute Health
Care Settings   243**
Sophia F. Dziegielewski and Diane Holliman

**Chapter 10   Long-Term Health Care and Restorative
Health Settings   267**

Part V   Conclusion

This page intentionally left blank

Foreword

There have been very few comprehensive and up-to-date books on health social work published in the past decade. Dr. Dziegielewski's second edition is not only the most comprehensive book in the field to date but is also the most informative, timely, and extremely well written. In the area of health care practice, managed behavioral health care, first introduced in the 1990s, presents a new type of evidence-based health care delivery. As Dr. Dziegielewski explicates in this valuable second edition of her text, health care social workers are expected to demonstrate that the services they provide are both time-limited and evidence-based. She is keenly aware of the importance of acknowledging this fact and warns that without this recognition health care social workers will remain at risk of being replaced by other health care professionals or paraprofessionals. The book is also quick to pinpoint how incremental changes can involve compromising service agreements that are based on the needs or wishes of various political forces. This makes the role of the social workers as patient and family advocate essential in ensuring quality service delivery in an era of cost containment. Health care workers must take an active role in ethical practice while advocating for social action and social change (Strom-Gottfried & Dunlap, 1999). This translates to advocacy that seeks to help society understand the needs of the client while controlling and regulating the health care industry. The chapters in the second section of the book highlight how these efforts at advocacy are further complicated by staff reductions and changes. To remain competitve, however, Dr. Dziegielewski states that health care social workers need to be flexible, open, and ready to embrace the future. Yet she warns that, even with the implementation of an evidence-based practice approach, the health care social worker should never lose sight of the ethical and moral judgment needed to steer the profession toward the betterment of the clients being served.

Overall, this book advocates for a proactive stance, whereas, to be considered effective and efficient traditional helping must go beyond just helping the client. For the health care worker, similar to other practice areas in social work, evidence-based practice must also clearly measure the concrete and identifiable therapeutic gains achieved, in the shortest amount of time. These interventions must be socially acknowledged as necessary and therapeutically effective utilizing individualized treatment protocols (Franklin, 2002).

This second edition of the book continues to acknowledge the dramatic changes that have occurred within the field. Each chapter is clear in outlining the current state of practice as well as discussing future trends and developments. This book explicates the fact that health care practice is focusing less on formalized inpatient acute, tertiary, and specialty/subspecialty care, and moving more toward ambulatory and community-based care (Rock, 2002). This requires that health care practitioners constantly battle "quality-of-care" issues versus "cost-containment" measures, while securing a firm place as professional providers in the health care environment.

In closing, Dr. Dziegielewski clearly highlights the role of the social worker as the professional "bridge" that links the client, the multidisciplinary or interdisciplinary team, and the environment. She advocates for a proactive stance, encouraging health care social workers to increase their accountability, documentation skills, discharge planning skills, marketability and competitive edge by moving beyond the traditional definition and subsequent roles occupied in the past. In this second edition, this book once again provides a realistic portrayal of the current state of affairs for the health care social worker while actively presenting a vision for the future.

This is the fifth book to be thoroughly revised into a second edition out of the 40 volumes in the Springer Series on Social Work, which began in 1984. We have come a long way in the social work profession in the past 20 years, and I am delighted to welcome this futuristic second edition.

Albert R. Roberts, PhD, Social Work Series Editor
Professor of Social Work and Criminal Justice
Director of Faculty Development
Faculty of Arts and Sciences,
Rutgers University
New Brunswick, New Jersey

REFERENCES

Franklin, C. (2002). Developing effective practice competencies in managed behavioral health care. In A. R. Roberts & G. J. Grene (Eds.) *Social workers' desk reference* (pp. 1–9). New York, N.Y.: Oxford University Press.

Rock, B. (2002). Social work in health care in the 21st Century. In A. R. Roberts & G. J. Greene (Eds.) *Social workers' desk reference* (pp. 10–16). New York: Oxford.

Strom-Gottfried, K., & Dunlap, K.M. (1999). Unraveling ethical dilemmas. *New Social Worker, 6(2),* 8–12.

This page intentionally left blank

Prologue

During the early years of the Clinton presidency "a radical, historic shift in society's health care process took place before our astonished eyes, driven totally by market forces and entirely outside regulatory management" (Nieves, 1998, p. xiii).

Dr. Dziegielewski clearly points out that the three legs on which our health care system currently stands (or wobbles as the case may be)—cost containment, access, and quality—are in perpetual conflict; she notes that we can get any two legs working together but not all three. Something is always lost in a health care system structured this way. This book suggests how social work services can be offered in health settings under these current conditions.

Dr. Dziegielewski provides systematic overviews of the activities that make up professional social work. She gives much-needed emphasis to the interactions between people and the social systems in which they live, and offers conceptual schemes for making sense of the intricacies of these interactions. She seeks to "provide a basis for the integration of basic clinical evidence-based practice strategy with a direct link to cost containment in the health care practice area."

Included in each chapter are examples of good social work practice, models of intervention and social work thinking based on real social workers and events that demonstrate where a social work administrator, practitioner, and client are in their work together. Dr. Dziegielewski notes that all clinical interventions in today's health care environment should (a) be time limited; (b) stress mutually agreed-on goals by patients and social workers; (c) have a focus that is concrete, realistic, and obtainable; (d) be behaviorally linked, outcome based, and measurable; (e) emphasize patients' strengths; and (f) be changeable based on patients' and families' needs.

This seminal book gives social work practitioners a basis for examining the complex issues facing us and, we hope, a rough road map for finding solutions. Dr. Dziegielewski rightly believes social workers' efforts will result in better care for our clients and, when combined with the hard work of our colleagues and collaborators, will be our best chance of improving social health services for all Americans.

Andrew Weissman, PhD
Associate Professor
Department of Community and Preventive Medicine
The Mount Sinai School of Medicine
The Mount Sinai Medical Center
New York, New York

REFERENCE

Nieves, J. (1998). In G. Schames & A. Lightburn (Eds.), *Humane managed care* (p. xiii)? Washington, DC: NASW Press.

Preface

This book reviews the basic concepts related to the delivery of social work services in the health care setting. Health care social work involves aspects of practice that include direct work with clients and their families, whether it is in the home, community, hospital setting, clinics, or other health care institutions. With the advent of numerous health care changes, such as managed health care with its focus on behaviorally based outcomes and objectives, those working in health care service and delivery are continually presented with numerous challenges and opportunities.

This situation must be understood and embraced in order to survive and thrive in this fluctuating and complex environment. Social workers must either accept this challenge to change and reevaluate the services provided or lose the opportunity to be players in this new era of competition for the provision of outcome-based service delivery. They must be able to truly show that what they do is necessary and effective. Today, however, it is important to note that effectiveness must go beyond just helping the client. Effectiveness must also involve validation that concrete and identifiable therapeutic gain was achieved with the least amount of financial and professional support. This means that not only must the treatment that social workers provide be therapeutically effective; it must also be professionally competitive with other disciplines that claim similar treatment strategies and techniques. In health care today, the battle of completing "more service with fewer resources" continues to rage.

Simply stated, health care social workers need to embrace these changes and become PROACTIVE at all levels of practice. They need to:

P: *Present* and *position* themselves as competent professionals with *positive* attitudes in all health care service settings, regardless of the type of practice being provided.

R: *Receive* and acquire adequate training and continuing education in the current and future practice area of health care social work. *Research* time-limited treatment approaches that can provide alternatives for social workers struggling to provide quality of care service while cutting costs.

O: *Organize* individuals and communities to help themselves receive safe, accessible, and affordable health care services. *Organize* other social workers to prepare for the changes that are occurring, and develop strategies to continue to provide ethical cost-effective service.

A: Help *address* and identify the policies and issues that are relevant to providing ethical, effective, efficient, cost-effective service.

C: *Collaborate* with other health care professionals to provide services using an interdisciplinary team approach for addressing client concerns and needs. *Complement* orthodox medical practices and techniques by using holistic practices and alternative strategies that can help clients achieve increased health and wellness.

T: *Teach* others about the value and importance of using social work services and techniques. *Take time* to help themselves holistically and thereby prevent professional burnout. Remain productive and receptive professionals who can serve as good role models for clients and other professionals.

I: *Investigate* and apply innovative approaches to current client-care problems and issues. *Involve* all social workers and make them aware of the change process that needs to occur in the traditional ways that health care social work has been delivered in the past.

V: *Visualize* and work toward positive outcomes for all those who are affected by behavioral managed care strategies. *Value* the role of other health care professionals and support them as they face similar challenges and changes.

E: *Explore* supplemental therapies and strategies that clients can self-administer at little or no cost to treat chronic conditions and to further preserve and enhance health and wellness. Most important, *empower* their clients and themselves by stressing the importance of *education* for self-betterment as well as strategies for individual and societal change.

As health care social workers face the many changes that are in store for all health care providers, they need to remember that in this era of cost cutting and containment they can remain viable players. After all, social workers can provide unique treatments, and in some cases (to spur competition) similar treatments for less money. In the social workers' code of ethics we are sworn to provide reasonable fees and base our charges on an ability to pay. This makes the fees social work professionals charge very competitive when compared to those of psychiatrists, psychologists, family therapists, psychiatric nurses, and mental health counselors who profess they can provide similar services. Thus managed care agencies may be enticed to contract with social workers instead of other professionals to provide services that traditionally have fallen in the domain of social work practice. In this era of managed care, no aspects of taking a proactive stance can be overlooked.

This book advocates a proactive stance for health care social workers and is designed to serve as a practical guide for understanding and addressing the philosophy of practice in our current health care environment. Suggestions are made for achieving ethical time-limited, evidence-based social work practice in these settings. At the end of each chapter, a "future directions" section is provided that will help social workers understand what can be expected and how to prepare for the practice changes needed to remain viable clinical practitioners.

SOPHIA F. DZIEGIELEWSKI, PhD, LCSW

This page intentionally left blank

Acknowledgments

I am very grateful for all the help I have received from the many practitioners and educators in the field of health care social work across the United States who helped in writing this book and providing me with their firsthand experiences in the area of managed behavioral health care. These visionary social workers are not only dealing with the challenges of this changing environment, but they also must bear the burden of exploring and subsequently influencing how those changes will affect our future professional practice. In addition, I would like to thank my clients and the clients of these contributing social workers for helping us see the effects of these health care strategies within an individualized "person-in-environment" framework.

I would also like to express my sincere thanks to all the individuals who helped in the production of this book. First, I would like to thank the Springer Series Editor, Dr. Albert Roberts, my mentor and colleague. I would also like to express my sincere gratitude to Sheri W. Sussman, Springer Editorial Director, whose support and encouragement were invaluable; Ursula Springer, whose drive and energy I know and admire; Melodee McAfee and Valorey Baron Young for all their help with the numerous reads and rereads of this book; and, Cindy Arnold, my colleague and new friend, who gave me the inspiration to reach for the stars in terms of my capabilities. Special thanks to Pamela Lankas for her high standards of excellence in making this second edition of the book the best it can be.

Lastly, the time and effort necessary to complete a book impose burdens on those with whom we share our lives inside and outside the work environment. I would especially like to thank my husband, Linden Siri, for over 22 years of love, understanding, and support. In addition, I would like to thank my other family members, colleagues, and friends who understood and supported me when I said, "I can't because I have to work on this book." I have been blessed with many caring and supportive family members, colleagues, students, and friends and with that encouragement and support, all things really are possible.

Contributors

Breanne K. Anderson, MSW
Lake Mary, Florida

Depsy Bredwood, MSW
Palm Bay, Florida

Sherri Diebolt, MSW
Orlando, Florida

Delbert Ernest Duncklee, Jr., MSW
Orlando, Florida

Cheryl Green, PhD., MSW
University of Central Florida
School of Social Work
Orlando, Florida

Diane Holliman, PhD, LCSW, MPH
Social Work
Valdosta State University
Valdosta, Georgia

George A. Jacinto, MSW, LCSW
University of Central Florida
School of Social Work
Orlando, Florida

Joanna Kaevats, MSW
Hospice Social Worker
Indialantic, Florida

Alicia C. Kalinoski, MSW
Orlando, Florida

Kelly Richards, BSW
Indialantic, Florida

Patricia Sherman, MSW, LCSW
Department of Social Work
Kean University
Union, New Jersey

Dawn Townsend, MSW
Cocoa, Floridao

This page intentionally left blank

PART I

Understanding the Practice of Health Care Social Work

This page intentionally left blank

CHAPTER 1

The Changing Face of Health Care Social Work

HEALTH CARE PRACTICE IN TURBULENT TIMES

This book reviews the basic concepts related to the delivery of social work services in health care settings. Health care social work has generally involved aspects of clinical practice with clients and their families in hospital settings, clinics, and institutions. However, with the advent of the current form of managed health care that began in the 1990s, there have been changes never before experienced. These changes have altered the role of health care professional and have required social workers and the services they provide to continually prove that evidence-based services are truly necessary, effective, and cost-efficient (Mitchell, 1999). In this arena, however, it is important to note that effectiveness goes beyond just helping the client. Effectiveness must also involve validation concrete and identifiable therapeutic gain was achieved with the least amount of financial and professional support (DePoy & Gilson, 2003). This means that not only must the interventions that social workers provide be socially acknowledged as necessary, but they must also be therapeutically effective (Franklin, 2002). In addition, these services must be professionally competitive with those of other disciplines that claim similar treatment strategies and techniques. Client betterment must now be evidence-based in order to be acknowledged as effective (Donald, 2002).

WHAT IS EVIDENCE-BASED HEALTH CARE?

Evidenced-based health care is best understood as a "decision-making framework that facilitates complex decisions across disciplines and sometimes conflicting groups" (Donald, 2002, p. 1). In this type of practice the social worker must use methods that have been shown to be effective and that are based in research. Evidence-based practice involves recognition of treatment or intervention options as well as risk management considerations for individuals, families, and groups.

Over the last 10 years, the battle in the health care arena of "more with less" has continued to rage. Social workers have one strong weapon in this struggle, and it should not be underestimated. It is the traditionally held notion that "social workers can provide similar treatments for less money." In the social worker's code of ethics, we are sworn to provide reasonable fees and base our charges on an ability to pay (National Association of Social Workers, 1996). This makes the fees social work professionals charge very competitive when compared with those of psychiatrists, psychologists, family therapists, psychiatric nurses, and mental health counselors who profess they can provide similar services. For this reason, managed behavioral care agencies may contract with social workers instead of other professionals to provide services that traditionally have been in the domain of social work practice (Dziegielewski, 2002). With the right marketing, this strength can help social workers gain additional ground, adding to their employment desirability.

Armas (2002) reported that according to the latest U.S. Census Bureau an additional 1.4 million people were without health insurance in 2001, over the previous year, as a result of increased unemployment and employers cutting benefits to save costs. This resulted in over 41 million people, or 14.6% of the U.S. population who lacked health coverage for all of 2001. In turbulent times, this is just one of the problems that health care social workers must help clients face.

This book is designed as a practical guide to help social workers understand the philosophy of the current health care environment and to illustrate how evidence-based social work practice can be delivered in various settings. The concept of "future directions" is always highlighted because providing social workers with a possible view into the future can help them understand what can be expected and can provide insight into how to prepare for practice changes needed to remain viable in the health care setting.

CASE STUDY

The following scenario is becoming a common practice situation that health care social workers must address.

Ms. Martha Edda had been living with her family for approximately a year. Before that, she had lived independently in her own apartment. Ms. Edda had to leave her apartment after she was found unconscious by a neighbor. The apartment was unsafe and filled with rotted food, urine, and feces throughout. On discovery, Ms. Edda was immediately admitted to the hospital. Originally, she was believed to have had a stroke. Later, she was formally diagnosed with a neurological condition called vascular dementia. Doctors believed that she was in the moderate to advanced stages, since Ms. Edda, at age 62, had pronounced movement and memory difficulties.

After discussion with the hospital social worker, it became obvious that Ms. Edda needed a supervised living arrangement. Joan, Ms. Edda's daughter, admitted openly how guilty she felt about what had happened to her mother, but did not think she could handle her at home. The social worker reminded Joan that the family would be able to benefit from Ms. Edda's receiving services from a home health care agency, and that a community day care program could be explored. After convincing her family to give it a try, Joan took her mother home.

Once in the home, Ms. Edda did receive home health care services. However, much to her daughter's surprise, all services stopped after just 2 months. Ms. Edda's daughter had relied heavily on these services, particularly the nurses' aides who helped with Ms. Edda's baths. Ms. Edda weighed 170 pounds and could not get into or out of the tub by herself. To help address this problem, Joan recruited the help of her husband, who reluctantly agreed. Unfortunately, Ms. Edda could not get into the adult day care center in the area because there were no spots available. She was placed on a waiting list. Ms. Edda required help with all of her activities of daily living, and her daughter feared leaving her at home alone during the day. So Joan quit her job to help care for her.

On the morning of January 12, Joan found her mother lying face down in her bed. She had become incontinent of bowel and bladder, was unable to speak, and her features appeared distorted on the left side of her face. When Joan could not arouse her, she began to panic and called an ambulance. Ms. Edda was immediately transported to the emergency room.

In the emergency room, they began to run numerous tests to see if Ms. Edda had had another stroke. Plans were made to admit her to the hospital, but there were no beds available. Based on the concern for supervised monitoring and possible bed availability in the morning, an agreement was made to keep her in the emergency room overnight. In the morning, she was admitted to the inpatient hospital. While in the hospital, Ms. Edda remained incontinent and refused to eat. She was so confused that the nurses feared she would get out of bed and hurt herself. She was therefore placed in restraints for periods throughout the day.

After 2 days, most of the medical tests had been run and were determined to be negative. Ms. Edda's vital signs remained stable. The physician thought that her admission in the hospital could no longer be justified, and the social worker was notified of the pending discharge. When the call was placed to prepare Ms. Edda's family for her return home, the social work case manager was told that the family would not accept her, and that they wanted her placed in a nursing home. The social worker was concerned about this decision because she knew that Ms. Edda did not have private insurance to cover her nursing home stay, and she was too young for Medicare eligibility. This meant that an application for Medicaid would have to be made. This state-funded program had a lower reimbursement rate, and most of the privately run nursing homes drastically limited the number of clients they would accept to fill these beds. After calling around, the social worker was told no beds were available.

When the social worker related her discharge problem to the physician, he simply stated, "I am under pressure to get her out, and there is no medical reason for her to be here—discharge her home today." Because it was after 4:00 p.m. and the administrative offices had closed for the day, the social work case manager planned to try to secure an out-of-area placement the following day.

When the physician returned at 6:00 p.m., he wanted to know why the client had not been discharged. The nurse on duty explained that a nursing home bed could not be found. The physician became angry and wrote an order for immediate discharge. The nurse case manager called Ms. Edda's family at 6:30 p.m. and told them about the discharge. Ms.

Edda's family was angry and asked why she was not being placed in a nursing home. The nurse case manager explained to the family that discharge orders had been written, and she was only trying to do her job. Ms. Edda's daughter insisted on speaking to the discharge physician before picking up her mother. A message was left for him, and at 8:00 p.m. her call was returned. The physician sounded frustrated when he told the family that all medical emergencies had been addressed, and she had to leave the hospital now. Ms. Edda's daughter became furious and yelled, "If she is still incontinent and in restraints, how do you expect me to handle her?" Seeing how upset she was, the physician softened his voice and said, "I will put the nurse on the phone to update you on her condition. In addition, the social work case manager will call you in the morning to arrange home health care services."

When Ms. Edda's daughter arrived at the hospital, her mother was hooked to an intravenous line, wearing a diaper, and still in restraints. Pleased to see the client's family member, the nurse sent for a wheelchair, unhooked the intravenous tubing, removed the restraints, and helped place her in the wheelchair for transport to the family's car.

Although this situation may sound unbelievable, unfortunately, situations similar to this one continue to occur. This case study is an accurate depiction of the events that occurred. With Joan's perseverance, she was eventually able (several months later) to get her mother placed in a nursing home. The strain, however, was so great on Joan that she ended up requesting that she be placed on medication to combat depression. Joan also began to fight with her husband and children over numerous issues related to the time required for her mother's care and the loss of the second source of family income. Like most American families, her paycheck was used not only to supplement basic needs (rent and food), but also for any sources of family luxury (movies and dining out). It is clear that in situations such as this, the price of this seemingly "cost-effective" strategy far exceeded the dollar emphasis placed on it. Sadly, in this situation, the client and her family become the *silent victims*.

For all professionals working in the health care area, reports of such cases are becoming increasingly more common. There was a calm (possibly cold) desperation reflected in the tones of many professionals involved in this case. Feelings of desperation and frustration are not uncommon when many professionals, not only social workers, feel trapped within a system where clients trust the professionals to have power to intercede on their behalf (i.e., to heal and to help). For health care social workers, the belief continues that they are regulated and snared within a system that does not allow them to exercise what they believe is the best ethical course of action. It appears apparent that ethical conflicts will continue to become more acute (Galambos, 1999) as social workers will need to balance quality of care with service limitations. Originally, it was postulated that a health care delivery team (physicians, nurses, social workers, physical therapists, etc.) with specialized roles could best meet the needs of each client while in the health care setting. However, when professionals are feeling frustrated, this degree of specialization can also provide a barrier, creating client–health care worker separation.

The emphasis placed on team member specialization (i.e., these are my specific job duties and responsibilities) can influence individual members to avoid taking overall responsibility for client welfare. This avoidance can create a type of shock absorber, affectionately known in the business as the client "buff and turf." During "buff and turf," only surface concerns related to the client are addressed. The real issue is left untouched, and the case is referred to the next professional on the health care delivery team. For example, in this case, the nurse avoided responsibility by stating that she was only doing her job. Later, the physician commented superficially and handed the telephone to the nurse for the problematic details. The social worker also had a role in addressing this situation. Other professionals on the health care team may view her primarily as "in charge of securing placement services." For example, some nursing professionals believe that nurses involved in discharge planning should take more of an administrative role; others see the nurses as people who teach patients and families complex postdischarge treatments, such as breathing treatments, decubitus and skin care, feeding tubes, and home injections (Penrod, Kane, & Kane, 2000). This puts the responsibility of placement on the shoulders of the social work provider, ignoring the inadequacy of the placement limitations and available options. In cases like this, it is important to note that the reality of the situation is that none of these professionals had the power to take control over what was happening; however, the client, the family, and possibly the community still believed they did or should have.

Cases like this force professionals to question the services they give, how they are being given, and why they are giving them. Many also question the system and what is happening to "patient care" as they knew it. The question remains: Is what is really happening now different from what would have occurred ten years ago? The answer for many social workers is "yes." For example, ten years ago Ms. Edda (see the case study earlier) would have been kept in the hospital until a bed could be found. Although this alternative might be best to help the overall family situation, is it really an efficient and effective use of an expensive hospital stay? One point remains evident—there are problems in the current system, and there does not appear to be an easy solution to this dilemma. Little emphasis is placed on community support (Meenaghan, 2001). Health care social workers can be assured that in these turbulent times more changes in the delivery of health care services will result because of cost containment, which is considered the primary method of controlling excessive health care costs (Alperin, 1994).

TODAY'S HEALTH CARE SOCIAL WORKER

Name: Mary O. Norris, MPH, LCSW
List State of Practice: Florida
Professional Job Title: Clinical Social Worker

Duties in a typical day:
I am director of a department comprising 40 clinicians who provide services at five hospitals. Our department's goal is to provide clinical interventions to both inpatients and outpatients. The corporation's case management department does discharge planning at all sites except at our children and women's hospital.

Arriving early in the mornings to work allows me to gather my thoughts and set priorities for the day. The schedule usually includes attending committee meetings, meeting with supervisors to decide how to handle issues and working on various projects. There is also the usual complement of voice mails and e-mails that need responses.

What do you like most about your position?
Developing our department for the last five years has always been considered a calculated risk. Thus, it is most rewarding now to witness the growth of line staff and watch them flourish in the

practice of their clinical skills. Equally satisfying is seeing social workers being recognized for the clinical expertise they bring to the health care team.

What do you like least about your position?
Although I enjoy the coordination and sense of satisfaction I get in team building, I miss providing direct patient and family care.

What words of wisdom do you have for the new health care social worker who is considering working in a similar position?
It is essential to have sufficient "hands-on" experience. Complementing this background should be additional education in administration so as to have the requisite theoretical and analytic skills. For me, having the dual degree of Master in Public Health and Master in Social Work has been invaluable. Further professional commitment is demonstrated by membership in a professional organization such as the Society for Social Work Leadership in Healthcare. Membership provides a wealth of networking opportunities and mentors to assist in the leadership of a department.

What is your favorite social work story?
While working as a clinical social worker on a pediatric pulmonary team, I counseled a young man with cystic fibrosis. When we first met he was extremely shy and nonverbal. During these 3 years of clinical interventions, we worked on body image, self-esteem, and sexuality issues. By the time I left this position, he had become verbal and self-disclosing regarding the many issues surrounding the impact of his chronic illness.

Several months after relocating to another city, the chief of pulmonology called me to notify me that the patient was hospitalized and was asking to see me. It seemed he was in the end stages of his disease and the team was uncertain if he truly comprehended the gravity of his situation. After having spent time at his bedside and with his family, I was preparing to leave. During the entire visit, he had never alluded to what issues were behind his request for my visit. Finally, he yelled out in a labored breathing "everyone out but Mary." He said he needed to ask me something but could not. After I explored with him his impending death, he verbalized his comfort level with dying; however, he was still unable to explain why he wanted to speak with me. I proceeded to ask him several questions, trying to understand his obviously intense issues. After verbalizing several possible concerns, I hoped to "hit" upon the right topic. Finally, I suggested he write down his thoughts. He then handed me a written note on a piece of brown paper towel. The note simply said, to my surprise, "please ma'am take off your shirt. Thank you." He said, "Mary, you know I have never been with a woman. I know I am dying, and I just want to be with one before I do."

"I am so flattered to have you ask me this." I responded. "I am your social worker, not your girlfriend." We talked a little more, and I told him good bye. He died during the night. When I went back to the pulmonary team, they were all anxious to know if he knew he was dying. My response was, "Believe me, he knows!"

EFFECT OF THE ENVIRONMENT ON HEALTH CARE DELIVERY

To understand the current practice of health care social work, we must first examine the environmental context of general health care delivery. This high-pressure health care environment requires that the following factors, different and contradictory as they may be, are expected to coexist. Table 1.1 lists and briefly describes the five factors.

The first factor to be considered is the public demand for quality service and "state-of-the-art care" (Shortell & Kaluzny, 1994). Politicians, consumers, and consumer advocates all agree that the American health care system is desperately in need of repair and reform (McKinney, 1995; Mizrahi, 1995). Americans are watching this transition and the resulting provision of health care with hesitancy and trepidation in fear of ending up with "less for more." American people are demanding quality service, but they are not willing to support increased costs in a system they believe is plagued by waste.

In addition to quality service, clients also expect to be able to gain access to state-of-the-art technology. Clients expect links between medical knowledge and technology in the provision of quality service. Therefore, health care delivery systems are expected to hire and retain the most qualified personnel, as well as purchase the most sophisticated equipment. The pressure to secure these services is great because

TABLE 1.1   Factors That Influence Health Care Delivery

Factors	Results
Quality of service and technological advances	Constant updating of training and equipment required to provide state-of-the-art care
	Constant updating for providers in terms of utilization of technology (e.g., computers, Internet)
Number and variety of professionals in competition	"Buff and turf" service delivery
	Organizational competition
Organizations that deliver services	Strive to survive and progress
Preserving quality of care	Pressure to provide "more for less"
Cost-containment	Cost-based service delivery is given primary consideration rather than quality client care

without these ingredients health care agencies cannot effectively compete for "covered" or "reimbursable" client resources.

The second factor related to the problems found in health care delivery is associated with (and among) the professionals who actually deliver health care services (Shortell & Kaluzny, 1994). An important aspect that must be considered when trying to understand this conflict is in the increased numbers of health care professionals in practice. The number of these professionals has increased dramatically over the years (Freudenheim, 1990). The health care industry alone is the nation's third largest employer, preceded by government (nonhealth) and retailing (Hernandez, Fottler, & Joiner, 1994).

In addition, not only have the numbers and types of health care professionals increased, but so also has their education level. In 1990, 4.9 million individuals in health delivery required some type of professional training or a college degree. This seems unbelievable when compared with the previous 200,000 health care professionals in 1900 (Ginzberg, 1990). According to the U.S. Bureau of the Census (1991), two thirds of all individuals employed in the health care industry are considered nontraditional allied health or support personnel. Here we find that the number of social workers has grown along with physician assistants, nurse practitioners, multiskilled health workers, laboratory technicians, occupational therapists, and physical therapists. This causes the position of the social worker to be viewed as just one of many "adjunct" professionals involved in health care delivery.

To compare salaries of **social workers in health care** with those in other professions such as:

- clinical nurse specialist
- staff nurse RN
- recreational therapist
- case manager
- counselor
- physician family medicine

Try this Web address: *http://aolsvc.salary.aol.com/*

After addressing the increased number of professionals providing health care service delivery, to avoid confusion, an examination of similar or duplicating functions that many of these professionals perform must be made (Buppert, 2002). This is particularly relevant for those directly providing services in the allied health fields of which social work is part (Lister, 1980). Often the roles that social workers perform overlap with these other disciplines (Davidson, 1990; Dziegielewski & Leon, 2001). For example, today nurses are often asked to run therapeutic support groups in the health care setting. This invitation remains contradictory to the traditionally held belief that most group leadership is the realm of the social work professional (Toseland & Rivas, 1984). Based on the increased number of allied health care professionals and the overlapping of skills, tasks, and roles, one point remains certain: all trained professionals will be forced to continue to compete and strive to find a solid niche in this new and emerging managed health care market.

The third factor that compounds the problems found within current health care delivery involves not only the individual providers, but also the organizations of delivery. Managed health care has created a competition for survival never before experienced. Previously, most health care organizations focused their attention on expanding and increasing marketability through services provided. Today, the ideal organization for health care delivery must base service delivery on insurance reimbursement while providing all levels of competitive evidence-based care to their defined population (Shortell & Kaluzny, 1994; Donald, 2002).

Each health care delivery organization must ensure that, at a minimum, at least two things are done to make it viable. The first is to take the necessary steps to ensure its own *survival*; the second is to be able to record *progress* toward the agency's and society's mission (Shortell & Kaluzny, 1994). Striving to survive and progress creates an air of competition that was originally designed to provide quality and competitive services for all. To compete, a variety of major strategies have been incorporated (Hernandez, Fottler, & Joiner, 1994). These include (a) provision of low-cost traditional health services; (b) provision of superior service through technology or client service; (c) specialization into certain areas of practice (i.e., centers of excellence); (d) diversification outside of the traditional bounds of health care delivery (i.e., wellness centers); and (e) creation of new and ingenious ways to relabel the traditional service to be more reflective of the greater society. For example, recently under the influence of managed care policies, many organizations have begun to look toward presenting their service in a new and different light. A societal and political paradigm shift has occurred, transforming health care from what we knew (e.g., focused on fixing problems or curing illness) toward wellness, resulting in a greater emphasis on the spirit and a continuum of health care services—not illness care services (Shortell & Kaluzny, 1994).

As with all societal change, people and the culture are slow to respond; therefore, this paradigm shift will require changes be implemented at the most basic levels. For example, there is little debate that in the traditional medical mode, the individual who receives the services has traditionally been referred to as the "patient." In health care social work, this caused many social workers to stop using words like *client* when referring to the individuals served and to adopt the dominant label used in the medical environment. This use and acceptance of the term *patient* is obvious when reading articles in the social work health care literature (Alperin, 1994; Brown, 1994; Coursey, Farrell, & Zahniser, 1991; Cowles & Lefcowitz, 1992).

To reflect consistently this societal paradigm shift away from the medical model in which the receiver of services is viewed as "sick," a wellness outcomes-based cost-effective approach is being emphasized today. For all health care professionals, referring to an individual service recipient as the "patient" is now in need of revising. The term *patient* is in conflict with the wholeness and prevention strategy that is advocated by most organizations to increase marketability in this competitive environment Terms now being utilized include *client* (a term familiar to social work professionals), *service consumers* or *patrons* (to represent those buying or purchasing a service), *product recipients* or *individual recipients* (those receiving a direct service), and *covered persons* (reflecting those who have some type of medical insurance coverage) Those in favor of the euphemism covered persons argue that it is not used just to indicate medical coverage but to indicate the universal care perspective and the assurance that comes with an individual having the security of medical coverage Therefore, "covered entities" are referred to as the health care providers that serve "covered persons " No matter what the final determination is, the influence it will have in enhancing the survival and progress of the organization, and its marketability, so to speak, most assuredly will be considered As for social workers practicing in the health care arena, they will probably soon follow suit and use the same terms to identify the recipient defined by managed health care plans After all, as one of the allied health care professionals providing service, it is important to conform for uniformity and provider eligibility

The fourth and fifth factors are a combination often hailed as the two most powerful forces driving managed health care delivery today (Shortell & Kaluzny, 1994) These factors involve the balance between preserving the quality of care delivered while maintaining cost control Usually these factors are considered equal in the political discussion of health care delivery, however, under most of the capitation or fixed fee models being proposed, revenue schemes that increase quality of care while increasing the cost of health care fail to garner support (Flood, Shortell, & Scott, 1994, Hernandez, Fottler, & Joiner, 1994, Ross, 1993)

Along with other professionals, many health care social workers feel the pressure to use for cost containment It is my expectation that, in the future, continued emphasis will be placed on cost containment at the expense of quality of care (Dziegielewski, 1996, 1997, Schneider, Hyer, & Luptak, 2000) Therefore, the role of the social work professional in actively advocating for the provision of quality services cannot be overstated (Dziegielewski, 2002, Franklin, 2002, Gibelman, 2002, Rock, 2002) Colby and Dziegielewski (2001) warn, however, that social workers need to do more than simply ensure the provision of "micro" (individually based) or "mezzo" (environmentally based) quality services They urge social work professionals to be active in the "macro" aspect of practice by monitoring policies and programs that will affect not only the clients they serve directly but also all Americans. Advocacy of this type means actively identifying and supporting state and federal legislation that provides basic standards of quality care. Services that allow universal accessibility, affordability, and service comprehensiveness need to be endorsed (National Association of Social Workers, 1994), while culturally sensitive practice is maintained (National Association of Social Workers, 2001).

THE ROLE OF MANAGED HEALTH CARE

In the early 1990s, the debate that secured its place in the forefront of the social and political agenda was that of health care delivery. The cost of health care delivery had been defined as a national crisis. Many thought that several of the key causes of this inflation were beyond control. Several reasons postulated for pushing health care costs beyond direct control included the increasing number of Americans reaching "old" age that would require services, the technological advances within the society, and the unregulated and varied cost of the services provided (Edinburg & Cottler, 1995). Other societal and professional factors included the fact that (a) many health care consumers were considered medically uneducated and unknowledgeable about medical services; (b) Americans were sensitive and resistant to paying more for the delivery of medical services; (c) the insurance industry was highly fragmented, with managerial administrators and leaders who were trained in a different environmental context that did not include "standardized cost containment techniques"; (d) there were simply too many hospital inpatient beds with the pressure to have them filled; (e) there was a focus on acute illness rather than a more holistic, wellness, or preventive perspective; (f) there was insufficient medical outcomes-based data that focused the benefit as the end result of service; (g) there were difficulties separating quality-of-life issues from technological advances, causing heroic attempts to implement expensive procedures without regard to quality of continued life; and (h) the medical community had been rocked by numerous malpractice suits that resulted in fear and pressure to ensure fewer complaints (Edinburg & Cottler, 1995; Shortell & Kaluzny, 1994).

Even though many of these societal and technological factors were considered difficult to address and change, concern about future predictions of the cost of health care delivery continued to send shivers down the spines of the entire American population. Health care costs were estimated at more than $640 billion in 1990 (Shortell & Kaluzny, 1994), and at that current rate, accrual was expected to reach $1 trillion (Hernandez, Fottler, & Joiner, 1994) to $1.5 trillion by the year 2000 (Skelton & Janosi, 1992). In 2002, the National Institutes of Health could receive a funding increase of $3.7 billion for the fiscal year that began October 1, with an additional expectation to double the agency's funding over five years under a bill approved by a U.S. Senate subcommittee (Reuters Health Information, 2002). To fuel the concern further, it was believed that as the years progressed, the baby boomers who would reach their 70s and 80s in the year 2030 would bring health spending to an astonishing peak at $16 trillion, or 30% of the gross domestic product (Burner, Waldo, & McKusick, 1992).

To add to this concern for cost containment, in the late 1970s and into the middle 1980s, it was estimated that the number of individuals without health insurance in the United States increased from 28.7 million to 35.1 million (United States Bureau of the Census, 1984). This left an estimated 37 million Americans who experienced health risks with an inability to afford needed health care (Roland, Lyons, Salganicoff, & Long, 1994). This fact particularly disturbed insurance companies, which complained of bitter upsets, and in 1988 the nation's top twelve health insurers reported financial losses of $830 million (Edinburg & Cottler, 1995).

In review, the 1980s represented a time when the nation was in the midst of economic stagnation and recession (Mizrahi, 1995); the alternate health care reform strategies suggested to alleviate this unprecedented burden were all of a "solution-based" or "evidence-based" nature (Donald, 2002). To address this situation, a course of action was considered successful if it ultimately resulted in a decision-making framework that supported efforts toward cost control, cost containment, or cost reduction.

In the early 1990s, the message of concern was clear, and the social climate was rich with politicians' verbal responsiveness to the American peoples' concern for reform. This acknowledgment was reflected in the election strategy of many of the candidates seeking office. It was not uncommon for many of the campaign platforms to present possible solutions designed to address health care reform. In fact, President Bill Clinton in his 1992 election, made health care reform his highest domestic priority (Mizrahi, 1995). Numerous proposals were considered, from single-payer-system approaches to limited policies for universal health care coverage.

After the 1992 presidential election, the victor, democratic President Bill Clinton, proceeded to address his campaign goal by establishing a task force to complete a plan for health care reform. The model emphasized was different from the single-payer approach that he had originally supported early in his campaign. This later approach involved a type of managed competition in which purchasing alliances were formed that would have the power to certify health plans and negotiate premiums for certain benefit packages (*The President's Health Security Plan*, 1993). Since employer–employee premiums would finance payment for these plans, the actual consumer out-of-pocket cost could vary based on the benefit package chosen. Title XVIII, Medicare, a federal entitlement program to pay for physician and hospital services for disabled individuals or others age 65 or older, remained a separate program. Title XIX, Medicaid, a means-tested program based on provision of medical services for low-income Americans, was included in the plan (Mizrahi, 1995). One possible economic reason for the attraction to include Medicaid in this reform process was that between 1990 and 1991 one third of the increase in the total U.S. expenditures was based on states' use of this program (Letsch, 1993).

The future of most health care delivery (70% of all coverage) is to be provided by managed health care plans (Edinburg & Cottler, 1995). In this system, managed care plans will cover preauthorization for service by qualified consumers; precertification for a given amount of care with concurrent review of the treatment and services rendered; continued determination of the need for hospitalization through a process of use review; and predischarge planning to ensure that proper aftercare services are identified and made available (Hiratsuka, 1990).

Five major types of managed care programs for health care delivery follow, all of which may employ social work professionals (Wagner, 1993). The first is *managed indemnity plans*. In these plans, traditional coverage is offered; however, the cost of the plan is directly related to the usage needs and requirements of the subscriber. A second type of managed care plan is the *preferred provider organization* (PPO). Here employers or insurance carriers contract with a select group of health care delivery providers to provide certain services at preestablished reimbursement rates. The consumer has the choice of whom to contact to provide the service; however, if the option of using a provider not on the provider list is chosen, higher out-of-pocket expenses will result.

A third type of managed care plan is the *exclusive provider organization*. This plan type is generally considered more restricted than the PPO because the consumer does not have the choice to go elsewhere, and services must be provided and received by the contracted organization or partnership. Employers often choose this type of health care delivery as a cost-saving measure. If a consumer does go outside of the system, reimbursement is generally not obtained (Wagner, 1993). The use of these facilities is the only way to gain reimbursable access to specialty care services (surgery, etc.).

A fourth type of managed care program is the *point-of-service plan*. Usually at the initiation of coverage, a choice is made whether to request a PPO format or an indemnity/HMO format for delivery of services. Thus the consumer can go outside of the provider system with minimal additional cost (Wagner, 1993).

The fifth type of managed care program is probably both the oldest and the most commonly related to the idea of managed care, the *health maintenance organization* plan (HMO). These plans provide service for a prepaid fixed fee. The organizations provide both health insurance and health delivery in one package. If a consumer must go beyond the traditional services offered by the HMO, the HMO determines where these covered services will be obtained. Five common types of HMO models for service delivery are staff models, where the physicians are employed directly by the HMO (i.e., a type of closed model); group models, where contracts are held with multispecialty groups of physicians (i.e., a type of closed model); network models, which result in a greater choice of physicians because any specialty physician who has the proper credentials can join (i.e., an open panel plan because enrollment is not limited to contracted staff or a group); individual practice association models, where the physician becomes a member but can still retain his or her own professional office; and direct contract models, where physicians are contracted to provide services on an individual basis (Edinburg & Cottler, 1995). It is important to note that the concept of using managed care plans through the use of health care organizational providers is not a new one. This type of delivery was originally formulated to provide efficient, comprehensive, and high-quality health care services (Shortell & Kaluzny, 1983).

CHAPTER SUMMARY AND FUTURE DIRECTIONS

In summary, the complexity and diversity required to define simply the current concept of managed health care in the area of health service delivery cannot be underestimated. In today's health care market, a specific definition of the term *managed health care* simply does not exist (Edinburg & Cottler, 1995). Unfortunately, attempts at a standard definition continue to change, and the term has expanded and broadened in complexity. Generally speaking, one characteristic remains consistent across all evidence-based managed care provision strategies: these strategies are designed to provide an array of features that will ultimately balance quality of care with cost containment, allowing this type of health care to survive and progress (Donald, 2002). In addition, directives and principles relevant to managed care that extend beyond it remain strong. These factors include evidence-based practice principles, brief goal-directed treatment, outcome measures, primary and preventive care, and case management (Rock, 2002). This will require that social workers continue their practice emphasis in this area, becoming proficient in formulating care plans and addressing the person as a whole, integrating health and mental health as well as mixing mind and body influences toward the achievement of comprehensive client care (Dziegielewski, 2002).

For health care social workers in the managed care environment, practice expertise will be measured through the use and development of technology-based interventions. This requires that intervention skills incorporate the use of computer-based data systems, telephone counseling, multimedia educational tools, and the Internet (Franklin, 2002).

In health care practice, computers are now often used for assessments, progress notes, routine correspondence, and reports (Gingerich, 2002). Social workers, like other health care professionals, will need to utilize this technology and employ these techniques to help clients to secure the services they need.

In closing, the intention of this first chapter is to set the stage for enlightenment regarding some of the concepts, ethical dilemmas, and resulting problems that a health care social worker can confront while ensuring service delivery. Health care social workers need to be aware of the many societal, philosophical, and technological trends that have occurred over the last ten years, and how the history of runaway health care expenses has influenced current expectations for future service delivery. These influences, combined with requirements for evidence-based practice, have truly transformed health care delivery (Donald, 2002). Changes relevant to controlling costs through managed behavioral health care have required that social workers be flexible, and there are new and varied expectations of what they will be required to perform. For today's health care social work professional, issues and problems similar to those experienced by Ms. Edda (see the case study earlier) are not unusual; unfortunately, unless health care social workers strive to understand and anticipate current and future trends in service delivery, cases like the one presented will become more common.

REFERENCES

Alperin, R. M. (1994). Managed care versus psychoanalytic psychotherapy: Conflicting ideologies. *Clinical Social Work Journal, 22,* 137–148.

Armas, G. C. (September 30, 2002). More people lose health insurance: The Census Bureau blamed the trend on the recession. *Orlando Sentinel,* Monday, *Associated Press,* A9.

Brown, F. (1994). Resisting the pull of the health insurance turbary: An organizational model for surviving managed care. *Clinical Social Work Journal, 22,* 59–71.

Buppert, C. (2002). NPs cannot order, certify, or recertify home care, or perform plan oversight. *Green Sheet, 4*(7), 1–3.

Burner, S. T., Waldo, R. R., & McKusick, D. R. (1992). National health expenditures: Projections through 2030. *Health Care Financing Review, 14,* 1–29.

Colby, I., & Dziegielewski, S. F. (2001). *Social work: The people's profession.* Chicago: Lyceum.

Coursey, R. D., Farrell, E. W., & Zahniser, J. H. (1991). Consumers' attitudes toward psychotherapy, hospitalization and after-care. *Health and Social Work, 16,* 155–161.

Cowles, L. A., & Lefcowitz, M. J. (1992). Interdisciplinary expectations of medical social workers in the hospital setting. *Health and Social Work, 17,* 58–65.

Davidson, K. W. (1990). Role blurring and the hospital social worker's search for a clear domain. *Health and Social Work, 15,* 228–234.

Depoy, E., & Gilson, S. F. (2003). *Evaluation practice: Thinking and action principles for social work practice.* Pacific Grove, CA: Brooks/Cole.

Donald, A. (2002). Evidenced based medicine: Key concepts. *Medscape Psychiatry & Mental Health ejournal, 7*(2), 1–5. http://www.medscape.com/viewarticle/430709.

Dziegielewski, S. F. (1996). Managed care principles: The need for social work in the health care environment. *Crisis Intervention and Time-Limited Treatment, 3,* 97–110.

Dziegielewski, S. F. (1997). Time limited brief therapy: The state of practice. *Crisis Intervention and Time Limited Treatment, 3,* 217–228.

Dziegielewski, S. F. (2002). *DSM-IV-TR™ in action.* New York: Wiley.

Dziegielewski, S. F., & Leon, A. (2001). *Social work practice and psychopharmacology.* New York: Springer Publishing Co.

Edinburg, G. M., & Cottler, J. M. (1995). Managed care. In R. L. Edwards (Ed.), *Encyclopedia of social work* (19th ed., Vol. 2, pp. 1199–1213). Silver Spring, MD: National Association of Social Workers.

Flood, A. B., Shortell, S. M., & Scott, W. R. (1994). Organizational performance: Managing for efficiency and effectiveness. In S. M. Shortell & A. D. Kaluzny (Eds.), *Health care management: Organizational behavior and design* (3rd ed., pp. 316–351). Albany, NY: Delmar.

Franklin, C. (2002). Developing effective practice competencies in managed behavioral health care. In A. R. Roberts & G. J. Greene (Eds.), *Social workers' desk reference.* (pp. 1–9). New York: Oxford.

Freudenheim, M. (1990, March 5). Job growth in health care areas. *New York Times,* p. 1.

Galambos, C. (1999). Behavioral managed health care. *Health and Social Work, 24*(3),191–198.

Gibelman, M. (2002). Social work in an era of managed care. In A. R. Roberts & G. J. Greene (Eds.) *Social workers' desk reference* (pp. 16–22). New York: Oxford.

Gingerich, W. J. (2002). Computer applications for social work practice. In A. R. Roberts & G. J. Greene (Eds.), *Social workers' desk reference* (pp. 23–28). New York: Oxford.

Ginzberg, E. (1990). Health personnel: The challenge ahead. *Frontiers of Health Care Management, 7,* 3–22.

Hernandez, S. R., Fottler, M. D., & Joiner, C. L. (1994). Integrating strategic management and human resources. In M. Fottler, S. Hernandez, & C. L. Joiner (Eds.), *Strategic management of human resources in health service organizations* (2nd ed., pp. 3–25). Albany, NY: Delmar.

Hiratsuka, J. (1990). Managed care: A sea of change in health. *NASW News, 35,* 3.

Letsch, S. W. (1993, Spring). National health care spending in 1991. *Health Affairs, 2,* 94–110.

Lister, L. (1980). Expectations of social workers and other health professionals. *Health and Social Work, 5,* 41–49.

McKinney, E. A. (1995). Health planning. In R. L. Edwards (Ed.), *Encyclopedia of social work* (19th ed., Vol. 2, pp. 1199–1213). Silver Spring, MD: National Association of Social Workers.

Meenaghan, T. M. (2001). Exploring possible relations among social sciences, social work and health interventions. In G. Rosenberg & A. Weissman (Eds.), *Behavioral and social sciences in 21st century health care* (pp.43–50). New York: Haworth Social Work Practice Press.

Mitchell, C. G. (1999). Perceptions of empathy and client satisfaction with managed behavioral health care. *Social Work, 43(* 5), 404–411.

Mizrahi, T. (1995). Health care: Reform initiatives. In R. L. Edwards (Ed.), *Encyclopedia of social work* (19th ed., Vol. 2, pp. 1185–1198). Silver Spring, MD: National Association of Social Workers.

National Association of Social Workers. (1994). *Guidelines for clinical social work supervision.* Washington, DC: Author.

National Association of Social Workers. (1996, August). *Code of ethics* (Adopted by NASW Delegate Assembly, August 1996). Washington, DC: Author.

National Association of Social Workers. (2001). *NASW standards for cultural competence in social work practice.* Retrieved from: *www.naswdc.org/pubs/standards/cultural.htm.*

Penrod, J. D., Kane, R. A., & Kane, R. L. (2000). Effects of post-hospital informal care on nursing home discharge. *Research on Aging, 22*(1), 66–82.

Reuters Health Information. (2002). U.S. Senate subcommittee approves health spending bill. *Reuters Medical News:*http:www.medscape.com/viewarticle/43860.

Rock, B. (2002). Social work in health care in the 21st century. In A. R. Roberts & G. J. Greene (Eds.), *Social workers' desk reference* (pp. 10–16). New York: Oxford.

Roland, D., Lyons, B., Salganicoff, A., & Long, P. (1994). A profile of the uninsured in America. *Health Affairs, 13,* 283–287.

Ross, J. (1993). Redefining hospital social work: An embattled professional domain [Editorial]. *Health and Social Work, 18,* 243–247.

Schneider, A. W., Hyer, K., & Luptak, M. (2000, Nov). Suggestions to Social Workers for surviving in managed care. *Health and Social Work, 25* (4), 276.

Shortell, S. M., & Kaluzny, A. D. (Ed.). (1983). *Health care management: A text in organization theory and behavior.* New York: Wiley.

Shortell, S. M., & Kaluzny, A. D. (1994). Forward. In S. M. Shortell & A. D. Kaluzny (Eds.), *Health care management: Organizational behavior and design* (3rd ed., p. XI). Albany, NY: Delmar.

Skelton, J. K., & Janosi, J. M. (1992). Unhealthy health care costs. *Journal of Medicine and Philosophy, 17,* 7–19.

The President's health security plan. (1993). New York: Times Books/Random House.

Toseland, R. W., & Rivas, R. F. (1984). *An introduction to group work practice.* New York: MacMillian.

U.S. Bureau of the Census. (1984). *Current population survey.* Washington, DC: Government Printing Office.

U.S. Bureau of the Census. (1991). *Statistical abstract of the United States*. Washington, DC: Government Printing Office.

Wagner, E. R. (1993). Types of managed care organizations. In P. R. Kongstvedt (Ed.), *The managed health care handbook* (2nd ed., pp. 12–21). Rockville, MD: Aspen.

GLOSSARY

Exclusive provider organization: This form of a managed care plan is generally considered more restricted than the PPO. Consumers do not have the choice to go elsewhere. Services must be provided and received by the contracted organization or partnership. Many times this plan is referred to as the "gatekeeper" because use of the services provided is the only way to gain reimbursable access to specialty care services.

Health care delivery organizations: In today's health care environment, these organizations are considered responsible for providing low-cost traditional and specialized health services; incorporation of technology into the service provided; diversification outside the traditional bounds of health care delivery (i.e., wellness centers); and new ways to label traditional service to be more reflective of environmental demands.

Health maintenance organization plans: These plans provide service for a prepaid fixed fee. These organizations provide both health insurance and health delivery in one package. If a consumer must go beyond the traditional services offered by the HMO, the HMO determines where these covered services will be obtained. Five common types of HMO models for service delivery are staff models (physicians are employed directly by the HMO), group models (contracts are held with multispecialty groups of physicians), network models (where enrollment is not limited to contracted staff or group providers), individual practice association models (physicians become members, but can still retain their own office and consumers), and direct contract models (physicians are contracted to provide services on an individual basis).

Length of stay: This is the actual time used or allotted (usually specified in number of days) for a consumer to receive a needed health care service.

Managed care: An organized system of care that attempts to balance access, quality, and cost-effectiveness.

Managed care programs: Programs designed to provide an array of features that balance quality of care with cost-containment strategies.

Managed indemnity plans: A type of managed care program where generally traditional coverage is offered; however, the cost of the plan is directly related to the usage needs of the subscriber.

Preferred provider organizations: Here employers or insurance carriers contract with a select group of health care delivery providers or service organizations to provide certain services at pre-established reimbursement rates. The consumer has the choice of whom to contact to provide the service; however, if a provider not on the provider list is chosen, higher out-of-pocket expenses will result.

Primary and preventive care: Client care that is focused on ambulatory and community-based care approaches as well as physicians' offices and health maintenance organizations.

Prospective payment system: This is a system of reimbursement for what is determined the average length of stay or duration of care for an individual with a certain medical or psychiatric diagnosis.

QUESTIONS FOR FURTHER STUDY

1. What changes do you predict for the field of health care social work because of the pressure to balance cost containment with quality of care?
2. Based on what you know of the social work profession, what new areas of practice "marketability" would you suggest for social work professionals to consider?
3. What do you believe is critical information to allow social workers to balance social work ethics with the reality of the practice environment?

WEBSITES

www.hmopage.com
www.NoManagedCare.org
www.tiac.net/biz/drmike/managed2.html

CHAPTER 2

Evolution of the "New" Health Care Social Work

THE PROFESSION OF HEALTH CARE SOCIAL WORK

No text on health care social work practice would be complete without a review of the profession's struggle to define the historical and current role of the health care social worker. What is most disturbing in today's practice environment is the fact that many individuals outside the social work discipline continue to remain unsure of what it is the health care social worker does. In addition, social workers themselves often battle over what constitutes "health care" social work. Establishing and agreeing upon a unified definition of health care social work remains critical for survival in today's behavioral managed health care environment. The current practice of health care social work is reflective of the environment where change and constant restructure are the usual state of affairs. Today, health care practice can present challenging times for all health care professionals (Donald, 2002; Imperato, 1996), not just social workers. Changes in the scope of practice, the roles social workers assume, and the expectations of both clients and practitioners have occurred quickly; and many times professionals feel trapped and lost in this whirlwind of activity.

In this turbulent, ever-changing environment, professional social workers must constantly balance "quality-of-care" issues versus "cost-containment" measures for the clients they serve (Dziegielewski, 1996, 2002). This delicate balance must also be reached in a time when the social worker's role and current position in the health care setting are tenuous at best. As social workers, we continue to remain skeptical as to whether quality of care will actually be able to win in a system that was originally characterized by social welfare institutions that represented the nonprofit motive (Poole, 1996).

The most important aspect of the profession of social work that makes it unusual when compared with other disciplines is that it involves helping individuals, families, and groups. This unique perspective, stated in its most simplistic form, is that of recognizing the importance of the "individual in the situation" or the "person in the environment" (Hepworth, Rooney & Larsen, 2002; Skidmore, Thackeray, & Farley, 1997). Today, however, for the health care social worker, recognizing the cultural uniqueness of an individual or person within an environmental context or situation can be much more complicated than what was traditionally perceived (Lum, 2003).

This perspective requires that the health care social worker go beyond the traditional confines of the health care institution and consider the needs of the individual, family, group, or community regarding their unique situations or environments. In the turbulent health care environment, the practice of the health care social worker must not only concentrate on providing important concrete services that clients need to function effectively within their environments, but also try to anticipate future changes in those environments to ensure that services remain effective and helpful. In addition, the health care social worker, also affected by the environment, must ensure that he or she continues to be able to maintain his or her own position as a service provider.

DEFINING HEALTH CARE SOCIAL WORK PRACTICE

Recently, I consulted with a colleague who has been a health care social worker for fifteen years. She had been asked to justify her position and the health services she rendered in the home health care environment—a job she had been doing for the last eight years. She knew the services she provided, but thought that these tasks needed to be presented in a perspective that made her duties different and marketable when compared with the nurses and other professionals working with clients. She feared that if she could not do this, budget cuts would force her duties to be turned over to the nurses and physical therapists, and she would lose her job. She also believed that as of late she was receiving fewer referrals, and thus was unable to provide adequate care to clients in need. Although the nurses often visited clients, they were generating fewer social work consults. When my social worker friend asked the nurses why this was happening, she was told that no clear need for a social work assessment could be established, based on the nurses' increased role in determining service use criteria. Her concern escalated when one of the agency's clients attempted suicide in response to the recent death of his wife. Although the client was being seen regularly by the service for medication injections, no referral was made to the social worker—even after the wife's death.

This social worker's concern is real. The competition for professional legitimacy has increased, and social workers are forced to compete for a place in the health care arena. Questions that seek to establish what social workers do, different from the services of other professionals, are becoming more common. Developing an answer to satisfy these questions is now necessary. This social worker, like many others, is being forced to justify her current and continued role as a vital member of the health care delivery team. The traditionally held belief that what social workers do is different, necessary, and unique from other counseling professionals continues to be questioned; the environmental climate of maintaining quality of care and cost containment is demanding that it be answered.

To help address this issue and the unique contributions social work brings to the practice of health care, a clear linkage between social work and the other related disciplines needs to be established. Traditionally, the role of social work has been to advocate for the poor, the disadvantaged, the disenfranchised, and the oppressed (Hepworth, Rooney, & Larsen, 2002; National Association of Social Workers, 1996, 2001). Historically, this has been accomplished by promoting and enhancing client well-being in a societal or environmental context. In this book, as in most of the social work literature, the term *client* is considered inclusive and may involve individuals, groups, families, organizations, or communities.

According to the National Association of Social Workers (1996) as stated in the revised Code of Ethics:

> The primary mission of the social work profession is to enhance human well-being and help meet the basic needs of all people, with particular attention to the needs and empowerment of people who are vulnerable, oppressed, and living in poverty. A historic and defining feature of social

work is the profession's focus on individual well-being in a social context and the well-being of society. Fundamental to social work is the attention to the environmental forces that create, contribute to, and address problems in living . . .

These activities may be in the form of direct practice, community organizing, supervision, consultation, administration, advocacy, social and political action, policy development and implementation, education, and research and evaluation. (p. 1)

Considering this definition, it becomes obvious that the general role of the social work professional in dealing primarily with the poor and the disadvantaged has expanded over time. For the health care social worker, in particular, it now involves working with diverse populations that can include those who are homeless, suicidal, homicidal, divorced, unemployed, mentally ill, medically ill, or drug abusing and delinquent, just to mention a few. In addition, the health care social worker must always strive to achieve restoration, enhanced wellness, the provision of concrete services, and prevention. Strategies to assist clients must address all of these areas, since many times these factors are considered intertwined and interdependent (Skidmore, Thackeray, & Farley, 1997).

TODAY'S HEALTH CARE SOCIAL WORKER

Name: Christopher L. Getz, MSW, PA
List State of Practice: Washington
Professional Job Title: Clinical Social Worker/Physician Assistant

Duties in a typical day:
I deal with people who have suffered a major tragedy surrounding a disease. I provide educational training to the client and his or her family members on the medical aspects of the disease and how to learn to live and cope with the disease process. I often act as advocate, to help the client get the necessary supports to improve the quality of his/her life.

What do you like most about your position?
I really enjoy working with the wide diversity of client problems and issues. I enjoy helping clients learn how to best cope with the disease process, encouraging empowerment each step of the way.

What do you like least about your position?
I often work long hours. At the end of the day, although I feel satisfied with what I have accomplished, I sometimes wish I could have done more.

What "words of wisdom" do you have for the new health care social worker considering work in a similar position?
In the area of medical social work, it is important to completely understand the process of the disease, from both a medical and psychosocial point of view. It is critical for the social worker to help the client to adjust and work through his or her feelings. Social workers need to help clients anticipate and prepare for the future. In terms of a progressive disease, acceptance and preparation are critical factors leading toward client empowerment and change.

THE UNIQUENESS OF HEALTH CARE SOCIAL WORK SERVICE PROVISION

CONTINUING EDUCATION

Given their understanding of the human condition, most social work health care professionals agree that, in general, the profession of social work is different from most of the other helping professions. Today, however, this assumption has come under direct attack. There are two important reasons for this attack: (a) in our current system of health care delivery, the number of practicing health care professionals has risen dramatically (Freudenheim, 1990; Shortell & Kaluzny, 1994); and (b) these professionals often perform the same or similar tasks (Lister, 1980). Often the roles and tasks that health care social workers perform overlap with those of practitioners from other disciplines (Davidson, 1990).

This will continue to make survival in the health care arena difficult for health care social workers, especially if we do not openly acknowledge and embrace the competition created by the circumstances noted earlier. For example, in a discussion at a National Association of Social Workers branch meeting, the issue of providing health care social work professionals with an ongoing series for continuing education was addressed. Many of the social workers at this meeting thought that if the state was going to require continuing education, then social workers should be able to obtain these hours through "related" workshops or seminars. In principle, this would make it easier for social work professionals to expand their choices of workshops and allow them to learn from other professionals.

As the task of establishing speakers and exploring topics for presentation began, a statement was made by one of the members and rapidly escalated into a heated discussion. Simply stated, the member asked, "How can we truly say that what we do as health care social workers is different from these other disciplines when we choose to receive most of our continued educational training from them?" This comment caused a lengthy debate. Some social work members stated that they appreciated this "additional" information, whereas others said it was not "additional" at all—it was "required" for effective practice. Regardless of what side was taken, most agreed that as social workers battle for a place in the health care delivery system, this "lack of uniqueness" concerning the skills and techniques often employed could be used against them. This makes the argument that social workers provide services not provided by other professionals a complicated one.

The disagreement and mixed emotions shared in this small meeting are not uncommon. Many states continue to struggle with continuing education requirements for social workers. How much is needed? Who should be eligible to provide programs? In this meeting a resolution was reached; however, it was not unanimous. These social workers recommended that continuing education should be required of all social work professionals, and this education could be provided by social workers or "other professionals." Thirty hours were recommended, with a minimum of fifteen being provided by social work professionals only. Although this policy recommendation was made for all areas of social work practice, most workshop presenters and topics under consideration were from the health care area.

For health care social workers in particular, the issue of the "uniqueness of social work services" remains a problem that we are forced to address. The competition for service delivery is fierce, and health care social workers must clearly establish that (a) what they do works; (b) they can do it quickly and in the most cost-effective way possible; and (c) what they do is different, contributing uniquely to the health and well-being of the clients served (Dziegielewski, 1997b).

RELATED HELPING DISCIPLINES

As stated in chapter 1, many other disciplines in the health care arena are doing the tasks that have traditionally been considered the role of social worker. In turn, social workers are also doing some of the tasks that have traditionally belonged to other disciplines. This complicates the ability to clearly establish a definition of what the health care social worker does as different and unique from the other related disciplines.

For example, most individuals know the difference between nursing and social work; however, in today's health care environment this distinction is no longer clear. Not only is there a blurring of roles between these two professions regarding the delivery of health care services, but there is overlap. Many nurses are now delivering services that were traditionally the role of the social work professional.

The role of the nursing professional is rapidly changing. In the past, nurses generally focused on the direct provision of medical and health-related services from the medical model perspective. Traditionally defined, a nurse was a person who was specially trained to care for sick or disabled persons (*Webster's Dictionary and Thesaurus*, 1993). It is this traditional role that secured them a place in health care along with physicians as essential personnel. Most of the psychosocial issues regarding patient care were either consulted with the social worker or left directly for the social worker to address. Today, however, this simplistic definition of the role of the nurse and of the social worker has clearly changed. No longer can the roles and tasks performed by social workers and nurses be so clearly differentiated. Nurses are now doing much more varied tasks than what would have been previously considered as "unusual nursing methods" of practice.

For example, for over a century "discharge planning" has been a part of the practice of health care social work as well as nursing. Historically, both disciplines recognize the need for formalized services that reflect discharge planning and have often worked together to provide subsequent aftercare activities. To date, studies (Egan & Kadushin, 1995; Holliman, Dziegielewski, & Teare, in press; Holliman, Dziegielewski, & Datta, 2001; Kulys & Davis, 1987; Sheppard, 1992) have looked at the differences between social work and nursing and the overlap of activities that often occurs. This role sharing has recently been noted as prospective payment systems have assigned discharge planning activities increased status, and overlapping and convergence of social work and nursing tasks has led to turf battles. The overlap and sharing between the two disciplines has led to the question of the exact role of the social worker and the nurse. To answer this question, Egan and Kadushin (1995) surveyed social workers and nurses to ascertain what generic hospital social service tasks should be done by social workers, nurses ,or both. Both social workers and nurses agreed that social workers were better qualified to provide concrete services such as setting up home equipment, arranging nursing home placement, and helping patients understand insurance and finances. However, both social workers and nurses saw themselves as qualified to perform the tasks of supportive counseling (Holliman, Dziegielewski, & Teare, in press).

In addition some studies have focused on systematic differences between the two groups. For example, Sheppard (1992) studied the communication styles of social workers and nurses during their interactions with physicians. Sheppard found that nurses contacted physicians more frequently than social workers, and the reason for contact often differed. Nurses generally contacted physicians about the patient's condition and treatment. Social workers contacted physicians less frequently; and when they did, they addressed the case's outcome, the final treatment plan, or family issues.

Bennett and Beckerman (1986) believed that the 1970s brought a change of status regarding the professionals who performed discharge planning. These authors pointed out that the "drudges of yesteryear" (i.e., those social workers who did not avoid assignments to medical and surgical services) had been transformed into major players. Carlton (1989) and Ross (1993) commended social workers for their ability to work with elaborate systems, and claimed that social workers were the best-qualified professionals to do discharge planning. Cox (1996), in a study of discharge planning with patients suffering from dementia, found that social workers were the team members most involved and influential with discharge decisions and nursing home placements. Atkatz (1995) found that social workers were commonly involved in discharges with the homeless because of the problematic placement issues with this group. Social workers were also frequently involved in cases of discharge planning with HIV/AIDS patients (Fahs & Wade,

1996; Marder & Linsk, 1995), the mentally ill (Gantt, Cohen, & Sainz, 1999; Tuzman, 1993), and infants with special care needs (Gentry, 1993). These studies support the importance of including social workers in discharge planning, especially when multiproblem cases occur and there is a lack of available community resources.

From the nursing perspective, several sources have claimed that nurses are the most qualified discharge planners because their medical training allows them to complete physical assessments, provide medical information with referrals, and assess the quality of health care resources and facilities (Lusis, 1996; McWilliams & Wong, 1993; Nurse specialists make discharge planning pay" 1994; Steun & Monk, 1990; Thoms & Mott, 1978; Worth, 1987).

McHugh (1994) and Spataro (1995) agree that although discharge planning remains a priority in nursing, the perceptions of what this requires vary. Some nursing professionals believe that nurses involved in discharge planning should take more of an administrative role; and others see the nurse's role as teaching patients and families complex postdischarge treatments such as breathing treatments, decubitus and skin care, feeding tubes, and home injections (Lusis, 1996; Penrod, Kane, & Kane, 2000).

The primary debate in the area of discharge planning focuses on who should be doing it, and what should be done. Turf battles between social work and nursing have increased over the last decade, as health care resources have become more limited. In summary, despite the continuous debates about who should do discharge planning, there is no empirical evidence that one group is more qualified than the other. Holliman, Dziegielewski & Teare (in press) conclude that despite role conflict and overlap, both social workers and nurses are able to make unique and substantial contributions in health care.

In addition to health care, many nursing professionals have advocated strongly for all nurses to be aware of the mental health aspects of practice, advocating for a new holistic approach to practice (Carson & Arnold, 1996). These professionals believe that nursing needs to expand and actively reach for a more comprehensive stance from which to base practice intervention strategy. According to these professionals, the idea that individuals are more than the sum of their parts must be incorporated into every aspect of professional nursing service. "In Mental Health Nursing, we therefore look at the total person, not just feelings and thoughts, but interaction of those feelings and thoughts with biological, social, cultural, and spiritual aspects of the person" (Carson & Arnold, 1996, p. xiii). These authors may be considered somewhat radical in their approach; however, they clearly reflect what is happening in the field. Whether it be the sheer numbers of nurses available to practice or the significant shifts in ideological thought among nurses practicing in the field, the profession of nursing is changing. Many of these changes have and will continue to affect the field of social work and the health care social work provider.

In this era of behavioral managed health care, nurses and physicians who are referred to as critical providers of medical services have a great deal of power in establishing a firm place in the delivery of health care services. Social workers, like many other allied professionals, are not considered essential. Therefore, nurses, in particular, can and often do compete for jobs or direct services that were usually done by social work professionals.

This means that nurse professionals are now, in addition to their traditional medical duties, initiating individual therapy, group therapy, crisis therapy, family therapy, mind–spirit therapies, health counseling and therapy, social work supervision, administrative services, and numerous other services that were usually considered the domain of the health care social worker.

After reviewing the services provided by helping professionals in the health care area, one sees that there is a great deal of overlap of roles and functions. With all the overlap, it is easy to see where confusion can originate as to the actual differences between the services these professionals provide. However, on careful examination, one ingredient remains conspicuously weak in the professions described, but prominent within social work. It is assistance to better the human condition, with the primary emphasis being placed on the environment that influences, surrounds, and reinforces it.

In summary, the greatest single factor that makes the professional health care social worker unique is the long-uncontested professional interest in the of "person in the situation" or the "person in the environment." This stance has long been our heritage or, more practically stated, our "guiding light for practice." Many of our basic texts describe it, and it is clearly reinforced in the classroom setting as well as in direct practice.

It is important to note that in today's practice environment, social workers are not the only ones aware of the importance of addressing clients within the environmental context. The importance of including a "person-environment stance" has not gone unrecognized within the other disciplines. Therefore, many of the traditional premises central to the field of social work (e.g., the total equals more than the sum of the parts) have been adopted by other health-related helping professionals for inclusion in their practice. These professionals now use many of the same principles and ideas of social work, further complicating or blurring the differences between the disciplines and the uniqueness of the roles that each professional provides.

TOWARD A DEFINITION OF CLINICAL HEALTH CARE SOCIAL WORK

Clinical social work in the health care setting is an area of practice that has sometimes been referred to as *medical social work*; it is not uncommon to see these terms used interchangeably. The *Social Work Dictionary* defines medical social work as a form of practice that occurs in hospitals and other health care settings and that facilitates good health and prevention of illness, as well as helps physically ill clients and their families to resolve the social and psychological problems related to disease and illness (Barker, 1995). To highlight the concept of facilitating good health further, wellness with its emphasis on promoting and maintaining a sense of client well-being has recently gained in popularity. In this definition, it is also important to acknowledge the role of the medical social worker in sensitizing other health care professionals to the social-psychological aspects of illness (Barker, 1995). In practice, the health care social worker addresses the psychosocial aspects of the client, alerts other team members to these needs, and facilitates service provision. Additionally the social worker not only represents the interests of the client, but also is expected to be reflective of the "moral conscience" for the health care delivery team.

As defined in this book, clinical health care social work practice includes a full range of social work services. These services include social work assessment or diagnosis, goal establishment, interventive foci, methods, and referral. It is important to note, however, that whenever possible, brief or time-limited intervention methods are strongly recommended for future practice survival (Dziegielewski, 1997a). When using time-limited interventions, no single theory or standard for practice application should govern a social worker's attempts to help an individual, group, family, or community resolve the problem being addressed. Further, many of the services that today's health care social workers are forced to provide can no longer be considered traditional. Many times the health care social worker is forced to see a client only briefly, or she or he may be unable to do more than concrete service referral and provision. Today's health care social worker must remain flexible and open to change, but there will always be exceptions.

In summary, the clinical health care social worker should always remember that clinical social work in the health field is a mutual process of face-to-face interventions in which the professional social worker provides social work services to clients, including services on behalf of those clients, who use them to resolve mutually identified and defined problems in client social functioning precipitated by actual or potential physical illness, disability or injury. (Carlton, 1984, p. 6)

Keeping this traditional definition in mind, the struggles that social workers must face in the health care area today should not be underestimated. Often the health care social work professional is viewed as "just" one of many providers. This makes purpose justification regarding service provision a daily struggle. Yet, it has become obvious that a clear statement of purpose and role performance is expected if one is to compete for and maintain a seat at the health care delivery table.

Establishing a clear definition of health care social work practice, either today or in our past, has not been an easy task. Health care social workers must remain flexible in the delivery of services. As a profession, this flexibility needs to be maintained not only to help our clients, but also to adjust to the environment in which our clients exist and need to be served.

ROLE OF THE HEALTH CARE SOCIAL WORKER IN MANAGED CARE

The current state of social work practice in the health care setting mirrors the turbulence found in the general health care environment. Medical social workers, like other health care professionals, are being forced to deal with numerous issues that include declining hospital admissions, reduced lengths of stay, and numerous other restrictions and methods of cost containment. Struggling to solve these issues has become necessary because of the inception prospective payment systems, managed care plans, and other changes in the provision and funding of health care (Davis & Meir, 2001; Johnson & Berger, 1990; Ross, 1993; Simon, Showers, Blumenfield, Holden, & Wu, 1995). Previous research has linked not receiving services to higher rates of high-risk patient relapse (Coulton, 1985). Social workers are being forced to discharge clients from services more quickly, and clients are being returned to the community in a weaker state of rehabilitation than ever before (Bywaters, 1991).

With so many changes in the social environment, there is little consistency in the delivery of health care social work and a great emphasis on cost containment (Davis & Meier, 2001). When health care administrators are forced to justify each dollar billed for services, there is little emphasis placed on the provision of what some term as "expendable services," such as mental health and well-being services, thorough discharge planning, and so on.

Unfortunately, the services that social workers perform are often placed in this category, and, as a result, they often feel the brunt of initial dollar-line savings attempts (Dziegielewski, 1996, 2002). As discussed earlier, just the sheer numbers of allied health care professionals who are moderately paid provide an excellent hunting ground for administrators pressured to cut costs. These administrators may see the role of the social worker as adjunct to the delivery of care, and may decide to cut back or replace them with concretely trained nonprofessionals simply to cut costs. These substitute professionals do not have either the depth or breadth of training that the social work professional has, which can result in substandard professional care. For example, a trained paraprofessional in hospital discharge planning may simply facilitate a placement order. Issues, such as the individual's sense of personal well-being, ability for self-care, or family and environmental support, may not be considered. Therefore, the employment of this type of paraprofessional can be cost-effective but not quality care driven. If personal/social and environmental issues are not effectively addressed, clients may be put at risk.

The client who is discharged home to a family that does not want him or her is more at risk of abuse and neglect (Kemp, 1998). A client who has a negative view of self and a hopeless and hapless view of his or her condition is more likely to try to commit suicide. Many paraprofessionals or members of other professional disciplines can differ from social work professionals because they do not recognize the importance of culture and environmental factors. The deemphasis or denial of this consideration can result in the delivery of "cheap" but substandard care.

As administrators strive to cut costs by eliminating professional social work services, the overall philosophy of wellness has been sacrificed for a concentration on cost cutting. It is important to note, however, that many times these types of staff reductions are not personal attacks on social work professionals. Changes and cutbacks in the delivery of services and those who provide them are often done to address an immediate need—cost reduction. The fluctuating and downsizing of social work professionals, as with other allied health professionals, may simply reflect the fluctuating demands of the current market (Falck, 1990, 1997).

Ross (1993) points out that health care employees who are at the greatest risk of losing their place in the delivery of health care services are those who (a) do not create direct hospital revenues; (b) are not self-supporting parts of the health care delivery team; (c) hold jobs where productivity is not easily measured or questionable; (d) provide service where the long-term benefit for cost of service is not measured; and (e) engage in a service where the professional's role is often misunderstood, challenged, and underrated in the system. Unfortunately, social workers, along with other allied professionals who participate in the health care delivery system, often meet these criteria (Dziegielewski, 1996). Therefore, it is important for social work professionals to be viewed as an essential part of the health care delivery team, providing both needed direct clinical services as well as fiscal support for the agency setting (Dziegielewski, 2002).

In closing, it is important not to confuse the social worker who works in managed care with the concept of providing case management in the health care setting (Davis & Meier, 2001). In the traditional provision of case management services, the goal is to get the client the best and most cost-effective treatment based on client need (Edinburg & Cottler, 1990), whereas, in behavioral managed health care the role of the social worker as a case manager is to help cut costs by discouraging any unnecessary services or procedures (Shorter, 1990).

CHAPTER SUMMARY AND FUTURE DIRECTIONS

The problem of developing a definition of health care social work as described in the beginning of this chapter is not an uncommon one. Originally, the roots of the health care social worker, similar to those of the social work profession, were generally linked to serving the poor and the disfranchised. However, over the years the role of the health care social worker has expanded tremendously. This makes defining exactly what social workers do a difficult task. Clarity of definition has been further complicated by changes in scope of practice, the diverse roles of social work, and the expectations within the client–practitioner relationship. This turbulent environment requires that social work professionals constantly balance "quality-of-care" issues with "cost-containment" measures for clients, while securing a firm place as professional providers in the health care environment.

In this chapter, a general definition of the role of the health care social worker was presented along with a discussion of role ambiguity and confusion. Some of the differences between health care social workers and the other related disciplines were outlined. In summary, the major distinguishing factor found was the practice-based environmental stance that has historically reflected the roots of social work practice. Therefore, health care social work needs to be viewed as the professional "bridge" that links the client, the multidisciplinary or interdisciplinary team, and the environment. Now, more than at any time in the past, it is important to define clearly the similarities and differences between the professions. The numbers of health care professionals in practice have risen dramatically; and these professionals who often perform similar or duplicating functions are competing for limited health care jobs.

For future marketability and competition, it is believed that social workers need to move beyond the traditional definition and subsequent role of the health care social worker. In the area of clinical practice, new or refined methods of service delivery need to be established and used. Social workers are encouraged to become managers, owners of companies, employees, administrators, supervisors, clinical directors, and case managers so they can help influence specific agency policy and procedure. They also need to make themselves aware of basic programs beyond their own individual practice that can affect health care service delivery. The specific recommendations, techniques, and guidelines discussed in the following chapters will be useful in helping health care social workers equip themselves with the tools in practice, administration, and supervision that they will need to secure a seat at today's table for health care delivery.

In closing, several steps are suggested to help social work professionals survive the numerous changes presented with managed care.

First, social workers need to market the services they provide and link them to cost-effectiveness. Social work is an old profession in the competition scheme when compared with many of the newer health care delivery professions. Traditionally, social workers helped the poor and disenfranchised (Hepworth, Rooney & Larsen, 2002), both of which are not considered desirable client populations in the managed care context. This is not to suggest that social workers abandon their roots simply to appear more marketable in the scheme of managed care. Rather, we should consider professional self-marketing and emphasize the myriad services that we actually do provide.

It is essential to link the provision of each service the health care social worker provides with the cost saving it creates (Dziegielewski, 1996, 1997b). For example, traditional services, such as hospital discharge planning, should emphasize dollars saved in the overall prospective payment reimbursement system. Dollar amounts should be calculated to justify of overall savings because of service provision. A second example of saving costs through prevention can involve the home health care social worker. Home visits can assist families and clients in the home to acquire needed counseling to defuse stressed situations, can provide needed social support, and can provide access to services to maintain community placement. The cost-cutting feature of living in the community is phenomenal when compared with institutionalized care of patients. Options like these are facilitated by the provision of effective social work services.

A new mind-set needs to be established with service provision. Each service needs to be competitive, and emphasis must be placed on income generated or cost savings incurred (Dziegielewski, 1996). Many times, even without direct income being generated, services can be valued based on the costs they can save the organization.

A second thing that health care social workers can do to compete successfully in the managed care market is to present their professional roles as essential ingredients to the success of the health care interdisciplinary team. For this to happen, the process must start with the individual social work professional. Each social worker, with each service provided, whether it be discharge planning, referrals, or direct clinical work, needs to make the client aware that the service being provided or coordinated is being done by a social work professional. Laypeople may mistake social workers for nurses or teachers, or even call them counselors. Many times we become so task-oriented that we forget this simple but essential point. Tell them you are a health care social worker.

As you work with the health care team, you also must make them aware of your importance in the overall success of the team. Thinking of the services you provide in a cost-saving prevention perspective will also help with gaining professional recognition. You help the other team members to be able to complete their jobs, and in addition, you help save them time and money.

A third aspect in the survival of social work in the health care delivery scene rests in the larger environment. Here, social workers need to support and lobby for political and social recognition of the value of social work services from both a quality-of-care and cost-effectiveness basis. In this constantly changing environment, it is important for social workers to be visible and ready to secure their current position as well as additional positions that may come open. For example, social workers may choose to fight for limited prescription privileges as a cost-cutting quality-of-care standard for practice (Dziegielewski, 1997a). Lobbyists, well aware of social work's goals and missions, need to be strategically placed as these managed care decisions are being made. Managed care planners need to be made aware of and enticed to include the services that social workers can provide.

Lastly, the role of the social worker in behavioral managed health care needs to continue to grow beyond what is considered traditional. Social workers need to continue to assume varied positions, such as managers, owners of companies, employees, administrators, supervisors, clinical directors, and case managers (Edinburg & Cottler, 1995). Once in these positions, social workers will have power to help influence specific agency policies and procedures. They also need to make themselves aware of basic programs and services that are available beyond their own individual practice that can affect overall wellness and service delivery. The profession of social work is strong enough to compete, but there is no time for hesitancy. The plans for tomorrow are being outlined today. These plans outline the delivery of services in which health care social workers can and need to remain an integral part.

REFERENCES

Atkatz, J. M. (1995). Discharge planning for homeless patients. *DAI* 55(11), 363A (University Microfilm No. AAC9509698).

Barker, R. L. (1995). *The social work dictionary* (3rd ed.). Washington, DC: National Association of Social Workers Press.

Bennett, C., & Beckerman, N. (1986). The drama of discharge: Worker/supervisor perspectives. *Social Work in Health Care, 11,* 1–12.

Bywaters, P. (1991). Case finding and screening for social work in acute general hospitals. *British Journal of Social Work, 21,* 19–39.

Carlton, T. O. (1984). *Clinical social work in health care settings: A guide to professional practice with exemplars.* New York: Springer Publishing Co.

Carlton, T. O. (1989). Discharge planning and other matters. *Health and Social Work, 14*(1), 3–5.

Carson, V. B., & Arnold, E. N. (1996). *Mental health nursing: The nurse patient journey.* Philadelphia: Saunders.

Coulton, C. J. (1985). Research and practice: An ongoing relationship. *Health and Social Work, 10,* 282–292.

Cox, C. B. (1996). Discharge planning for dementia patients: Factors influencing caregiver decisions and satisfaction. *Health and Social Work, 21*(2), 97–104.

Davidson, K. W. (1990). Role blurring and the hospital social worker's search for a clear domain. *Health and Social Work, 15,* 228–234.

Davis, S. R., & Meier, S. T. (2001). *The elements of managed care: A guide for helping professionals.* Pacific Grove, CA: Brooks/Cole.

Donald, A. (2002). Evidenced based medicine: Key concepts. *Medscape Psychiatry & Mental Health ejournal, 7*(2) 1–5: http://www.medscape.com/viewarticle/430709.

Dziegielewski, S. F. (1996). Managed care principles: The need for social work in the health care environment. *Crisis Intervention and Time-Limited Treatment, 3,* 97–110.

Dziegielewski, S. F. (1997a). Should clinical social workers seek psychotropic medication prescription privileges? Yes. In B. A. Thyer (Ed.), *Controversial issues in social work practice* (pp. 152–165). Boston: Allyn & Bacon.

Dziegielewski, S. F. (1997b). Time limited brief therapy: The state of practice. *Crisis Intervention and Time Limited Treatment, 3,* 27–228.

Dziegielewski, S. F. (2002). *DSM-IV-TR™ in action.* New York: Wiley.

Edinburg, G. M., & Cottler, J. M. (1990). Implications for managed care in social work in psychiatric hospitals. *Hospital and Community Psychiatry, 41*, 1063–1064.

Edinburg, G. M., & Cottler, J. M. (1995). Managed care. In R. L. Edwards (Ed.), *Encyclopedia of social work* (19th ed., Vol. 2, pp. 1199–1213). Silver Spring, MD: National Association of Social Workers.

Egan, M., & Kadushin, G. (1995). Competitive allies: Rural nurses' and social workers' perceptions of the social work role in the hospital setting. *Social Work in Health Care, 20*(3), 1–23.

Fahs, M. C., & Wade, K. (1996). An economic analysis of two models of hospital care for AIDS patients: Implications for hospital discharge planning. *Social Work in Health Care, 22*(4), 21–34.

Falck, H. S. (1990). Maintaining social work standards in for profit hospitals: Reasons for doubt. *Health and Social Work, 15*, 76–77

Falck, H. S. (1997). The social work career in health care: Assessments, predictions, and some advice. *Newsletter of the Society for Social Work Administrators in Health Care, 23*(4), 1–6.

Freudenheim, M. (1990, March 5). Job growth in health care areas. *New York Times*, p. 1.

Gantt, A. B., Cohen, N. L., & Sianz, A. (1999). Impediments to discharge planning effort for psychiatric inpatients. *Social Work in Health Care, 29*(1), 1–14.

Gentry, L. R. (1993). The special caretakers program: A hospital solution to the boarder baby problem. *Health and Social Work, 18*(1), 75–77.

Hepworth, D. H., Rooney, R. H., & Larsen, J. (2002). *Direct social work practice: Theory and skills* (6th ed.). Pacific Grove, CA: Brooks/Cole.

Holliman, D., Dziegielewski, S. F., & Datta, P. (2001). Discharge planning and social work practice. *Journal of Health Care Social Work. 32*(3), 1–19.

Holliman, D., Dziegielewski, S. F., & Teare, R. (in press). Differences and similarities between social work and nurse discharge planners. *Health and Social Work.*

Imperato, P. J. (1996). Keeping care in health care reform. *Journal of Community Health, 21*, 155–158.

Johnson, R. S., & Berger, C. S. (1990). The challenge of change: Enhancing social work services at a time of cutback. *Health and Social Work, 15*, 181–190.

Kemp, A. (1998). *Abuse in the family: An introduction.* Pacific Grove, CA: Brooks/Cole.

Kulys, R., & Davis, M. A. (1987). Nurses and social workers: Rivals in the provision of social services? *Health and Social Work, 12*(2), 101–112.

Lister, L. (1980). Expectations of social workers and other health professionals. *Health and Social Work, 5*, 41–49.

Lum, D. (2003). *Culturally competent practice.* Pacific Grove, CA: Brooks/Cole.

Lusis, S. A. (1996). The challenges of nursing elderly surgical patients. *AORN Journal, 64*(6), 954–958.

Marder, R., & Linsk, N. L. (1995). Addressing AIDS long-term care issues through education and advocacy. *Health and Social Work, 20*(1), 75–80.

McHugh, R. (1994). *Hospital staff nurses' perceptions of their role and responsibility in the discharge planning process. DAI32*(05), 1373. (University Microfilms No. AAC1356729)

McWilliams, C. L., & Wong, C. A. (1993). Keeping it secret: The costs and benefits of nursing's hidden work in discharge patients. *Journal of Advanced Nursing, 19*(1), 152–153.

National Association of Social Workers. (1996, August). *Code of ethics* (Adopted by the National Association of Social Workers Delegate Assembly, August 1996). Washington, DC: Author.

National Association of Social Workers. (2001). NASW Standards for cultural competence in social work practice. Retrieved from: *www.naswdc.org/pubs/standards/cultural.htm.*

Nurse specialists make discharge planning pay. (1994). *American Journal of Nursing, 94*, 9.

Penrod, J. D., Kane, R. A., & Kane, R. L. (2000). Effects of post-hospital informal care on nursing home discharge. *Research on Aging, 22*(1), 66–82.

Poole, D. L. (1996). Keeping managed care in balance. *Health and Social Work, 85*, 163–165.

Ross, J. W. (1993). Redefining hospital social work: An embattled professional domain. *Health and Social Work, 18*(4), 243–247.

Sheppard, M. (1992). Contact and collaboration with general practitioners: A comparison of social workers and community psychiatric nurses. *British Journal of Social Work, 22*(4), 419–436.

Shortell, S. M., & Kaluzny, A. D. (1994). Forward. In S. M. Shortell & A. D. Kaluzny (Eds.), *Health care management: Organizational behavior and design* (3rd ed., p. 11). Albany, NY: Delmar

Shorter, B. D. (1990). Managed care/case management: What, why and how to cope. *Discharge Planning Update, 10*, 1–19.

Simon, E. P., Showers, N., Blumenfield, S., Holden, G., & Wu, X. (1995). Delivery of home care services after discharge: What really happens. *Health and Social Work, 20*, 6–14.

Skidmore, R. A., Thackeray, M. G., & Farley, O. W. (1997). *Introduction to social work* (7th ed.). Boston: Allyn & Bacon.

Spataro, J. (1995). An investigation of staff nurses' and nurse managers' knowledge and sense of responsibility for discharge planning. *MAI 33*(04), 1231. (University Microfilms No. AAC1359746)

Steun, C., & Monk, A. (1990). Discharge planning: The impact of Medicare's prospective payment on elderly patients. *Journal of Gerontological Social Work, 15*(3/4), 149–165.

Thoms, R.L., & Mott, R. (1978). A new role for the RN: Discharge coordinator. *Hospital Progress, 59*(2), 38–40.

Tuzman, L. (1993). Clinical decision making for discharge planner in psychiatric settings. *DAI50*(09), 320. (University Microfilms No. AAC9000681)

Webster's dictionary and thesaurus. (1993). Ashland, OH: Landoll.

Worth, A. (1987). Community nurses and discharge planning. *Nursing Standard, 21*(8), 25–30.

GLOSSARY

Allied health care workers: Professionals involved in health care delivery. The individual, group, family, or community is the focus of intervention.

Clinical social work practice: Often referred to as medical social work (see *medical social work*).

Family counseling: A practice methodology that centers on the "family" as the client or unit of attention.

Health care practice: Activities that are designed to enhance physical and psychological well-being.

Health care social work: The practice of social work that deals with the aspects of general health, specifically in the areas of wellness, illness, or disability. The social work professional can address these issues through working directly with individuals, groups, families, or communities, or to effect broader social change.

Health care social worker: Is seen as the professional "bridge" that links the client, the multidisciplinary or interdisciplinary team, and the environment.

Hospital social work: Historically defined as the provision of social services in the medical setting. Currently, refers to the delivery of social work services in hospitals and related health care facilities.

Medical social work: A form of social work practice that occurs in health care settings with the goal of assisting those who are physically ill, facilitating good health, and preventing illness.

Nursing: A field of practice versed in medical matters and entrusted with caring for the sick.

Practice of social work: The application of social work knowledge, theories, methods, and skills to provide professional, sound, ethically bound, culturally sensitive social services to individuals, groups, families, organizations, and communities.

Psychology: The profession and science concerned with the behavior of humans and related mental and physiological processes.

Public health: Tasked with prevention of disease and maintenance of health in the population.

QUESTIONS FOR FURTHER STUDY

1. In your own words, state several concrete differences between what nurses do and social workers do in the health care setting.
2. What do you believe can make health care social work practice an integral part of health care delivery?
3. What characteristic of social work practice makes it the most marketable in today's health care practice arena?
4. How do you believe health care social work will be defined in the future?

WEBSITES

www.ahcpr.gov
Health care research and policy information.

www.policy.com/vcongress/pbor/index.html
Information on Patient Bill of Rights.

www.patientadvocacy.org
Information on patient advocacy.

CHAPTER 3

The Many Faces of Social Work Practice

HISTORICAL ROOTS OF HEALTH CARE PRACTICE

Health care social work has generally dealt with the social factors that influence health, mental health, and illness and disease. Throughout history, clinical health care social work has often been called *medical social work*. As a practice that tries to create an environment favoring general health and wellness, medical social work can be viewed as one of the oldest and well-established fields of professional social work practice.

ALMSHOUSES

Health care social work can be traced back as far as the 1700s to the almshouses, which were places of refuge for poor, medically sick, and mentally ill patients of all ages. They were frequently referred to as the "poorhouses" or places of death. These philanthropic institutions were often scarcely funded. They primarily housed only society's outcasts, particularly those who were poor or incapacitated or who suffered from contagious diseases. Individuals who had any form of family support were cared for at home. In these early days, health care was considered a private matter, and individuals and their families were expected to take care of themselves. Therefore, the almshouse was used as an "option of last resort," providing a type of indoor shelter and relief for the destitute. It was one of the earliest practice areas for health care providers. The health care workers who provided caretaking services in the almshouses often became ill themselves, since, like

48

the occupants of the almshouse, they were subjected to poor sanitary conditions and numerous contagious diseases.

In 1713, William Penn founded the first almshouse in Philadelphia; in 1736 a second almshouse was founded at Bellevue Hospital in New York. The almshouse in Bellevue usually housed the mentally ill and later became one of the most famous mental health hospitals in the state of New York. Throughout history, the almshouse has been noted as a community-based institution, often viewed as the forerunner of today's hospital (Nacman, 1977). Service within these institutional settings remained standard until the 1800s, when slowly the services needed for sick individuals began to be viewed separately from services needed to house the poor (Colby & Dziegielewski, 2001).

Individuals who could afford medical care did not want service from these institutions, and philanthropic gifts were used to start new and more proficient facilities for providing care (Nacman, 1977). The poor were eventually separated out, and although "indoor" relief was still provided, they were expected to live and work in special facilities. In many cases, the government actually contracted with private individuals to feed and provide shelter and clothing for these individuals in exchange for contracted labor services. Soon children were also removed from the almshouses by the efforts of the Children's Aid Society. These children were later placed in orphanages. In 1851, the mentally ill were also removed and sent to improved facilities, primarily through the crusading efforts of Dorthea Lynde Dix. Basically, the "holding tank" nature of the almshouse was replaced with more segregated forms of institutionalized care such as orphanages and other residential facilities.

When the Revolutionary War began, soldiers needed to receive adequate medical care in order to return to battle. New York Hospital ,designed to treat the military, was the first hospital to actually begin to provide systematized training to medical students. By 1840, hospitals originally founded by philanthropy were beginning to specialize and provide care to certain populations or for particular diseases (Nacman, 1977).

It was around this time that "indoor" forms of social welfare relief, in which the individual had to live within the institution to get services, were replaced by "outdoor" forms of relief in which the poor were provided with concrete supplies, goods, and services while living in their own homes.

CHARITY ORGANIZATION SOCIETIES

With the delivery of health care outside of the institution came the emergence of charity organization societies. The first American Charity Organization Society began in Buffalo, New York, in 1877. These groups are considered important in the historical development of health care social work because they provided the basis for the modern social service agencies of today. The workers they employed are often considered to be some of the first to deliver social services in the home setting to poor and disenfranchised individuals. These service workers were referred to as "friendly visitors." The charity organizations and the workers who represented them, however, were not objective. Many times they previously defined who was worthy of assistance and who was not. For example, children and elderly were believed to be unable to control their situations, whereas younger adults could. The ideology subscribed to here was primarily one of social Darwinism, in which only the strongest and best people would survive. The friendly visitors were usually upper-class people whose mission was to reform or redeem the poor. They had specific predetermined plans for fixing the problems they encountered. Each organization set its own limits and parameters and handled situations as it saw fit. This form of health delivery had several weaknesses: (a) there was no systematized way of delivering services, and duplication of services often occurred; (b) most services delivered were on a "one-time" basis, and no education or teaching was provided to negate future problems; and (c) the service workers were not professionally trained, and many times acted on predetermined notions of client worth and aptitude. Often these early health care workers believed that the clients they served were at fault. In many cases, the client was seen as responsible for the problem because it was believed that the problem originated "within the client," not within the system. In turn, little advocacy for improvement of public health standards was noted, although some referrals for direct medical intervention did occur.

HOSPITAL SOCIAL WORK

Hospital-based social work practice has been in existence since the late nineteenth century, when early social service professionals were sought to help connect the client's environmental system with the hospital where care was rendered. These early social workers reached beyond the traditional bounds of the hospital to educate the patient and the general public about environmental factors that influence health (Cabot, 1915). Connecting the institution, the person, and the environment is a common theme throughout the history of hospital social work.

Johns Hopkins Hospital established its first social work program in 1907; the first social worker to be employed there was Helen B. Pendleton (Nacman, 1977). Because of internal conflicts at the hospital, Ms. Pendleton did not stay in this position long, and another social worker soon took her place. At the same time, Massachusetts General Hospital assigned a social worker to the neurological clinic; 4 years later, New York State began to support after-care programs for discharged patients. The inclusion of these early health care social workers is important because they highlighted the need and laid the groundwork for the addition of professional social work services. They were often responsible for the care, maintenance, storage, and return of the medical record as well as for determining who was eligible to receive indigent care. Generally, medical records were not treated as confidential, and information regarding content was distributed on a need-to-know basis. Often these social workers were moralistic and paternalistic regarding worker–client interactions.

In these early days, health care social work services were generally performed by hospital nurses. These nurses were often considered convenient choices for employment because they were easily accessible, already knew agency procedure, and were aware of community resources. Later, however, it was established that more specialized training understanding social conditions was needed. To address this need for specialized training in social work, the School of Philanthropy was developed in 1898. This organization was designed to outline rules and guidelines for the profession; however, it did not actually influence formal social work education until 1932, when the schools that formally taught social work joined together to establish curriculum rules.

In 1918, the National Conference of Social Work in Kansas City helped to form the American Association of Hospital Social Workers. This was the first professional social work organization in the United States (Carlton, 1984). The formation of this association clearly established the acceptance of health care social work as a legitimate form of social work services. As the role of health care social work expanded beyond the traditional bounds of the hospital, a name change for the organization was initiated to make it more inclusive. To reflect this expansion, in 1934 the name of this organization was changed to the American Association of Medical Social Workers. Actually, it was the American Association of Medical Social Workers that constituted one of the seven professional social work associations that merged together in 1955 to form the National Association of Social Workers.

In the 1920s, Flexner, a prominent scholar of the time, fueled the debate as to whether social work was a profession when he said it was not. This debate prompted social workers to try to clearly define what they did and the role they played among the helping professions (Austin, 2001; Thyer, 2002). In the 1930s "removing patients" or discharge planning was devalued and described as an administrative or clerical function (Bartlett, 1940). Therefore, from 1920 to1970, the trend was for social workers with the least formal education to provide concrete services and discharge patients, while those with more skill would focus on more abstract, and presumably more difficult and more specialized, functions such as counseling (Davidson, 1978; Kadushin, 1989; Steun & Monk, 1990).

In 1928, the American College of Surgeons developed and included a minimum standard of service provision for social service departments. In the 1920s and 1930s, the United States military started to add social workers to its ranks. Regardless of theoretical orientation or exact role performed, social workers and the services they provide have since been considered necessary. Reflected in service commitment through the National Association of Social Workers, as well as through other professional groups (e.g., the Association of Health Care Social Workers, the Association of Clinical Social Workers, and the Council on Social Work Education), health care social workers have maintained an active role in the policies, procedures, and services required by today's demanding health care environment.

During the time period from 1920 to1980, rising health care costs caused great concern, and different ways to address and reduce these costs were explored. As the role of the hospital expanded ,so did the need for hospital social work, and departments headed and staffed by professional social workers emerged within hospital administrative structures.

In 1983 diagnosis related groups (DRGs) was phased into hospitals as a prospective reimbursement system whereby hospitals billed according to diagnosis rather than according to the costs of services. With these specific treatment guidelines and expected time limits, pressure increased for hospitals to discharge clients as expediently as possible.

It was during this time that discharge planning became recognized as a vital function within the hospital. Therefore, the professionals who performed the tasks that facilitated timely discharge were considered essential to the health care delivery team (Holliman, 1998). With the pressure to reduce costs, however, attempts to eliminate what might be considered nonessential professional staff also emerged. The resulting fear of job loss helped to increase the competition among disciplines already serving as part of the client-care team. The competition between social work and nursing amplified, and nurses started to show an increased interest in discharge planning activities. Unfortunately, in the 1990s downsizing to reduce costs caused many services that were considered nonessential to be eliminated, and in some cases hospital social work departments were eliminated (Dziegielewski & Holliman, 2001; Holliman, Dziegielewski, & Datta, 2001). Hospital social workers were generally recognized for their supportive interventions (i.e., counseling and adjustment), rather than for direct placement. This cost-saving administrative decision had many ripple effects in the social work profession. It limited the availability of social work supervision and continuing education for social worker discharge planners (Holliman, Dziegielewski, & Datta, 2001).

PULLING IT ALL TOGETHER

Carlton (1984) defines health care social work in its broadest sense by referring to it as "all social work in the health field" (p. 5). Thus, he believes that it includes more than just basic clinical practice. Although the concentration in this book is primarily on the clinical practice of health care social work, it is important to note that the concept of health care social work can be much broader. It can include, at a minimum, practice in relation to institutional, community, state, and federal health policy; program planning and administration; preparation, supervision, and continued training for social workers and other allied health professionals in the health field; and social research (Carlton, 1984).

Difficulty in trying to define this branch of social work is not new, and problems with establishing exactly what the health care social worker does have for a long time been a thorn in the side of health care administrators who justify funding. Because of the varied and situation-dependent circumstances each social worker must deal with, it becomes easy to understand how difficult it is to predict exactly what a health care social worker will do in practice. Health care social workers in particular are known for their ability to "fix what is broken" and to do this with an incredible sense of urgency and competence in the most cost-effective manner possible. Given the complexity of the human situation, sometimes this task is not as simple as it might sound. Therefore, it remains difficult to say exactly what health care social workers do. Now, imagine having to "do it" in a constantly changing environment (Davis & Meier, 2001). Unfortunately, this is the world in which the health care social worker often struggles to best meet the needs of clients.

TODAY'S HEALTH CARE SOCIAL WORKER

Name: Ricardo Oliver, BSW
List State of Practice: Florida
Professional Job Title: Senior Case Manager

Duties in a typical day:
Answer and return calls to health care professionals, other case managers, peers and colleagues, and referral sources for existing or potential clients. I also visit hospitals, rehabilitation centers, nursing homes, and Adult Congregate Living Facilities (ACLFs) and client homes to perform initial intake interviews and assessments. I also complete home visits and make recommendations for home modifications to maximize independence. I also assist in securing services and durable medical equipment for the clients the facility serves.

What do you like most about your position?
Meeting with clients and helping to empower them to become more independent or secure. I also like to work with clients and assure them I will make every attempt possible to meet their needs.

What do you like least about your position?
My greatest disappointment is that I do not have the power to bend the guidelines enough to meet the individualized needs of each client. I do not like having to deny services or to talk with families when their relative has died.

What "words of wisdom" do you have for the new health care social worker who is considering working in a similar position?
Don't let the job get to you and don't take it home with you. Get ready for stressful situations because in this field you can expect them to occur.

What is your favorite health care social work story?
I once had a client who had a brain injury as well as spinal cord injuries. She was in a motor vehicle accident while vacationing in Florida. In the accident she lost her spouse and became a single mother of two minor children who were both in Pennsylvania. Her injuries were very severe, and with the help of the Brain Injury Association of Florida we were able to get her started on relearning her own activities of daily living (ADLs). Once she was able to take care of herself, she had to relearn how to be a parent. After years of hard work, my proudest moment was when she went back home to Pennsylvania and once again began to assume the role of mother of her children. In this case interagency coordination was essential, and close contacts were kept between her treatments in Florida and her children that were staying with relatives in Pennsylvania. This interagency teamwork allowed her to be retrained and reunited with her family.

ROLES OF THE HEALTH CARE SOCIAL WORKER

The Social Work Dictionary (Barker, 1995) describes the term *health care worker* as "a generic name for all the professional, paraprofessional, technical and general employees of a system or facility that provides for the diagnosis, treatment and overall well-being of patients" (p. 164). However, there is a clear distinction between the terms *health care worker* and *allied health care worker.* To distinguish between the two terms, clearly one must remember that (a) *health care workers* usually refers to nonprofessional staff involved in health care delivery, and (b) *allied health care workers* refers to the professionals involved in health care delivery. The health care workers are generally those nonprofessionals who work in health care, such as home health aides, medical records personnel, nurses' aides, orderlies, and attendants (Barker, 1995).

Allied health professionals, do not include physicians and nurses, but do include professional personnel of hospitals and other health care facilities. Physicians and nurses are not considered allied service providers because their service is considered essential to any basic medical care. Allied health care providers include audiologists, dietitians, occupational therapists, optometrists, pharmacists, physical therapists, psychologists, social workers, speech pathologists, and others.

It is under the label *allied health professional* that the health care social worker generally performs most of his or her duties in the health care arena. It is believed that health care social workers serve this area well because of their broad-based training on the biological, psychological, and social factors (i.e., the biopsychosocial approach) that can affect a client's environmental situation.

PROVISION OF CORE CLINICAL SERVICES

Today, the role of the health care professional has been clearly established. Social workers can now be found in every area of our health care delivery system. Table 3.1 summarizes the core services provided to individuals, families, and groups, which include (a) case finding and outreach, which primarily relates to helping clients and their families to identify not only the health care services that they need but also how to obtain them; (b) preservice or preadmission planning that is designed to anticipate barriers to accessing care; (c) assessment, especially about the need for the provision of social work services and planning for continued health and well-being; (d) concrete service provision, as in admission and discharge from service planning; (e) psychosocial evaluations, which assess clients from a biopsychosocial perspective with cultural considerations appropriately highlighted; (f) identification of clear goals and specific objectives that need to be accomplished during health care service delivery; (g) direct clinical counseling that reflects the therapeutic intervention strategy for individuals, families, and groups and that considers the biopsychosocial perspective; (h) assistance with short-or long-term planning, where clients and their families are helped to anticipate their current and future service needs; (i) direct assistance with preventive remedial and rehabilitative measures; (j) information and education through instruction on significant health issues and problems that will assist clients, their families, and significant others; (k) training and support for

TABLE 3.1   Core Services Provided by Health Care Social Workers

Service	Description
Case finding and outreach	Identify and assist clients to secure services they need
Preservice planning	Identify and subsequently help client/family to plan and gain access to health care services
Assessment	Identify clients in need of service, and screen to identify health and wellness issues
Concrete service provision	Assist client/family to meet current and posthealth service needs, such as admission, discharge, and after-care planning and services
Psychosocial evaluations	Gather information on client biopsycho-social, cultural, financial, and situational factors for a formal psychosocial assessment plan or report
Identification of goals and objectives	Establish mutually negotiated goals with specific objectives to address client health and wellness issues
Direct clinical counseling	Help client/family to deal with situation and problems related to health intervention needed or received
Assistance with short- or long-term planning	Help client understand, anticipate, and plan for services needed based on current or expected health status
Information and health education	Provide instruction on areas of concern regarding client/family health and wellness
Assistance with wellness training	Help clients to establish a plan to secure continued or improved health status based on a holistic prevention model
Referral services	Provide information regarding services available and direct connection when warranted
Continuity of care	Assist client/family to be sure proper connections are made with the linking of all services needed considering the issue of multiple health care providers

(continued)

TABLE 3.1 *(continued)*

Service	Description
Client advocacy	Teach and assist clients how to obtain needed resources, or, on a larger scale, advocate for changes in policy or procedure that can have the direct or indirect benefit of assisting the client

continued health and wellness program development and participation; (l) referral service, which includes helping clients gain access and learn how to use these services; (m) continuity of care for the client as connections are made to other health care service providers; and (n) client advocacy, which means teaching clients how to obtain needed resources or, on a larger scale, advocating for changes in policies or procedures that can have a direct or indirect benefit.

As listed, the core clinical skills of the health care social worker can involve more than what has traditionally been called "discharge planning." Health care is a changing environment where even the classic definition of discharge planning has been altered. Social workers are not only coordinating discharges and services; they are providing oversight for the multidisciplinary or interdisciplinary teams to be sure that clients are getting the services they need. Furthermore, once the team agrees that a client is ready for discharge, it is often the social worker who is held responsible for ensuring that transfer forms are completed, client and family education has been done, and the records that support continued care are ready for transfer (Mankita & Alalu, 1996).

The role of the clinical social worker in the health care setting is a complex one. The responsibilities are often varied, and health care social workers must be willing to assume the roles needed plus remain flexible enough to advocate for change strategies that represent the best interests of the client.

The rest of this chapter will discuss supervisory, administrative, and community-based services, which go beyond what is generally considered the core of health care social work; however, all social workers must remain aware of and participate in these tasks and functions, particularly in this era of managed care.

PROVISION OF SUPERVISION

Supervision in the field of social work has a long, rich history. Kadushin (1976) provided a basic definition of a supervisor:

> An agency administrative staff member who is given authority to direct, coordinate, enhance, and evaluate on-the-job performance of supervisees for whose work he [or she] is held accountable. In implementing this role the supervisor performs administrative, educational, and supportive functions in interaction with the supervisee in the context of a positive relationship. The supervisor's ultimate objective is to deliver to agency clients the best possible service, both quantitative and qualitatively, in accordance with agency policies and procedures. (p. 21)

This general definition applies well to the field of health care social work. However, one must add "flexibility" because of the many ongoing changes in health care and how these changes can affect the health care practice environment. In the health care field, so many programs are under cost-containment restraints. This can lead to many reorganizations, cutbacks, and ultimately reductions in the work force (Braus, 1996). Davis and Meier (2001) warn that this can be a particular problem for health and mental health workers because they are continually forced to modify practice provisions based on third-party payers who refuse to cover some services or who have issues with length of stay. This makes the role of the social worker and thus the supervisor difficult, because "whatever these programs are called, they all involve reductions in funding that can result in fewer programs or resources, more restrictive service policies, closing and reorganization of physical offices, and loss of jobs by attrition or firing" (p. 269). Thus, training for successful health care social work in today's environment must emphasize a clear focus on controlling the rising costs of medical care (Caper, 1995).

It is believed that the allied health professionals trained in this way will clearly reap the greatest rewards in this managed health care environment. However, the flexibility and the changes required for practice survival that deviate from the traditional delivery of social work services often create a stressful environment for the supervisor, the supervisee, the organization, and the client or family being served.

Sheafor, Horejsi, and Horejsi (1997) believe that *supportive supervision* in human service organizations cannot be overemphasized. This type of supervision can help to address areas such as staff morale, and work-related anxiety and worry. If these factors are left unaddressed, they can lead to decreased job satisfaction and commitment to the agency. Supportive supervision can help to build worker self-esteem and emotional well-being. In health care social work this is important, and it can help to reduce employee burnout (Resnick & Dziegielewski, 1996; Sheafor, Horejsi, & Horejsi, 1997).

The National Association of Social Workers (1994) recommends that supervision be a combination of case presentations and education about these cases in a protected environment. The supervisee is to provide information to the supervisor about assessment, diagnosis, and proper treatment of the client. The supervisor, in turn, provides oversight, guidance, direction in assessing, diagnosing, and client treatments, while doing so in a nonthreatening environment that is conducive to learning. In a survey completed by Kadushin (1992), supervisees identified the need for uninterrupted supervisory sessions in current supervisory settings. This is particularly problematic in the health care area, where frequent changes based on program cutbacks can lead to organizational stress and forced decisions that may not be based on the best interests of the client or his or her family.

Levin and Herbert (1995) further warn that there are not clear guidelines about what constitutes the tasks of medical social workers at the MSW and BSW level, both of which often provide services in the health care setting (Holliman, Dziegielewski, & Teare, In Press). This lack of a clear definition means that supervisors need to be careful in assigning cases and tasks to be performed. When clear definitions do not exist, it is possible to assign tasks that are beyond the competence of the social worker and that can compromise client care and create worker stress (Levin & Herbert, 1995).

In today's health care environment, the health care social worker is often called on to serve in the role of mediator (Berkman, 1996). The social work supervisor does not take any side; he or she takes a stand of neutrality (Shulman, 2002). Advice and direction need to be given about how best to handle client care issues for the supervisee, the multidisciplinary or interdisciplinary professionals, the agency, and community. This may mean that the supervisor must be able to recognize conflicts that are not overt and help the supervisee to address them in the most professionally ethical and moral way possible. As an advocate, the supervisor must be willing to assist with the development of needed services to clients, their families, and significant others, while not losing sight of the common ground that links the supervisee to administration (Shulman, 2002). The supervisor must also serve as liaison to the community on behalf of the client. This last role will help to ensure that connections are made and contacts initiated.

The last area in which supervision in the health care setting is essential is in health education and health promotion programs. This is not a new area for social work; however, counseling that focuses on this perspective alone is. Because of the importance of this function for health care social workers, other areas of this book have been devoted to the specifics of teaching health and wellness issues in the medical setting. Supervisors need to be aware that this type of counseling was not generally stressed in the practice arena of most social work training programs. Thus supervisors must learn how to conduct this type of treatment and, in turn, help those who are being supervised to use it (see Table 3.2).

ADMINISTRATION AS A CORE SERVICE

Generally, administrative duties are not considered in the core practice area of health care social work. This chapter cannot cover all that is involved in this role. However, health care social workers who serve as administrators have a direct relationship to service provision that cannot be overlooked. For social work administrators, like other health care administrators, there have been competing management philosophies and issues that must be addressed. On one side, administrators have been told to increase the participation of professional staff members in agency decision-making processes as well as to improve psychological commitment and involvement with the organization. This is evidenced in recent literature that introduces and emphasizes the use of quality circles and total-quality-management principles for building a corporate culture that includes individual and management goals for the good of a corporation.

On the other side, financial and economic pressures have caused health care agencies to become concerned about securing adequate numbers of clients to justify service. This means increasing competitiveness and maximizing reimbursement potential. This often forces

TABLE 3.2 Core Health Practice Supervisory Skills

Service	Description
Direct social work supervision	Provide direct professional social work supervision through direction, guidance, and education on case service delivery and counseling
Direct supervision	Provide direct professional supervision through direction, guidance, and education in case service delivery as a contributor to the interdisciplinary or multidisciplinary team
Administrative supervision	Educate and advise social work supervisees on policy and program issues
Consultation	Provide consultation services to other social workers and to multidisciplinary and interdisciplinary professionals
Education	Assist and participate in training professionals to administer health education and health promotion programs

workers to be terminated while increasing the workloads of those who stay. A "more-with-less" mentality prevails that is not conducive to increased quality of life for employees. Often employee development and other "services" considered on the fringe are curtailed.

Given this paradoxical situation, social work health care administrators often feel trapped. Administration and funding agencies often send double messages to the administrator. This leaves the health care administrator with *limited power* that is often not viewed that way. Professionals and other service employees often believe that the administrator is capable of and responsible for sorting and balancing the true "reality" of the situation, and administrators feel trapped in the middle and unable to base their decision primarily on the provision of quality client care.

Noting that human services administrators do not operate in a vacuum is important. They are often forced to respond to pressures in the environment that can influence the decisions that they make and the guidance they provide about formation and implementation of policy and procedure. Although administrators provide consultation to agency boards and funding bodies on how to enhance service delivery to clients and organizations, they are limited. Often it is the boards and organizational personnel that oversee them that have the power to replace them. This is why it is essential that administrators work to develop procedures for ensuring procedural justice, due process, and ethical decision making. To help the administrator refine and develop new and improved programs to service client needs, quality assurance or continuous quality improvement are recommended. This is one way that an administration can ensure that services provided are meeting professional and efficient standards. Administrators need to advocate and serve as liaisons to help with the development of needed services for clients, their families, and significant others (see Table 3.3).

PROVISION OF COMMUNITY OUTREACH

Health care social work services from a community perspective are considered the third area of nontraditional core health care social work services. Community organization involves an intervention process to help with social problems and to enhance social well-being through planned collective action. The health care community organizer strives to help address community problems or areas where quality of life can be enhanced (Sheafor, Horejsi, & Horejsi, 1997; Jackson, 2001). Services addressed from a community perspective include (a) service outreach including identification of unmet needs, with emphasis placed on creating programs to service clients in unserved areas; (b)identification of the service needs for at-risk populations; (c) consultation services to other social workers and multidisciplinary and interdisciplinary professionals; (d) participation and instruction in health education and health promotion programs to serve the community better; (e) policy and program planning to ensure that the needs of clients are addressed; and (f) liaisons with the community on the behalf of the client. This last role will help to ensure that connections are made and contacts initiated (see Table 3.4). From a community perspective, health primarily involves availabilty and access to quality care. For health care social workers, community practice involves acknowledging whether hospitals and clinics and the services they provide are available to the

TABLE 3.3 Core Administrative Services

Service	Description
Agency consultation	Provide consultation to agency administrators on how to enhance service delivery to clients and organizations
Program development	Assist the agency to refine and develop new and improved programs to service client needs
Quality improvement	Assist the agency to be sure that continuous quality services are provided that meet professional and efficient standards
Service advocacy	Assist the agency in recognizing the needs of clients and help to develop new or needed services
Agency liaison	Serve as liaison to the agency on behalf of the client, ensuring connections are made between the client, the supervisor, and the community

clients in the area, as well as advocating for clients in terms of prevention and wellness (Kirst-Ashman, 2000).

CHAPTER SUMMARY AND FUTURE DIRECTIONS

Social workers, whether in the role of clinical practitioner, supervisor, administrator, or community organizer, are challenged to understand and anticipate the trend within our current health care system and the effects this trend will have on their current and future practice. Incrementalism, which is often reflective of current health care planning, involves compromising and engaging in agreements based on the needs and wishes of various political forces. The essential outcome that is often used to measure success, regardless of the type of service delivered to individuals, couples, families, or communities, is cost containment. It is essential that every health care social worker comprehend that control of rising health care costs will ultimately be considered his or her responsibility, whether he or she has the ultimate power to control this trend or not. Often, quality-of-care issues will be surrounded and ultimately influenced by a cost-containment strategy. This is not to reduce the importance of professional practice placed on quality control; however, to survive, all health care social workers will be

TABLE 3.4   Core Community Services

Service	Description
Service outreach	Identify unmet needs and services that are not available to clients; advocate for programs and services
At-risk service outreach	Identify clients who are at risk of decreased health or illness; advocate to secure services for them
Community consultation	Provide consultation services to communities to assist with the development of community-based services
Health education	Participate and instruct communities on developing and implementing health education programs
Policy and program planning	Assist in formulation and implementation of health care policies and programs that will help to meet client needs
Liaison to the community	Serve as a contact or connection person between the client and his or her family and the community

expected to help contain costs regardless of the role they are expected to perform (Caper, 1995).

This emphasis on cost-containment increases the importance of two primary aspects of health care social work practice. First, there must be increased emphasis on the macro–health care practice. This perspective calls for greater social action and social change. To accomplish this, social workers must (a) seek to understand the nature of the problem fully, (b) analyze trends, (c) collect and synthesize the data, and (d) communicate these data in a way that is understandable to health care administrators (Sheafor, Horejsi, & Horejsi, 1997). With this format in mind, social workers must work actively to make society understand its responsibility to create and regulate the health care industry. Believing that the health care system will eventually solve its own problems is ludicrous. Health care social workers, no matter what role they choose for practice delivery, must help to develop and present a format for approaching the problems in our current system and for establishing means for addressing them.

The second area that must be ingrained into all areas of health care social work practice is *advocacy* that leads to client empowerment. In advocacy social workers will help to identify and build on client's strengths, while helping clients to negotiate what can be a confusing and fragmented health care system. It is important for health care social workers to relinquish the mind-set that "managed care and the policies dictated by it are all bad." The benefits of managed health care can be pronounced for both clients and providers. Managed care and the implementation of these external fiscal controls can benefit our clients by providing (a) enhanced and more accessible and accountable mental health treatment; (b) enhanced client outcomes by forcing concentration on specific goals and objectives in therapeutic treatment; (c) time limits that can force the concentration and identification of external and environmental supports to allow continued therapeutic gains; and (d) deterrence of long-term therapy that can result in decreased long-term medication supplementation. Reducing the economic drain on the health care dollar in American business can only benefit the larger society (Browning & Browning, 1996).

Despite these stated benefits of managed health care, there are also many pitfalls. As a health care social worker, it is important to advocate for clients by assisting health care agencies in recognizing clients' needs. The social worker must help to develop new or needed services within a managed care framework. Advocacy that leads to empowerment requires that the health care social worker teach and assist clients in how to obtain needed resources. In addition, on a larger scale, it requires that she or he advocate for changes in policy or procedure that can have the direct or indirect benefit of assisting the client to receive the services needed.

REFERENCES

Austin, D. M. (2001). Flexner revisited [Special issue]. *Research on Social Work Practice, 11* (1), 1–3.

Barker, R. L. (1995). *The social work dictionary* (3rd ed.). Washington, DC: National Association of Social Workers.

Bartlett, H. M. (1940). *Some aspects of social casework in a medical setting.* Chicago: American Association of Medical Social Workers. Reprinted by the National Association of Social Workers, 1958.

Berkman, B. (1996). The emerging health care world: Implications for social work practice and education. *Social Work, 41,* 541–549.

Braus, P. (1996). Who will survive managed care? *American Demographics, 18,* 16.

Browning, C. H., & Browning, B. J. (1996). *How to partner with managed care.* Los Calamitous, CA: Duncliff's International.

Cabot, R. C. (1915). *Social service and the art of healing.* New York: Moffat, Yard.

Caper, P. (1995). The next shift: Managed care. *Public Health Reports, 110,* 682–683.

Carlton, T. O. (1984). *Clinical social work in health care settings: A guide to professional practice with exemplars.* New York: Springer Publishing Co.

Colby, I., & Dziegielewski, S. F. (2001). *Social work: The people's profession.* Chicago: Lyceum.

Davidson, K. (1978). Evolving social work roles in health care: The case of discharge planning. *Social Work in Health Care, 4*(1), 43–54.

Davis, S. R., & Meier, S. T. (2001). *The elements of managed care: A guide for helping professionals.* Belmont, CA: Brooks Cole.

Dziegielewski, S. F., & Holliman, D. (2001). Managed care and social work: Practice implications in an era of change. *Journal of Sociology and Social Welfare, 28(* 2), 125–138.

Holliman, D. (1998). *Discharge planning in Alabama hospitals.* DAI-59–09A 3647 Ann Arbor: UMI: Unpublished Dissertation.

Holliman, D., Dziegielewski, S. F., & Datta, P. (2001). Discharge planning and social work practice. *Journal of Health Care Social Work. 32(* 3), 1–19.

Holliman, D., Dziegielewski, S. F., & Teare, R. (in press). Differences and similarities between social work and nurse discharge planners. *Health and Social Work.*

Jackson, R. L. (2001). *The clubhouse model: Empowering applications of theory to generalist practice.* Pacific Grove, CA: Brooks/Cole.

Kadushin, A. (1976). *Supervision in social work.* New York: Columbia University Press.

Kadushin, G. (1989). Social workers' views of their roles as discharge planners with elderly patients in acute care hospitals. *DAI51*(01), 295. (University Microfilms No. AAC 9015750)

Kadushin, A. (1992). What's wrong, what's right with social work supervision? *Clinical Supervisor, 10,* 3–19.

Kirst-Ashman, K. K. (2000). *Human behavior, communities, organizations & groups in the macro social environment.* Pacific Grove, CA: Brooks/Cole.

Levin, R., & Herbert, M. (1995). Differential work assignments of social work practitioners in hospitals. *Health and Social Work, 20,* 21–30.

Mankita, S., & Alalu, R. (1996, spring). Hospital social work: Challenges, rewards. *New Social Worker,* pp. 4–6.

Nacman, M. (1977). Social work in health settings: A historical review. *Social Work in Health Care, 2,* 407–418.

National Association of Social Workers National Council on Practice of Clinical Social Work. (1994). *Guidelines for clinical social work supervision.* Washington, DC: Author.

Resnick, C., & Dziegielewski, S. F. (1996). The relationship between therapeutic termination and job satisfaction among medical social workers. *Social Work in Health Care, 23,* 17–35.

Sheafor, B. W., Horejsi, C. R., & Horejsi, G. A. (1997). *Techniques and guidelines for social work practice* (4th ed.). Needham Heights, MA: Allyn & Bacon.

Shulman, L. (2002). Developing successful therapeutic relationships. In A. R. Roberts & G. J. Greene (Eds.), *Social workers' desk reference* (pp. 375–378). New York: Oxford University Press.

Steun, C., & Monk, A. (1990). Discharge planning: The impact of Medicare's prospective payment on elderly patients. *Journal of Gerontological Social Work, 15*(3/4), 149–165.

Thyer, B. A. (2002). Developing discipline specific knowledge for social work: Is it possible? *Council on Social Work Education, 38*(1), 101–114.

GLOSSARY

Advocacy: When professional activities are aimed at educating, informing, or directly defending or representing the needs and desires of individuals, families, or communities through direct intervention or empowerment.

After-care: Continued treatment, or social and physical support of client convalescence.

Allied health care providers: These professionals are often considered adjunct in the delivery of medical services. Professionals in this area include audiologists, dietitians, occupational therapists, optometrists, pharmacists, physical therapists, psychologists, social workers, and speech pathologists.

Allied health care workers: Professionals involved in health care delivery.

Almshouses: Places of refuge for society's poor, medically sick, and mentally ill of all ages. Historically, referred to as the "poorhouse" or place of death. Considered the forerunner of the hospital.

Charity organization societies: Privately or philanthropically funded agencies that delivered social services to the needy. Often considered the forerunners of today's nonprofit social service agencies.

Clients: The individual, group, or family or community that is the focus of intervention.

Clinical social work practice: Often referred to as medical social work (see *medical social work*).

Continuing education: Training provided to professionals to update or enhance their skills and knowledge in the field.

Family counseling: A practice methodology that centers on the "family" as the client or unit of attention.

Friendly visitors: General workers and health care workers that represented the charity organization societies.

Devaluation: When a director attributes exaggerated negative qualities to an employee.

Health care practice: The activities conducted that are designed to enhance physical and psychological well-being.

Health care social work: The practice of social work that deals with general health, specifically in the areas of wellness, illness, or disability. The social work professional can address these issues by working directly with individuals, groups, families, or communities, or under through the auspices of broader social change.

Health care social worker: The professional "bridge" that links the client, the multidisciplinary or interdisciplinary team, and the environment.

Hospital social work: Historically defined as the provision of social services in a medical setting. Currently, it refers to the delivery of social work services in hospitals and related health care facilities.

Medical social work: A form of social work practice in health care settings with the goal of assisting those who are physically ill, facilitating good health, and presenting illness.

Nursing: A field of practice versed in medical matters and entrusted with caring for the sick.

Practice of social work: The application of social work knowledge, theories, methods, and skills to provide professionally sound, ethically bound, culturally sensitive social services to individuals, groups, families, organizations, and communities.

Public health: Tasked with prevention of disease and maintenance of health in the population.

Quality care: Quality care reflects the degree of excellence required in service provision. Excellence is directly related to the degree of consensus and conformity that can be reached in the society providing the service.

QUESTIONS FOR FURTHER STUDY

1. What are the primary differences between what health care social workers see as their role and what other professionals see?
2. How have the historical roots of health care practice influenced social work practice as we know it today?
3. What do you believe can make health care social work practice an integral part of health care delivery?
4. What characteristic of social work practice makes it the most marketable in today's health care practice arena?
5. How do you believe health care social work will be defined in the future?
6. How has the role of the supervisor changed over the years?
7. What makes the role of the supervisor in the health care setting unique to other areas of social worker supervision?
8. What changes can social work professionals expect regarding the provision of core clinical skills?

WEBSITES

The Clinical Social Work Federation
An organization for social workers in the health care and/or mental health fields.
http://www.cswf.org/

Health Care and Social Work
Accesses online articles from the above journal.
http://www.naswpress.org/publications/journals.html

Health Care and Social Work Jobs
Job openings in the field.
http://www.quintcareers.com/healthcare_jobs.html

The National Association of Social Workers
Considered the premier organization for social workers.
http://www.naswdc.org

Social Work and Health Care
Features 864 recent developments in social work and health care.
http://www.polyglot.lss.wisc.edu/socwork/SW8641/course.html

CHAPTER 4

Standards, Values, and Ethics in Clinical Health Care Practice

Sophia F. Dziegielewski and George Jacinto

PROFESSIONAL STANDARDS IN THE HEALTH CARE SETTING

One primary function of the National Association of Social Workers (NASW) is to help establish, define, and describe standards for professional practice. In 1977, NASW and the Joint Committee of the American Hospital Association, in a joint effort, published a standard for hospital social workers. Later, based on need, more refined criteria were established that were viewed as reflecting all health care settings. This revised set of criteria was published by NASW in 1980 and makes up the current *Standards for Social Work in Health Care Settings* (NASW, 1992). With today's growth and change within the health care field, it is expected that further revision of these standards will soon be completed. Although NASW publishes these standards, it openly admits that their application is a voluntary process. The standards can only improve practice and service delivery if they are adopted and carried out by health care social workers and their employers.

According to the standards of health care practice proposed by NASW (1992), the primary principle that must be considered in service delivery is that social work services need to be an integral part of every health care organization. Further, it is essential that these services be made available to the population groups that social workers generally serve, which include individuals, families, significant others, special population groups, communities, health-related programs, and educational systems.

In an attempt to provide continuity of care within a comprehensive format, all social workers employed in the health care arena are strongly encouraged to follow the guidelines established by NASW in 1992 for health care professionals. These standards include the following: (a) promotion and maintenance of physical and psychosocial well-being; (b) promotion of conditions essential to ensure maximum benefit from short-or long-term care services; (c) prevention of physical and mental illness; (d) promotion and enhancement of physical and psychosocial functioning, with attention to the social and environmental impact of illness and disability; and (e) promotion of ethical responses to address the often conflicting value positions held by various parties in the health care settings (NASW, 1992, p. 3).

WRITTEN PLANS THAT DOCUMENT SERVICE PROVISION

According to the NASW *Standards for Social Work in Health Care Settings* (NASW, 1992), several core standards are required to ensure professional service provision. First, every health care organization needs to have a written plan for providing social work services. This written plan must be carried out as a contractual agreement involving, at a minimum, a graduate-level social worker experienced in health care. When available, professional licensure of the social work professional is recommended. The written plan should have a clear explanation of agency policy and procedures and how they can affect the health care social worker–client relationship. The written plan should also stipulate the types of services offered and how the delivery of organized services will be completed. Client confidentiality should always be ensured. Outreach services and client advocacy need to be made in an attempt to identify clients and families that could potentially require treatment. Specific decisions regarding the types of items needed in each proposed plan will depend on the health care facility employed and the specific circumstances of the case (Kagle, 2002).

SUPERVISION AND DIRECTION BY A GRADUATE-LEVEL SOCIAL WORKER

The second factor to be considered is that the provision of professional social work services should be administered under the direction of a graduate-level social worker from a school accredited by the Council on Social Work Education. The standards employed by this council ensure that a standard of care and continuity of training for the social work professional have been obtained (NASW National Council on Practice of Clinical Social Work, 1994). Here, the social work professional who is assigned the directorship of the social work program will ultimately be considered accountable to the chief executive officer of the administration. Although it may happen in today's practice environment, responsibility to another allied professional (e.g., a public health coordinator) or to a professional in a related discipline (e.g., nursing) has been traditionally discouraged.

The director of social work health care program services will have varied responsibilities within the agency setting. However, generally these responsibilities can be broken down into two areas: administrative and agency responsibilities and clinical and supervisory duties (Munson, 2002). As a health care administrator, the social worker will be responsible for agency planning, including the assurance that there is adequate space, budget, and deployment of social work personnel to cover the needs of the program being serviced (NASW, 1992). Social workers must advocate for adequate space, especially to ensure privacy when working with and advocating for the clients they serve (Gelman, 2002). In budgeting, social workers must become familiar with the technique of *line item budgeting*. This financial planning technique will allow the social work administrator to estimate a proposed expense for a given year and compare it with the year before.

In this time of limited resources, there is a constant struggle to balance need and cost-containment strategies that generally result in work force reduction (Lehr, McClean, & Smith, 1994). When working within a bureaucracy with specific tasks and goals and a clearly defined hierarchy, social workers may feel trapped. In times of flux and change, the bureaucracy may become more rigid. Policies and procedures may be adhered to more rigidly, and this may become a particular problem for social work administrators who want to create new and innovative programs and methods of service delivery.

Second, the social work director will often be responsible for the recruitment, selection, and retention of program personnel. This means that the director needs to strive to recruit and select work force personnel that reflect diversity. The standards set out by Title VII in the provision of the 1964 Civil Rights Act, which prohibits discrimination in hiring, placement, and so on on the basis of race, color, religion, sex, or national origin, should be met as well.

One of the most critical elements of the current health care environment is related to the changes that have occurred in the work force in the United States. With numerous cultural and demographic shifts, inclusion of women and persons of color in recruitment and retention efforts is essential. With reliance on equal opportunity and performance profiles, incorporation of these individuals into the management-success process is further encouraged.

Once an employee has been hired, it is the role of the health care social work director to ensure that an adequate employee orientation is provided. This orientation needs to help the employee to recognize clearly and understand what is expected of him or her in the job setting. The probable changing status of service, and the flexibility required of the employee, should be openly introduced into discussion. Providing the employee with an orientation checklist that the employee completes and signs will document in writing that the employee has fulfilled the requirements of the orientation process.

Today, in the health care work environment, it is common for *employment contracts* to be used. The actual form and content of these contracts can vary, but they provide either verbal or written communication regarding expectation of the job requirements and basic employer and employee rights (Lehr, McClean, & Smith, 1994). The director's dual role begins with assisting the employee to better understand what will be expected. Second, the director must safeguard the health care agency by updating and modifying contract inclusions, and must clarify any misleading or ambiguous agency policy or procedures that could be misconceived. Further, to help in this clarification effort, it is generally the social work director who is responsible for an outline of social work procedures and documentation of what is expected of the employees under his or her charge. All efforts to clarify employee contracts, agency policy and procedure, and any related documentation will reduce the number of claims that promises made during recruitment or hiring were not made or kept.

After the employee has joined the staff, evaluation by the social work director will be conducted. This evaluation often includes the creation of *professional supervisory profiles,* and should be conducted on a regular basis. It is helpful to structure both summative and formative evaluations of the employee. The formative evaluation provides the opportunity to provide ongoing informal feedback and correction with regard to the employee's performance. This affords the supervisor an opportunity to provide assistance in skill building and assimilation into the culture of the work environment. The summative evaluation, which commonly takes place at the end of the first six months, is a more global look at the employee's work during that period of time and documents the employee's progress in meeting the details of the position description. In reality, it should be noted that often the director may or may not have direct responsibility for this task. The director may be involved in the evaluation of members of the interdisciplinary team; however, input from a social work professional, particularly in the job evaluation and rating of another health care social worker, is strongly encouraged.

Social work administrators are warned against engaging in the practice of *assimilation*, especially regarding diversity. In this process, differences among employees are acknowledged to exist but are avoided by trying to steer away from diversity issues altogether, ignoring how they can affect job performance. In addition, social work directors must also be aware of and try to avoid a process referred to as the *halo effect*. Here, the director allows personal influences of one or more notable traits to influence the overall rating given (Barker, 1995). This can result in an unfair *devaluation* (attributing exaggerated negative qualities) or *idealization* (over-estimating individual attributes) of the employee. In evaluating employees, the *Hawthorne effect* should also be considered. This is when the employee reacts in a certain way because of his or her knowledge of being watched. What is then seen may not be truly relevant to job innovation or change.

Besides the administrative and supervisory responsibilities of the health care social worker, the clinical and professional supervisory duties cannot be forgotten. All social workers must maintain good-quality record-keeping services (Kagle, 2002) and clearly set standards for the evaluation of work (Reamer, 2002a, 2002b). Because these topic areas are beyond the scope of this chapter, the reader is referred to the section in this text on record keeping for more detailed information. Other clinical services include professional supervision, provision of continuing education, and client liaison services (see Tables 4.1 and 4.2).

TABLE 4.1   Responsibilities of Administrative or Agency Directors

Responsibility	Task to be performed
Planning	List budget, space, and use patterns of social work personnel
Selection of program personnel	Hire social work professionals, considering diversity and professional performance issues
Employee orientation	Ensure that the social work employee is oriented to agency policy, procedure, and services
Evaluation of program personnel	Complete supervisory job evaluations
Procedural documentation	List social work–related policies and procedures
Ensuring quality	Participate in continuous quality improvement and service-monitoring activities
Continuing education	Assist related disciplines in securing information on the role of the social work professional and provide direct training for other disciplines
Community education and training	Assist other disciplines and the public by providing education regarding health and wellness issues
Student education	Assist in the training and supervision of social work students
Agency-community liaison	Assist the agency to provide support and education within the community setting
Support and development of client-centered research projects	Evaluate and develop research proposals that address the needs of clients served

Source: Modified from NASW (1992). *NASW standards for social work in health care settings.* Washington, DC: Author.

ENSURING EFFECTIVE, EFFICIENT, AND QUALITY SERVICES

QUALITY ASSURANCE OR CONTINUOUS QUALITY IMPROVEMENT

Knowledge is essential for the director of social work service programs as well as for direct health care social work providers. In most health care organizations, this requires participating in either a voluntary or

TABLE 4.2 Responsibilities of Clinical or Supervisory Directors

Responsibility	Task to be performed
Clinical documentation	Maintain and oversee quality record keeping for services delivered
Clinical evaluation/revision and research	Use evidence-based measures to ensure practice efficiency and effectiveness Evaluate current methods of practice
Professional supervision	Ensure quality professional supervision is either provided directly or made available
Continuing education	Ensure that adequate educational opportunities (e.g., workshops, seminars, etc.) are made available to employees
Client liaison services	Ensure that adequate linkages are made for clients within and outside the agency

Source: Modified from NASW (1992). *NASW standards for social work in health care settings.* Washington, DC: Author.

mandated effort to ensure that the quality and cost-effectiveness of services are provided. Generally, one or more programs to ensure that this continues to occur is implemented through some type of use-review process, often referred to as *utilization review*. With the increased emphasis on quality of care and quality of life, utilization of the *case mix system* provides a venue for improving service quality. As part of the efforts of a health care agency to manage *quality improvement (QI)* or *continuous quality improvement (CQI)*, data on clinical outcomes are gathered and integrated in a problem-solving format. Once this structure for maintaining quality care is in place, the development of quality indicators is stressed, as it allows for the comparing of outcomes and best practice efforts. See Figure 4.1 for important factors for social workers in the utilization review process.

According to Heeschen (2000), the use of clearly defined quality indicators can improve the quality of many aspects of health care delivery. Utilizing these types of systems produces improved survey outcomes, increased reliability, allowance for verification, and utilization of existing data sources for reporting. Also, standardization increases efforts for all helping initiatives across numerous health care facilities to become more consistent in approaches to care. Health care

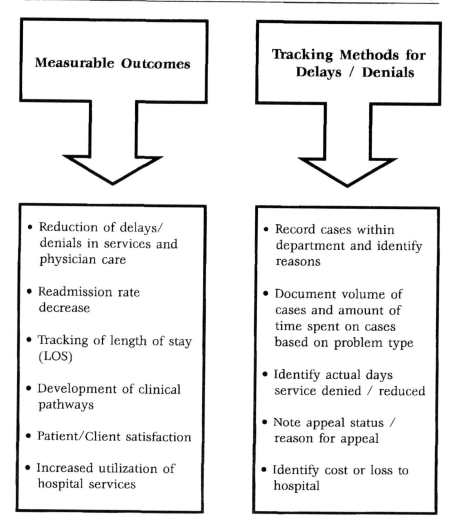

FIGURE 4.1   Factors in utilization review.

social workers are often mandated to participate in and be responsible for a wide array of quality assurance activities. These activities can include client satisfaction measurements, use of services, reimbursement reviews, risk management, and due process procedures.

No matter which activity or combinations of activities are used for assessing quality of services, it clearly is not an easy task. Furthermore, professionals and consumers may not necessarily agree on what constitutes "quality" care (Williams & Torrens, 1993). Clearly defined quality indicators can help with this problem (Heeschen, 2000). Therefore, clarification is necessary on what constitutes quality of care and at what level the society wishes it to be obtained and available to the people served. Today, this is further complicated by the realization that wellness or preventive services (which may have initial dollar costs associated with them) can head off problems that could be of future high cost to the provider.

Often health care social workers are asked to help with measurement of client satisfaction. These measures can be obtained through interviews or questionnaires. Social workers need to be active in the creation of these measures to ensure that the client being served perceives such measurements as nonthreatening and understandable. It is also important to note that, at times, funding bodies do not like receiving data regarding negative perceptions from clients served. The desire to satisfy funding bodies may cause reluctance to report accurate and clear reflections of the client's perceptions when they are of a negative nature. The role of the health care social worker is important in helping to document and convey information about patient satisfaction as accurately as possible, in order to assist the agency in implementing changes and strategy to address the problematic areas identified.

In most health care institutions, such as hospitals, the quality assurance process and use-review procedures are often combined. Generally, controls for use-review procedures specifically address services designed to monitor and provide appropriate incentives to enhance the delivery of health care services. Monitoring generally includes examining admission rates, providers, and services delivered; determining the appropriateness of inpatient admissions and usual length of stay; and determining the frequency of certain diagnostic and other therapeutic procedures (Williams & Torrens, 1993). Often use-review procedures can also be done across institutions to decide the appropriateness of the practice patterns at the agency (Heeschen, 2000).

Health care social workers need to be aware and remain active participants during quality assurance activities. In this process, they advocate for client needs by identifying policies and procedures that are in need of changing and program and service needs that are going unmet. Social workers must maintain an active role in this process to ensure that they continue to be viable players and service providers in the health care environment.

TODAY'S HEALTH CARE SOCIAL WORKER

Name: Julie Gray, MSW, LICSW
Current Position: Supervisor, Senior Health Specialists,
                     Evergreen Hospital Medical Center
City, State: Kirkland, Washington

Duties in a typical day
I manage and direct the daily operations of a geriatric medial practice owned by Evergreen Hospital. This includes providing supervision for physicians, a physician's assistant, social workers, nurses, medical assistants and support staff. I develop and manage the clinic budget. Additionally, I am responsible for process improvement projects in the clinic and for ensuring that the clinic meets all JCAHO and Washington State Department of Health standards.

What do you like most about your position?
The most enjoyable aspect of my job is helping our team develop an innovative model of geriatric medicine. One of our biggest challenges is to make certain the care we provide is cost-effective, while at the same time ensuring that the quality of care is not compromised. The obstacles seem enormous at times yet the rewards are great. Our stellar patient satisfaction scores keep me going on the rough days.

What do you like least about your position?
The least enjoyable aspect of being a clinic manager/supervisor is dealing with various facility problems like plumbing disasters and broken fax machines.

What "words of wisdom" do you have for the new health care social worker who is considering working in a similar position?
I highly recommend completing a practicum in a hospital setting as a discharge planner or emergency department social worker. I also suggest that students take a course in medical terminology. Medicine has its own language and system of abbreviations; it is imperative that social workers have a solid grasp of the terminology so they can communicate with the team. If you aren't a student but want to enter the field of medical social work, experience in areas such as domestic violence, crisis services, and long-term care creates

a basic foundation that will help you get your foot in the door. Be prepared to work weekends and holidays! For those wanting to manage a medical clinic, it is essential to have experience working in a clinic setting at some point in your career. Also, you must be able to demonstrate a career path in which you took on progressive leadership responsibilities. Social workers can capitalize on their people skills and their extensive experience working as part of a multidisciplinary team.

What is your favorite health care social work story?

I enjoy telling the story about walking one of our patients out to the waiting room. She was in her late 80's and talked a mile a minute about her adventures volunteering at the local senior center. "My friends at the senior center say I talk too much," she suddenly announced in the middle of a complicated tale. Eventually, I was able to ask if I could call anyone to drive her home. She waved me off, smiled, and said, "Don't worry honey, I have my cell phone." Then, she sat down, pulled out a phone from her large purse, and proudly called the taxi service. She died several months after my encounter with her. Whenever I am faced with a new challenge and start resisting change, I think about her energy and zest for life. She was frail, yet she lived life to its fullest and never feared embracing new technology.

PROVISION OF CLIENT EDUCATION

Education is another important area for health care social workers to develop. Not only is providing continual education important for social work and the related disciplines, but it is also important for health care social workers to help in providing direct training for other multidisciplinary and interdisciplinary team members. Health care social workers can help inform or educate individuals and fellow professionals regarding the seriousness of a problem, or how serious it might become if left unattended (Kirst-Ashman & Hull, 1993). When working as part of a team, education is only the first step to persuading, thus creating a dialogue toward advocacy for your client, the agency, and the community. Education as staff development nurtures not only the employees within the organization but also the representatives of the parent organization (Smith & Fottler, 1994).

All professionals need continuing enrichment and education. It is the responsibility of the employing agency not only to allow professionals to attend training but to also make it possible to attend, and sometimes to cover the cost. When training is provided, having documentation of completion placed in the employee's file for future reference is important.

Important roles for health care social workers include serving as providers and facilitators of community education and training. According to research, if a concern to increase wellness behavior exists, better-educated individuals are more likely to have general physicals, immunizations, tests, and procedures for preventive purposes than the less educated; more educated women, for example, are more likely to seek early prenatal care (Aday, 1993). Social work directors must also consider providing educational services to student social workers. Mentoring and training those students will prepare them for their careers.

PROVISION OF RESEARCH SUPPORT

The final responsibility of the health care directors and providers is to participate in research studies and projects that will help to better address the needs of the client. This area will be addressed in greater depth throughout the application chapters; however, the social worker with practice expertise is an excellent contributor to the establishment and implementation of research to measure both program and practice effectiveness.

VALUES, ETHICAL DILEMMAS, ROLE CONFLICTS, AND STRESS

CLIENT SELF-DETERMINATION AND CONFIDENTIALITY

Most people in this country highly value a person's right to self-determination and privacy. In fact, "every person has a right to determine for himself [or herself] when, how, and to what extent he [or she] wants to share (or have shared) information about himself [or herself] with others" (Loewenberg & Dolgoff, 1996, p. 76). Maintaining client's privacy or confidentiality requires that information learned regarding the client should not be openly disclosed (Loewenberg & Dolgoff, 1996; Loewenberg, & Dolgoff, & Harrington, 2000; Reamer, 2002a, 2002b).

Overall, confidentiality can be a complicated process, since there are certain circumstances in which breaching it is sanctioned by both state laws and professional standards. For example, in social work practice confidentiality may be breached with or without the client's consent to report incidences of neglect and abuse. Other circumstances include when a client may be a danger or harm to self or others, or when other compelling reasons exist, such as imminent harm to a client, or when laws require disclosure. In the health care arena, most professionals agree that there are situations in which breach of confidentiality is certainly justifiable and expected (Dunlap & Strom-Gottfried, 1998; Gothard, 1995). Yet the principles that surround maintaining confidentiality are important for gaining client trust and support (Edwards, 1999). For the health care social worker, this can be a complex issue with many factors that must be considered for sound ethical decision making.

One of the dilemmas encountered by social workers is the question of the *duty to warn*. In explaining duty to warn, the Tarasoff case is often cited (*Tarasoff* v. *Regents of the University of California*, 1976). Unfortunately, because interpretations of this case differ in regard to the therapist obligations for reporting, the exact course of action to be taken can be complicated. In practice, the exact definition of what constitutes duty to warn can vary from state to state. Some states say that there is a duty to warn the person who may be an intended victim of a violent crime, whereas other states do not. In some states there is a requirement for the disclosure of confidential information but this information can only be given to medical or law enforcement professionals when there is imminent danger of injury to the client or to others by the client. Generally, the most common assumption is that if the client presents a danger to self or other then the practitioner must take reasonable steps to avert the expected harm. Simply stated, if a client presents a threat of harm to self or others, the social worker is expected to act in some way. Because laws and expectations differ from state to state it is advisable to investigate alternatives in order to select the best course of action. It also may be helpful to consult with an attorney and make sure that the health care social worker is always covered under some type of malpractice insurance. Be sure to contact the malpractice insurance provider and ask for information concerning duty to warn. And, to verify the applicability to the state where the health care social worker is practicing, don't forget to check with the state licensing board. Furthermore, consult a mental health professional who is knowledgeable about the ethics of the mental health profession. Regardless of what the exact policy is in the practicing state, appropriate deliberation and consultation with other professionals must be carefully documented. This is especially important when there has been disclosure by a client to the social worker of a serious threat.

For the field, maintaining ethical practice (including confidentiality) has been at the forefront in social work—so important, in fact, that in 1996 the NASW ratified and modified the existing version of the Code of Ethics. This was the first substantial revision in almost twenty years, and only the third time the social work Code of Ethics had received major revisions throughout the history of NASW. These changes "significantly expanded ethical guidelines and standards for social work practice" (Reamer, 1998, p. 492). The importance and complexity of privacy and confidentiality are evident, since no less than eighteen separate paragraphs of the Code of Ethics are devoted to these issues (Dickson, 1998).

The 1996 NASW Code of Ethics provides lengthy standards with regard to privacy and confidentiality, clearly stating that social workers should "respect clients' right to privacy . . . and . . . should protect the confidentiality of all information obtained in the course of professional service, except for compelling professional reasons" (NASW Code of Ethics, 1996, Standard 1-1.07, p.10). A social worker should make every attempt possible to adhere to the rules of confidentiality, promoting self-determination, but should also be aware that there are some situations that should not be kept confidential (Kirst-Ashman & Hull, 1993). In most cases where maintaining confidentiality is an issue, consideration is needed to determine what is "sufficiently compelling to warrant a breach of confidentiality" (Kopels & Kogle, 1994, p. 2).

NASW CODE OF ETHICS, STANDARDS 1-1.07, PRIVACY AND CONFIDENTIALITY

(a) Social workers should respect clients' right to privacy. Social workers should not solicit private information from clients unless it is essential to providing services or conducting social work evaluation or research. Once private information is shared, standards of confidentiality apply.

(b) Social workers may disclose confidential information when appropriate with valid consent from a client or a person legally authorized to consent on behalf of a client.

(c) Social workers should protect the confidentiality of all information obtained in the course of professional service, except for compelling professional reasons. The general expectation that social workers will keep information confidential does not apply when disclosure is necessary to prevent serious foreseeable and imminent harm to a client or other identifiable person, or when laws or regulations require disclosure without a client's consent. In all instances, social workers should disclose the least amount of confidential information necessary to achieve the desired purpose; only information that is directly relevant to the purpose for which the disclosure is made should be revealed.

(d) Social workers should inform clients, to the extent possible, about the disclosure of confidential information and the potential consequences, when feasible before the disclosure is made. This applies whether social workers disclose confidential information on the basis of a legal requirement or client consent.

(e) Social workers should discuss with clients and other interested parties the nature of confidentiality and limitations of clients' right to confidentiality. Social workers should review with clients circumstances where confidential information may be requested and where disclosure of confidential information may be legally required. This discussion should occur as soon as possible in the social worker-client relationship and as needed throughout the course of the relationship.

(f) When social workers provide counseling services to families, couples, or groups, social workers should seek agreement among the parties involved concerning each individual's right to confidentiality and obligation to preserve the confidentiality of information shared by others. Social workers should inform participants in family, couples, or group counseling that social workers cannot guarantee that all participants will honor such agreements.

(g) Social workers should inform clients involved in family, couples, marital, or group counseling of the social worker's, employer's, and

agency's policy concerning the social worker's disclosure of confidential information among the parties involved in the counseling.
(h) Social workers should not disclose confidential information to third party payers unless clients have authorized such disclosure.
(i) Social workers should not discuss confidential information in any setting unless privacy can be ensured. Social workers should not discuss confidential information in public or semipublic areas such as hallways, waiting rooms, elevators, and restaurants.
(j) Social workers should protect the confidentiality of clients during legal proceedings to the extent permitted by law. When a court of law or other legally authorized body orders social workers to disclose confidential or privileged information without a client's consent and such disclosure could cause harm to the client, social workers should require that the court withdraw the order or limit the order as narrowly as possible or maintain the records under seal, unavailable for public inspection.
(k) Social workers should protect the confidentiality of clients when responding to requests from members of the media.
(l) Social workers should protect the confidentiality of clients' written and electronic records and other sensitive information. Social workers should take reasonable steps to ensure that clients' records are stored in a secure location and that clients' records are not available to others who are not authorized to have access.
(m) Social workers should take precautions to ensure and maintain the confidentiality of information transmitted to other parties through the use of computers, electronic mail, facsimile machines, telephones and telephone answering machines and other electronic or computer technology. Disclosure of identifying information should be avoided whenever possible.
(n) Social workers should transfer or dispose of clients' records in a manner that protects clients' confidentiality and is consistent with state statutes governing records and social work licensure.
(o) Social workers should take reasonable precautions to protect client confidentiality in the event of the social worker's termination of practice, incapacitation, or death.
(p) Social workers should not disclose identifying information when discussing clients for teaching or training purposes unless the client has consented to disclosure of confidential information.

(q) Social workers should not disclose identifying information when discussing clients with consultants unless the client has consented to disclosure of confidential information or there is a compelling need for such disclosure.

(r) Social workers should protect the confidentiality of deceased clients consistent with the preceding standards.

Extracted from NASW Code of Ethics, 1996, Standard 1–1.07, p.10.

In health care social work, as in all of social work practice, ethical decisions are not usually simple, right-or-wrong choices made without a great deal of thought. Instead, they generally involve choosing between two undesirable actions; neither choice may appear to be the correct one, yet some considerations will outweigh others. For example, decisions must be made if maintaining the client's right to self-determination may actually cause him or her harm (Strom-Gottfried & Dunlap, 1999). In social work practice, ethical decisions often must be made quickly, but with sufficient thought and attention to ensure that the right decision is made (Levy, 1993; Loewenberg, Dolgoff, & Harrington, 2000). Furthermore, although helpful as a guideline, the NASW Code of Ethics does not provide specific direction when professional values clash (Reamer, 1995).

The declared purposes for the Code of Ethics are to espouse ethical conduct and to control ethical violations by establishing guidelines of professional behavior (Berliner, 1989; Reamer, 1995). "The Code of Ethics cannot resolve all ethical issues or disputes or capture the richness and complexity involved in striving to make responsible choices within a moral community" (NASW Code of Ethics, 1996, p. 4). Instead, a code of ethics describes values, principles, and standards to which social workers "aspire and by which their actions can be judged" (NASW Code of Ethics, 1996, p.4).

To further examine confidentiality in the practice setting, two studies in the area exemplify how ethical dilemmas arise in the field of social work with both individuals and groups.

A study by Holland and Kilpatrick (1991), conducted in Atlanta and the surrounding area in 1989, attempted to identify "dimensions of ethical judgment" used by twenty-seven social workers (p. 138). All of the social workers held master's degrees in social work, and each had a different amount of experience in the field. Most of the social workers were female, and all were directly involved with clients. Holland & Kilpatrick (1991) contend that, in order to appropriately consider ethical dilemmas, social workers should be aware of, and not discount, their own and the clients' current circumstances. When ethical issues arise (e.g., fair distribution of resources or restrictions on divulging client information), "information and skill are not sufficient to solve them. These issues require thoughtful analysis in the context of participants' values and commitments" (Holland & Kilpatrick, 1991, p. 138).

Their study focused on analyzing various ethical issues to which social workers are regularly exposed in their duties. In addition to defining, addressing, and resolving the issues, the participant's background and associations were analyzed, as well as any professional happenings that might have affected the respondent. An interview format was used to explore how practicing social workers comprehend and handle ethical issues, and their responses were examined in an attempt to recognize "common themes and differences regarding these issues" (Holland & Kilpatrick, 1991, p. 139).

The results of this study identified three dimensions that seemed to be fundamental to the ways that social workers managed ethical dilemmas. First, decisions were often based on a continuum ranging from "an emphasis on means to an emphasis on ends" (Holland & Kilpatrick, 1991, p. 139). Reasons given for decisions made ranged from acknowledging laws and procedures to focusing on gaining positive outcomes for clients. In the second dimension, social workers made decisions based on interpersonal orientations that ranged from emphasizing client autonomy and freedom to stressing the importance of mutuality. For example, many respondents emphasized client self-determination over client safety, while others justified denial of client self-determination in order to protect the client from hurting him or herself (Holland & Kilpatrick, 1991). In the third dimension, authority for ethical decisions was explored. In this area responses varied from "reliance on internal or individual judgment to compliance with external rules, norms, or laws" (Holland & Kilpatrick, 1991, p. 140). Many respondents based their decisions on personal self-direction rather than agency policy, and other respondents were more likely to follow the policies and laws (Holland & Kilpatrick, 1991).

Holland and Kilpatrick (1991) concluded that decisions regarding ethical issues are most likely affected by prior experience, degree of professional developmental, and situational factors that include the immediate organizational or professional context, the characteristics of respondents'work roles, and the overall organizational culture. In closing, the authors observed that of the 27 respondents participating in their study, not one participant referenced the NASW Code of Ethics as a resource in helping make an ethical decision (Holland & Kilpatrick, 1991).

In a second study, Dolgoff & Skolnik (1996) investigated how 147 social workers made ethical decisions in the group setting. A survey instrument was used that consisted of background information and seven vignettes with competing ethical issues. Each vignette was followed by an open-ended question, allowing for an explanation of the action needed to resolve the dilemma. The seven vignettes consisted of ethical dilemmas involving group self-determination, primary responsibility to client, confidentiality, self-determination, informed consent, and authenticity. Also included was a list of sources that the participant would use to assist with the decision making. The choices included practice wisdom, Code of Ethics, another professional code, a particular philosopher or religious teaching, a book or journal article, or other sources.

These authors concluded that the primary method used by social workers in the group setting for making ethical decisions was practice wisdom, which was highly influenced by contextual elements and personal values. In addition, the majority of the respondents sought compromise solutions rather than a specific yes or no type of answer. Similar to Holland and Kilpatrick (1991), Dolgoff and Skolnik (1996) found limited use of the NASW Code of Ethics to assist with making ethical decisions; and additional instruction on the Code was suggested to better prepare students for ethical decision making. Although the two studies mentioned above do not specifically address confidentiality and self-determination, these studies do address ethical dilemmas in social work practice and how decisions are made.

In closing, when one looks specifically at issues of client self-determination and confidentiality, one sees that managed health care has clearly affected the practitioner–client relationship (Loewenberg, Dolgoff, & Harrington, 2000). At times contractors require that information be provided, in conflict with professional standards of confidentiality. Social workers may be placed in a dilemma regarding the NASW Code of Ethics and the contradiction encountered with information disclosure procedures of managed health care organizations

(Loewenberg, Dolgoff, & Harrington, 2000; Strom-Gottfried & Corcoran, 1998). In addition, technological advances have led to increased reliance of the industry on electronic data collection and storage, which has put the confidentiality of client information at risk (Strom-Gottfried & Corcoran, 1998). Regardless of the exact impact of the managed care practice principles and the technological advances often employed, the professional decisions made by professional social workers are never easy and straightforward. This can create a new dimension that needs to be factored into an already ambiguous decision-making process where social workers cannot help but be influenced by either organizational or managerial expectations. These requirements add a number of complex elements to decisions about releasing confidential information regarding clients. It is not surprising that social workers in this study and elsewhere would vary their approaches to maintaining confidentiality, since the legal system remains unclear regarding disclosure of confidential information (Behnke, Winick, & Perez, 2000).

In the health care setting, there are no simple answers or clear guidelines that address ethical dilemmas with regard to decisions that violate client self-determination or confidentiality. Maintaining client self-determination and autonomy is an issue that must be considered, but the primary stress must be placed on avoiding self-harm when a client is unable to meet his or her own care needs without assistance (Corey, Corey ,& Callanan, 2003). For the health care social worker, it is important to remember that each individual and situation are unique and deserve careful ethical decision making. Furthermore, the question remains unanswered as to whether the current process of ethical decision making is more representative of the "art" within the field of social work or the "science."

As stated earlier, all social workers are expected to regularly make difficult decisions that in many cases have no "right" or "wrong" answer. Previous studies show that important social work values such as client self-determination, ensuring client safety and maintaining confidentiality can constitute an ambiguous process where there may not be a "correct" answer. This information reminds all educators and practitioners, particularly those who serve as supervisors, of the importance of including analysis of personal values and life experiences as well as social work ethics, laws, or agency policies (Loewenberg, Dolgoff, & Harrington, 2000). If schools of social work and clinical supervisors spend little time on ethical content and decision making, social work students may be led to believe that they must learn about social work ethics on their own. Lack of information and training in this area can be a disservice to practitioners that will have ramifications in terms of decisions and resulting consequences.

In addition, there needs to be more discussion regarding the NASW Code of Ethics that focus on how the code can serve as a universal resource for practitioners facing ethical dilemmas.. The dearth of empirical literature regarding the issue of confidentiality suggests that more research is needed. Since practice decisions are rarely based on dichotomous principles (yes or no answers), future research should involve a number of choices over a continuum spanning from least to most desirable. The continuum fits well with the principle of self-determination because most individuals prefer selection from two or more choices when solving complex problems. In this turbulent environment client issues are often complex and multidimensional, and the greater knowledge and skill a practitioner is able to acquire in ethical decision-making the better.

CASE STUDY

Marg, a medical social worker, could barely hold back frustration as the nurse called her to facilitate the discharge of her client. The client, a 14-year-old girl, was admitted the previous night. She had taken an overdose of aspirin, and was kept in the hospital overnight for observation. The only thing holding up the discharge was Marg's signature on the discharge summary sheet. The client had been medically cleared, and all members of the team were expected to sign off on the order for proper discharge procedure to be implemented.

Marg thought about her day and the five other clients for whom she had to find placement. She thought about the 45 clients on her unit, many she had not even seen yet. It would be so easy to sign the discharge summary and move on to the next client. The nurse noticed Marg's hesitancy as she stood waiting for her to sign. "Her parents are in the waiting room; is there a problem?" asked the nurse. Marg knew what she wanted to ask, but she also knew what asking these questions involved.

"Was it a suicide attempt?" asked Marg.

"Yes, we think so," said the nurse.

"Has anyone talked to the client about it?" asked Marg.

"Yes, the physician did," said the nurse.

"Has anyone talked to the parents?" asked Marg.

"Yes, the physician explained that she is now fine medically, and suggested that they get some type of counseling. Do you want to talk to them about it?" asked the nurse.

Marg knew what answering this question meant. She had not had time to talk with her client or the family. The hospital did not make a referral to social work or psychiatry for an evaluation; and even if they had, the quick and abrupt discharge would not have given them enough time to complete an assessment. Marg had been trained to deal with issues of suicide, and she knew that a rushed or avoidant approach to the matter would never be enough. Marg was familiar with clients who had attempted suicide and others who had succeeded. Marg knew what needed to be done to get the counseling prevention process started. She was also realistic and knew the time involved and the pressure she was facing to release a medically cleared client. After thinking it over, her ethical and professional choice was made as Marg asked, "I really think I need to talk to the client and the family before they go. Can you give me some time?"

THE ROLE OF THE SOCIAL WORKER IN THE HEALTH CARE TEAM

In the case example, direct application to the health care setting is made, making it easy to see how complicated such ethical decision making can be, even by the most experienced clinicians. For health care social workers, awareness and skill in formulating ethical decisions are critical.

The situation Marg faced is common, and similar to numerous quick and minimally planned discharges this hospital social worker was forced to make. The ethical and professional responsibility Marg felt to advocate for and assist her client conflicted with the time demands placed by insurance reimbursement and use-review standards. The approach of the other professionals on the team further complicated the situation. Many professionals, like social workers, also feel this pressure, and a type of role blurring occurs (Davidson, 1990; Dziegielewski, 1996; Netting & Williams, 1996). Situations like this often result in a "buff and turf" of responsibility. The process of buff and turf occurs when professionals do not accept responsibility for solving aspects of the client's problem, and either address them on the surface or simply pass the problem to another professional on the team (Dziegielewski, 1996).

Although this case specifically involved a hospital social worker, ethical dilemmas such as this one are not unusual. All health care social workers need to realize and openly discuss the actual role of the health care social worker regarding performance expectations. What social workers believe is their role in the health care setting does not always match what other members of the team believe. Stated simply, often social workers and other professionals simply do not agree on the role of the health care social worker.

Often other health care professionals see the role of the social worker primarily as (a) helping the client to adjust into the environment he or she will be entering after service discontinuance; (b) performing instrumental tasks (e.g., providing assistance for transportation and location of nursing homes); (c) being active in concrete service provision; (d) focusing on the discharge of clients and on creating outcomes beneficial to reducing lengths of stay (Berkman, 1996); and (e) assisting in problem solving, including assessing client problems, examining possible solutions, informing and linking community resources, and assisting with applications to obtain additional concrete services.

Based on these expectations by other professionals, it follows that social workers often feel misunderstood in the health care setting, especially because they see their role as (a) providing general counseling skills to clients and their families; (b) confronting psychosocial problems and identifying and addressing behavioral or emotional factors; (c) assisting clients and families around ethical decision-making issues; and (d) assessing, treating, referring, and gathering resources. Therefore, social workers can and often do perceive their role differently from the other members of the health care delivery team (Davidson, 1990; Dziegielewski, 1996; Dziegielewski & Holliman, 2001) and increasing collaboration can only benefit this relationship (Sira & Szyf, 1992).

Although different expectations of the role of the health care social worker often exist, social workers still feel a need to be part of the system or the team in which they work. Resnick and Dziegielewski (1996), in a study of 144 health care social workers and other professionals who completed discharge planning, found that overall 86% of these professionals reported satisfaction with their jobs. It is important to note, however, that overall job satisfaction was linked to (a) finding purpose in what they did; (b) being able to see the outcome of one's work; (c) having contributed something to some patient's life; and (d) believing that what was done had benefited the client served (Resnick & Dziegielewski, 1996). Overall, Resnick and Dziegielewski (1996) found that if health care social workers knew they were providing a service that benefited their client, they were more pleased with their jobs and their own performance.

The role of the health care social worker can be a difficult and misunderstood one. Concrete suggestions to be considered in making the working environment more conducive to health care social work include the following.

First, developing creative and challenging ways for social workers to get feedback is important. Feedback after service discharge is sorely lacking in the health care arena. Some studies have shown that increased feedback can result in increased job satisfaction (Resnick & Dziegielewski, 1996). This can be accomplished through introducing mail-back surveys, scheduled telephone interviews, and concrete evaluation measures.

A second way to create a more conducive environment for health care social work is to facilitate and increase communication between referral sources and the health care service. This can be accomplished by implementing reply-transfer summaries that need to be returned to the original provider. In these situations, the receiving service would do a brief arrival note and return it to the sending service. For facility-based health care social workers, this can be further accomplished by introducing patient follow-up issues into medical rounds that are generally a part of most inpatient units. This way the service providers can see the "environmental" benefit of their labor, and may be more open to helping establish these gains for future clients. For health care social workers not part of an inpatient unit or interdisciplinary team, updates on referrals and client activities from the referee are considered essential.

The last suggestion is to facilitate increased communication with and between team members when an interdisciplinary team is involved. For example, when a social worker addresses biopsychosocial concerns with the client, this information should be related to the team. The team can then see the benefit of this interaction for the overall treatment process. The logic is simple: By understanding the role of the social worker more completely, other professionals will be more likely to support and encourage its inclusion in service delivery problems.

RECOGNIZING AND HANDLING STRESS

It is important to note that whatever the responsibility of the social work director or social work provider, stress is an important component that needs to be addressed. Many researchers believe that if social workers feel stressed, they are more likely to avoid the traditional patterns of expected behavior and indulge in more conservative and self-protective behaviors (Fottler & Smith, 1994; Hall & Mansfield, 1971; Staw, Sandelands, & Dutton, 1981; Whetten, 1981).

There are many areas in which health care social workers can manifest stress reactions. First, they may choose quick unrealistic strategies, or engage in anxiety-releasing behaviors to avoid dealing with more complicated problem-solving behaviors. Throughout their busy days, health care social workers deal with numerous health issues that could result in life or death situations for their clients. An immediate or quick discharge can result in numerous problems, as documented in several case studies throughout this book. The pressure to make such discharges must be addressed, and any means of professional stress reduction to avoid this scenario is encouraged (i.e., exercise, recreation that is non-work related, and time for self).

Second, discharge strategies need to always be in the best interest of the client, not the agency. If the client's best interest is not considered paramount it could result in decreased advocacy for the client and his or her family. In the managed care environment, the importance of advocacy for our clients cannot be overestimated.

Third, communication patterns can be decreased, deemphasized, or devalued in an attempt to quickly get a group consensus. Simply reducing the numbers of participants in decision making, or just letting the team decide without the social worker's input, can "speed things up." For example, often in "patient care" conferences, there can be a delayed initiative to involve the client or family members in the planning and discussion of treatment. Unfortunately, because of the time-consuming nature of this input, it may be discouraged, although it is mandated as part of care. In addition, a stressed health care social work director might assume a style of authoritarian management that would allow him or her to gain greater control over the other social workers and the subsequent events resulting from the decision process.

A fourth result of stress in the social work health care director or provider can be more rigid patterns of rule concentration or importance.

Here, the "rules" are identified and held responsible for decisions being made—not the decision maker (e.g., "I must go along with this because it is the rule"). This directly removes the responsibility from the director or provider and places the "rule" into a position where it cannot be easily addressed, changed, or reasoned with.

Lastly, the director or provider may be more likely to perceive routine tasks or decisions as more complicated and difficult to make than they actually are. This can result in procrastination or an increased emphasis on groupthink to solve quickly what seems overwhelming to the director or provider.

Stress is a normal part of life. In excess, however, it can make decision makers uncomfortable and inflexible in their decision-making role. In the health care field in particular, stress is a psychological hazard that can cause distress and difficulty.

CHAPTER SUMMARY AND FUTURE DIRECTIONS

In closing, it is important to note that many health care social workers in practice today are witnessing unprecedented changes. For example, in the hospital setting, many private hospitals and veterans' health centers are drastically changing the structure and responsibility for the provision of social work services. The traditional departments of social work that were located in each of these facilities have changed. Social workers are often being reassigned to units or wards, or directly into service provision areas (such as discharge planning). Often their supervisors are no longer social workers; rather, they are nurses or other health care administrative personnel.

The problems and limitations of this "splitting" are obvious. As a social work consultant, the most common complaint I have heard is that this splitting makes health care social workers feel that they are losing their identity and the strength that comes with having a solid departmental structure. Also, when they are referred cases, the problems are significant in terms of discharge planning or adjustment, making these types of referrals more time-and labor-intensive and much less cost-effective. Therefore, in the utilization review process where the emphasis is on service provision outcomes, it appears that social workers have lower productivity rates. Others report that they are losing the camaraderie and support of having other trained social work professionals to cover for them, reassign work, and so on. In addition, the lack of direct supervision can present a significant problem for some social workers, particularly those who need regular visits and documented supervision by a licensed social worker to secure their own licensing.

Unfortunately for many, structural changes such as these will dictate practice reality. Although this development may at first appear threatening, it can help open yet another door, and help the social worker gain recognition and increased importance as a part of the health care delivery team. The fact is simple, whether health care social workers like it or not: interdisciplinary teamwork is as much a part of the present as it is of the future (Abramson, 2002). By being physically located on the unit, social workers can be recognized as part of the team and not just outsiders providing a service. These social workers will gain easy, quick, and convenient access to the client and his or her family members. During the discharge process, in particular, this could be helpful. In addition to assisting the client, if the health care social worker adapts quickly to this change, she or he will be able to capitalize on the newness of the situation and assist all team members in building group spirit and cohesion. This, in turn, will lead to greater unification and support for direct service provision and referral.

MANAGED CARE: DOMAINS OF CHANGE

Cost Effectiveness and Payment	Services and Timing
Outcomes for Ensuring Quality	Roles and Structure

As stated earlier, the changes that have occurred in health care service provision and delivery through the inception of behavioral managed health care are unprecedented. Regarding the changes health care social workers will be expected to face in the future, the phrase "we have only just begun" seems most appropriate.

REFERENCES

Abramson, J. S. (2002). Interdisciplinary team practice. In A. R. Roberts & G. J. Greene (Eds.), *Social workers' desk reference* (pp. 44–51). New York: Oxford University Press.

Aday, L. (1993). Indicators and predictors of health services utilization. In S. J. Williams & P. R. Torrens (Eds.), *Introduction to health services* (4th ed., pp. 46–70). Albany, NY: Delmar.

Barker, R. L. (1995). *The social work dictionary* (3rd ed.). Washington, DC: NASW Press.

Behnke, S. H., Winick, J. D., & Perez, J. D. (2000). *The essentials of Florida mental health law: A straightforward guide for clinicians of all disciplines.* New York: W. W. Norton.

Berkman, B. (1996). The emerging health care world: Implications for social work practice and education. *Social Work, 41,* 541–549.

Berliner, A. K. (1989). Misconduct in social work practice. *Social Work, 34,* 69–72.

Corey, G., Corey, M. S. & Callanan, P. (2003). *Issues and ethics in the helping professions* (6th ed.). Pacific Grove, CA: Brooks/Cole.

Davidson, K. W. (1990). Role blurring and the hospital social worker's search for a clear domain. *Health and Social Work, 15,* 228–234.

Dickson, D. T. (1998). *Confidentiality and privacy in social work: A guide to the law for practitioners and students.* New York: Free Press.

Dolgoff, R., & Skolnik, L. (1996). Ethical decision making in social work with groups: An empirical study. *Social Work with Groups, 19*(2), 49–63.

Dunlap, K. M., & Strom-Gottfried, K. (1998). Maintaining the confidence in confidentiality. *New Social Worker, 5*(3), 10–11.

Dziegielewski, S. F. (1996). Managed care principles: The need for social work in the health care environment. *Crisis Intervention and Time-Limited Treatment, 3,* 97–110.

Dziegielewski, S. F., & Holliman, D. (2001). Managed care and social work: practice implications in an era of change. *Journal of Sociology and Social Welfare, 28*(2), 125–138.

Edwards, J. (1999). Is managed mental health treatment psychotherapy? *Clinical Social Work Journal, 27,* 87–102.

Fottler, M. D., & Smith, H. L. (1994). Managing human resources over the organizational life cycle. In M. Fottler, S. Hernandez, & C. L. Joiner (Eds.), *Strategic management of human resources in health service organizations* (2nd ed., pp. 3–25). Albany, NY: Delmar.

Gelman, S. R. (2002). On being an accountable profession: The code of ethics, oversight by board of directors, and whistle-blowers as a last resort. In A. R. Roberts & G. J. Greene (Eds.), *Social workers' desk reference* (pp. 75–80). New York: Oxford University Press.

Gothard, S. (1995). *Legal issues: Confidentiality and privileged communication. Encyclopedia of social work* (Vol. 2, pp. 1579–1584). Washington, DC: NASW Press.

Hall, D. T., & Mansfield, R. (1971). Organizational and individual response to external stress. *Administrative Science Quarterly, 16,* 533–547.

Heeschen, S. J. (2000). Making the most of quality indicator information. *Geriatric Nursing, 21,* 206–209.

Holland, T. P., & Kilpatrick, A. C. (1991). Ethical issues in social work: Toward a grounded theory of professional ethics. *Social Work, 36*(2), 138–145.

Kagle, J. D. (2002). Record-Keeping. In A. R. Roberts & G. J. Greene (Eds.), *Social workers' desk reference* (pp. 28–37). New York: Oxford University Press.

Kirst-Ashman, K. K., & Hull, G. H. (1993). *Understanding generalist practice.* Chicago: Nelson-Hall Publishers.

Kopels, S., & Kogle, J. D. (1994). Teaching confidentiality breaches as a form of discrimination. *Arete, 19*(1), 1–9.

Lehr, R. I., McClean, R. A., & Smith, G. L. (1994). The legal and economic environments. In M. Fottler, S. Hernandez, & C. L. Joiner (Eds.), *Strategic management of human resources in health service organizations* (2nd ed., pp. 26–57). Albany, NY: Delmar.

Levy, C. S. (1993). *Social work ethics on the line.* New York: Haworth Press.

Loewenberg, F. M., & Dolgoff, R. (1996). *Ethical decisions for social work practice.* Itasca, IL: F. E. Peacock.

Loewenberg, F. M., Dolgoff, R., & Harrington, D. (2000). *Ethical decisions for social work practice* (6th ed.). Itasca, IL: F.E. Peacock.

Munson, C. E. (2002). The techniques and practice of supervisory practice. In A. R. Roberts & G. J. Greene (Eds.), *Social workers' desk reference* (pp. 38–44). New York: Oxford University Press.

NASW National Council on Practice of Clinical Social Work. (1994). *Guidelines for clinical social work supervision.* Washington, DC: NASW.

National Association of Social Workers (NASW). (1992). *Standards for social work in health care settings.* Pamphlet, Silver Spring, MD: Authors.

National Association of Social Workers (NASW). (1996). *Code of ethics.* Silver Spring, MD: Authors.

Netting, F. N., & Williams, F. G. (1996). Case manager–physician collaboration: Implications for professional identity, roles and relationships. *Health and Social Work, 21,* 216–224.

Reamer, F. G. (1995). *Social work values and ethics.* New York: Columbia University Press.

Reamer, F. G. (1998). The evolution of social work ethics. *Social Work, 43,* 488–500.

Reamer, F. G. (2002a). Ethical issues in social work. In A. R. Roberts & G. J. Greene (Eds.), *Social workers' desk reference* (pp. 44–51). New York: Oxford University Press.

Reamer, F. G. (2002b). Risk management. In A. R. Roberts & G. J. Greene (Eds.), *Social workers' desk reference* (pp. 44–51). New York: Oxford University Press.

Resnick, C., & Dziegielewski, S. F. (1996). The relationship between therapeutic termination and job satisfaction among medical social workers. *Social Work in Health Care, 23,* 17–35.

Sira, Z. B., & Szyf, M. (1992). Status inequality in the social worker-nurse collaboration in hospitals. *Social Science Medicine, 34,* 365–374.

Smith, H. L., & Fottler, M. D. (1994). Training and development. In M. Fottler, S. Hernandez, & C. L. Joiner (Eds.), *Strategic management of human resources in health service organizations* (2nd ed., pp. 334–364). Albany, NY: Delmar.

Staw, B. M., Sandelands, L. E., & Dutton, J. E. (1981). Threat-rigidity effects in organizational behavior: A multilevel analysis. *Administrative Science Quarterly, 26,* 501–524.

Strom-Gottfried, K. J., & Corcoran, K. (1998). Confronting ethical dilemmas in managed care: Guidelines for students and faculty. *Journal of Social Work Education, 34*(1), 109–119.

Strom-Gottfried, K., & Dunlap, K. M. (1999). Unraveling ethical dilemmas. *New Social Worker, 6*(2), 8–12.

Tarasoff v. Regents of the University of California, 551 p.2d 344 (1976).

Whetten, D. A. (1981). Organizational responses to scarcity: Exploring the obstacles to innovative approaches to retrenchment in education. *Education Administration Quarterly, 17,* 80–97.

Williams, S. J., & Torrens, P. R. (1993). Assessing and regulating system performance. In S. J. Williams & P. R. Torrens (Eds.), *Introduction to health services* (4th ed., pp. 377–396). Albany, NY: Delmar.

GLOSSARY

Assimilation: When used regarding hiring and evaluation of employees, it refers to acknowledging that in the evaluation process differences based on diversity can exist and therefore can affect job performance, yet the director may either avoid or deny the existence of such factors when implementing decision making regarding the employee.

Budget: A record of funds, credits, and debts that is kept by an agency.

Bureaucracy: A formal organization with specific tasks, goals, and a clearly established hierarchy of decision making. Administrative and organizational procedures, rules, and regulations are clearly defined.

Bureaucratization: The recent pull for social organizations to become more rigid (centralized) in terms of policies and procedures.

Case mix system: Provides a standardized method or venue for improving service quality that is to be used across numerous agencies and service providers.

Continuous quality improvement (CQI): In this method, data on clinical outcomes are gathered and integrated in a problem-solving format.

Duty to warn: Although exact definitions can vary by state, this basically means that the social worker is expected to warn the intended victim of a violent crime.

Employment contracts: These contracts can vary, but basically they provide either verbal or written communication of job requirements and basic employer and employee rights. Requests for this type of contract are becoming more common in the health care field.

Equal Employment Opportunity Commission: Commission established by Title VII of the 1964 Civil Rights Act. Enforces equal employment opportunities.

Essential health care providers: Generally refers to physicians and nurses as they are viewed as necessary professionals in the health care arena.

Halo effect: When the director allows one or more notable traits to influence the overall rating given.

Hawthorne effect: When the prospect of change will occur simply because a subject is being watched.

Idealization: When a director allows an overestimation of individual attributes to influence employee decision making.

Incrementalism: Used in social planning, this involves compromising and reaching agreements based on the needs and wishes of various political forces.

Line item budgeting: Financial planning technique in which each proposed expense for a given year is identified and compared with the year before.

Professional supervisory profiles: This type of evaluation of the supervisee ncludes both formative information (ongoing formal feedback and correction) and summative information (documents progress).

Quality assurance: Organizational procedures to assess whether services or products meet required standards.

Quality improvement (QI): See *continuous quality improvement (CQI).*

Quality indicators: Concrete and measurable criteria that allow for the comparing of outcomes and best practice efforts.

Title VII: Provision of the 1964 Civil Rights Act that prohibits discrimination in hiring, placement, and so forth on the basis of race, color, religion, sex, or national origin.

Use review: A variety of mechanisms for monitoring and evaluating the provision of "quality care" provided. See *quality assurance.*

Utilization review: A [formal]review process that is conducted in health care facilities and that is designed to ensure quality of care.

QUESTIONS FOR FURTHER STUDY

1. What changes can social work professionals expect regarding the provision of core clinical skills?
2. What changes do you believe will be made in the standards for social work provision when they are revised?
3. What are some specific ways social workers can prepare for and address ethical decision making in the health care field?
4. What are appropriate ways to document disclosure of a client intent to harm self or others?
5. What are the different guidelines for ethical decision making offered by the various mental health associations?

WEBSITES

American Medical Association
The AMA promotes the art and science of medicine and the betterment of public health.
http://www.ama-assn.org

Health Resources and Services Administration
HRSA directs national health programs to vulnerable and in-need populations.
http://www.hrsa.dhhs.gov

The Institute for Mental Health Initiatives
IMHI is a nonprofit organization for mental health professionals that
makes mental health research accessible to the public.
http://www.imhi.org

The International Federation of Social Workers
An international organization of professional social workers.
http://www.socialworkers.org

National Council for Community Behavioral Healthcare
Advocates in Washington to advance the interests of members and
consumers.
http://www.nccbh.org/

National Institutes of Health
The NIH conducts research and communicates biomedical information.
http://www.nih.gov

National Institute of Mental Health
NIMH is the foremost mental health research organization in the
world.
http://www.nimh.nih.gov/

PART II

Foundation Skills Necessary in Today's Health Care Environment

This page intentionally left blank

CHAPTER 5

Concepts Essential to Clinical Practice

Sophia F. Dziegielewski and Cheryl E. Green

UNDERSTANDING THE BIOPSYCHOSOCIAL APPROACH

Although the practice of health care social work has evolved through the years, the core concept in health service provision has remained constant. This core concept serves as the foundation upon which all health care services are provided, and it emphasizes the implementation of a *biopsychosocial* approach to practice. This approach, in its many varied forms, has traditionally been viewed as the basis for social work practice in the health care area. It is an approach that helps the worker understand that the client's experiences result from the interactions among biological, psychological, and societal processes (Gilbert, 2002; Newman & Newman, 2003). The biopsychosocial approach considers three overlapping aspects of the client's functioning. The "bio" refers to the biological and medical aspects of a client's health and well-being. The "psycho" involves the psychological aspects of the client, such as individual feelings of self-worth and self-esteem. The "social" considers the social environment that surrounds and influences the client. When all three of these domains are assessed and addressed, the biopsychosocial model of practice intervention is being applied (Rock, 2002). For example, addressing all three aspects of the biopsychosocial model to the problem of "stress" is thought to be necessary to treat the problem comprehensively (Lawrence & Zittel-Palamara, 2002). In today's managed care environment, this traditional perspective continues to be used; however, as will be discussed later, all resulting information gathered is to be related to behavioral outcomes.

Regensburg (1978) referred to the biopsychosocial approach as the "wholeness, oneness and indivisibility of every human being" (p. 9). Engle (1977) further conceptualized the biopsychosocial model as a system-based approach clearly embedded in systems thinking; and Sperry (1988) applied it to treatment issues, calling it biopsychosocial therapy. Rock (2002) noted that the biopsychosocial model tries to integrate a view of the client as a person-in-situation, and indicated that this model recognizes that understanding biological factors is necessary but insufficient for "understanding a human person in a social world" (p. 11). Social workers need to remain mindful that the application of this type of model includes all three domains. Carlton (1984) has commented that, in the past, the "bio" in biopsychosocial has been virtually ignored by social workers. The remaining elements of "psycho" and "social" have been placed on a continuum, with the psychological aspects at one end and the social elements at the other. This artificial separation viewing the individual from the wholeness perspective. Concepts fundamental to social work, such as "person-in-situation" and "person-in-environment," foster this sense of wholeness, making this artificial separation inconsistent with traditional clinical practice.

Gilbert (2002) has pointed out that while many practitioners may recognize the importance of a biopsychosocial approach, few may really adopt this approach in either their clinical practice or their research because adopting this approach "calls for radical shifts in research, training and practice." In fact, Kiesler (1999) pointed out that this approach is often poorly formulated and poorly taught. However, having an understanding of these three factors is essential in understanding the human condition within the health care setting. Each part should be weighed equally; separation into its subsequent components is not as important as ensuring that each element gets the attention that it deserves. This is particularly true when that attention is needed for continued growth in the other areas. Treatment may focus on one domain during the initial stage of the intervention and shift to the other domains during subsequent stages as the therapeutic process evolves. For example, if someone is suffering from an acute medical condition that must be addressed or stabilized for continued survival, certainly the medical (or biological) aspect must be addressed first. However, the social and psychological aspects of this condition cannot be ignored; and once the medical needs of the patient have been met, these aspects need to be addressed. Some examples of psychological difficulties include feelings of depression, the realization of being forced to face one's own mortality, and the struggle with life-and-death issues. Examples of social problems that may need to be addressed include occupational, recreational, or significant other difficulties with family members. It is the balanced perception of these elements that makes the health care social worker's skills so necessary and unique.

Although most supporters of the biopsychosocial perspective propose the importance of these three primary areas, Rankin (1996) now advocates for the inclusion of a fourth area. This fourth area targets the spiritual needs of the patient. The modified term considers a *biopsychosocial-spiritual perspective*. In this perspective, the spiritual component "focuses attention on the essential being of the individual, the role of the transcendent in the person's life, and the spiritual qualities of the belief system that person holds" (Rankin, 1996, p. 516). Rankin believes that by considering the addition of this factor, the health care professional is able to consider a much broader concept of the client and the factors that can contribute to his or her development.

Biomedical Approach to Practice

The dominant model for understanding disease is generally referred to as the *biomedical model* (Wise, 1997). It derives its roots from basic scientific facts and focuses on the derivation of empirical evidence (Engel, 1977). From a traditional perspective, this model often considers disease as an entity yet does not directly recognize social behavior. This biological perspective, which represents the biomedical model, is basic to medicine and the other medical sciences (Gilbert, 2002; Rock, 2002; Spraycar, 1995). This biomedical approach can clearly assist the client by increasing understanding of the origin, signs and symptoms, medical diagnosis, treatment procedures and protocol, and prognosis for any physical health condition (Carlton, 1984). Many professionals in the medical field, particularly those in family medicine, have long argued that the biomedical approach is not enough. When the biomedical approach alone is used, emphasis is placed on curing or resolving the physical problem that has been experienced. Focus on physical phenomena, which are empirically verifiable (e.g., wasting of muscle, loss of weight, sweating, etc.), of a patient's illness, however, leaves out the systemic and interrelated nature of the problem. Many believe that to heal the patient, it is necessary to include the capacity to understand the person's inner world—the values, thoughts, feelings, and fears a person has as well as his or her perception of injury and the way it will affect current lifestyle (McWhinney, 1989).

Regardless of whether social workers believe in the use of a biomedical approach to practice or not, they must be fluent in the language that is used by those who follow that model. Social workers unable to understand medical terms or the jargon used in the medical field are at a significant disadvantage. The inclusion of this content in schools of social work is essential. Although there are complete dictionaries devoted to medical terminology, Tables 5.1 and 5.2 provide a brief primer to assist social workers in becoming more familiar with some of the basic terms, and medical conditions often used in the medical setting that are reflective of the biomedical approach to practice.

One of the major problems confronting a biomedical approach today relates to the process of the *deprofessionalization* of medical care. The essence of the biomedical approach to practice rests in the assumption that the professional possesses some type of special esoteric knowledge and skill that can be applied to the client. In the past, the physician–client relationship was rarely questioned. The physician was thought to possess some type of specialized knowledge that only he or she could access that would eliminate a client's pain or suffering. With the advent of increased education, however, much of this authority is called into question. The result has been an erosion of what used to be the blind obedience by the patient in the patient–doctor relationship (Kurtz & Chalfant, 1991). In addition, as already mentioned, a biomedical approach to health care delivery alone is not enough. The dominant conceptions of this model make incorporating the psychosocial aspects difficult (Meikle, 2002; Schlesinger, 1985). Further, the process of deprofessionalization is now forcing the few areas still practicing from this perspective to branch out. Therefore, the combination of all of these aspects into a "managed behavioral" biopsychosocial approach continues to be the one that is primarily used.

PSYCHOSOCIAL APPROACH TO PRACTICE

In this traditional approach to clinical health care practice, the professional seeks to establish a relationship with the client for the specific

TABLE 5.1   Medical Terminology

Medical term	Definition
Abdomen	The part of the trunk that lies between the thorax and the pelvis; can include the pelvic area
Acidosis	A state characterized by actual or relative decrease of alkali in body fluids in relation to acid content
Activities of daily living	The general performance of basic self- and family care responsibilities needed for independent living
Amputation	The cutting off of a limb or other body part
Amputee	A person with a amputated limb or part of a limb
Anatomical	Relating to anatomy
Anemia	Any condition in which the number of blood cells, the amount of hemoglobin, and the volume of packed red blood cells are less than normal
Anesthesia	A pharmacological agent that induces loss of sensation of nerve function or a neurological dysfunction
Antigen	Any substance that, as a result of coming in contact with appropriate cells, induces a state of sensitivity or immune response
Apgar rating	A score given to an infant to indicate its relative health
Aphasia	The inability to use language skills that were present in the past
Artery	Carries blood away from the heart (red rich color)
Carcin	Cancer
Carcinoma	A malignant neoplasm (a cancerous tumor)
Cardio, cardiac	Pertaining to the heart
Caries	Decay of the teeth (*cavity* is the lay term)
Cephal, cephalo	Relating to the head
Chondro	Cartilage, granular, gritty
Cirrhosis	Progressive disease of the liver
Cyst	Refers to the bladder, or an abnormal sac containing gas, fluid, or semisolid materia, with a membranous lining

(continued)

TABLE 5.1 *(continued)*

Medical term	Definition
Cyt, cyto, cyte	Cell
Degeneration	A worsening of mental, physical, or moral qualities
Derma	Skin
Dermatitis	Inflammation of the skin
Ecto	Outside
Endo	Within, inner
Entero	The intestines
Gloss	The tongue
Gyn, gync	Woman
Graph	A recording instrument
Hormone	A chemical formed in one organ or body part that moves to another (can alter functional activity)
Hema, hem, hemato	Blood
Hepato	Liver
Hist	Tissue
Hydro	Water, hydrogen
Hyper	Excessive, above
Hypo	Below, deficiency
Hystero	Uterus
Ia, iasis	A condition
Kin	Movement
Leuk	White
Lipo	Fat, lipid
Litho	A stone
Logy	Study of
Macro	Large
Masto	Breast
Micro	Small
Neur	Nerve
Node	A circumscribed mass of tissue
Oculo	Eye
Odont	Tooth
Oophor	Ovary
Orchi	Testis
Oste, ost	Bone
Path	Disease

TABLE 5.1 *(continued)*

Phos, phot, photo	Light
Phren	Diaphragm
Psyche, psych, psycho	The mind
Rhino	Nose
Rrhea	A flowing or a flux
Sacro	A muscular substance
Salpingo	Tube
Scler	Hardness
Scope	An instrument for viewing
Scopy	The use of an instrument for viewing
Somato	Relating to the body
Stom, stoma	Mouth
Therm	Heat
Thromb	Blood clot
Toxi	A toxin or poison
Tricho	A hairlike structure
Vaso	A duct or blood vessel
Vein	Carries blood toward the heart
Virus	An infectious agent that is capable of passing through fine filters that retain most bacteria

purpose of helping the client overcome specific social or emotional problems and achieve identified goals for problem resolution and well-being (Barker, 1995). The types of problems that clients often encounter (as recognized by this perspective) include interpersonal conflicts, psychological and behavior problems, dissatisfaction with social relations, difficulties in role performance, problems of social transition, inadequate resources, problems in decision making, problems with formal organizations, and cultural conflicts.

The tenets of psychosocial learning theory were postulated by Lewin in the late 1940s. Lewin (1947) described three phases that clients must successfully negotiate to learn and incorporate an event. These phases include (a) "unfreezing," where a client recognizes that there is a need to learn and becomes willing to incorporate this learning into current behavior; (b) "moving," where the client participates actively in the learning process; and (c) "refreezing," where the learned behaviors are incorporated and subsequently integrated into the behavior

TABLE 5.2 Medical Conditions

Medical condition	Brief definitions[a]
Acquired immunodeficiency syndrome (AIDS)	Generally a fatal disease caused by infection by the human immunodeficiency virus
AIDS dementia complex	Impairment of cognitive functioning because of infection related to the human immunodeficiency virus (HIV)
AIDS-related complex	An imprecise term that refers to the signs and symptoms of AIDS
Diabetes mellitus	A deficiency in the body that results in chronic inability to create insulin, which results in too much sugar in the blood and urine
Diarrhea	An abnormally frequent discharge of semisolid or fluid fecal matter from the bowel
Emphysema	A disease of the respiratory system that results in continued episodes of difficult breathing and breathlessness
Epilepsy	A chronic disorder characterized by paroxysmal neuronal brain dysfunction related to excessive activity and characterized by the development of seizures
Failure to thrive	A condition in which an infant's weight gain and growth are far below what is expected for that level of development and age
Hepatitis	Inflammation of the liver
Hypertension	High blood pressure
Migraine	A symptom complex occurring periodically and related to pain in the head
Mitral valve prolapse	A problem related to the mitral valve in the heart
Multiple sclerosis	A common demyelinating disorder of the central nervous system
Palsy	Paralysis or paresis

[a]These definitions have been simplified and in many cases presented within a brief nontechnical context.

scheme of the client. This perspective requires that the therapist "focus on interpersonal and social concerns in addition to intrapsychic concerns" (Barker, 1995, p. 304).

In completing a *psychosocial assessment*, the social worker summarizes the various issues that he or she sees as problems that need to be addressed. Often this assessment can include diagnostic labels, results of psychological tests, a brief description of the problem that needs to be addressed, assets and resources the client may have, the prediction or prognosis, and the plan designed to address the problem (Barker, 1995). The psychosocial assessment is not a static entity; the social worker must constantly change and update his or her appraisal to reflect progress on the issues the assessment is designed to address.

MANAGED BEHAVIORAL HEALTH CARE

The biopsychosocial approach has traditionally been used to integrate the biomedical and the psychosocial approaches to practice. Beginning in the 1980s, however, the demand for concrete-based services was required. This meant that a type of behavioral health care that focused on "outcomes" and performance standards derived in service provision was needed (Franklin, 2002). These clinical outcomes had to be related to the expected change that a client would experience based on services received. This new integrated type of "behavioral-based psychosocial approach" provides health care social workers with a theoretical base that can be used to support the services and interventions they provide. In addition, the focus on behavioral outcomes further attracts funding agencies, providing a basis for measuring service effectiveness and accountability. Like any method of practice, it does not answer every question or concretely address each possible situation. It is an abstraction or guideline that can be used to guide practice—in what could otherwise be a complicated process (Dziegielewski, 2002).

The use of the biopsychosocial approach based in behavioral outcomes continues to have merit in practice delivery. All other disciplines involved in health care delivery understand and recognize the importance of this approach. Because the biopsychosocial approach is valued by other professions, social workers are able to provide leadership in understanding the "psycho" and "social" factors impacting clients (Rock, 2002). Additionally, the emphasis in today's health care environment on maintaining health and wellness provides avenues for social workers to assume leadership roles (Dziegielewski, 2002). Here the input of the social worker can be viewed as essential in predicting, anticipating, and developing ways to address probable health issues that may arise. The value of this input is contingent on the value others place on the behavioral biopsychosocial perspective within the current chronic care model of treating illness.

Increasingly, acute conditions consisting of one single episode are no longer the focus of treatment (Shortell & Kalunzy, 1994). Today, there are believed to be a multiplicity of factors that contribute to health and wellness and that must be addressed. In addition to this, service can often be rushed; yet for the social worker, taking the time to establish rapport with the client can serve to speed up the therapeutic process (Shulman, 2002).

The managed behavioral biopsychosocial approach can provide a firm basis for health care social workers to practice in today's turbulent environment. This model is consistent with competent and ethical social work practice because it emphasizes client empowerment and self-determination in a system that usually fosters patient compliance (Netting & Williams, 1996). Because of competition from other allied health professionals, health care social workers, now more than ever, need to emphasize and rely on the strength of our practice profession— remaining active members in the planning process for the client.

Unfortunately, in adhering to this model, there are negative factors that need to be discussed. One problem embedded in this method of service delivery is the hierarchy of power that the approach assumes. The behavioral biopsychosocial approach continues to be housed within the medical model. In this medical model, the primary care physician is seen as the gatekeeper and typically has the discretion in planning and referral for the general welfare of the client. He or she is generally given service-entry decision-making power, whether it is based on an individual, multidisciplinary, or interdisciplinary team approach. Although these decisions are influenced by the factors that surround the client's situation (i.e., medical condition, service availability, reimbursement potential, and team members' suggestions), the entry to service and in many cases ultimate responsibility rests with the primary care physician. This power to make final decisions regarding client care can often allow him or her to determine the ultimate course of treatment. In this model, the health care social worker is bound by the physician's decision—even when these decisions involve psychological or social issues.

A second possible problem with the behavioral biopsychosocial model stems from the blurring and mixing of tasks that professionals who subscribe to this method of service delivery provide. Ambiguous role definition allows other professionals to see themselves as performing the same function as social workers (Holliman, Dziegielewski, & Datta, 2001). In some instances, this has led to other professionals actually being ascribed the tasks that were initially considered the role of the social worker. The problem with the psychosocial area of delivery is that the tasks performed do overlap and can be varied in relation to the client need. Therefore, social workers need to remain active in establishing their "turf" and the actual roles and services they perform (Dziegielewski, 1996).

COLLABORATION AMONG HEALTH CARE PROFESSIONALS

Social workers are only one part of a unified health care delivery team. They are expected to work together with other professionals to ensure that the best possible care is provided. In the health care arena every client, whether an individual, a family, or a group, must have an individualized plan for service delivery. The established plan that is reflective of the biopsychosocial approach to practice must address the needs of the client regarding the current problem as well as prepare for continued health and wellness.

One important way that social workers differ from other professions providing health care is their training. Social workers are generally trained to provide a large range of professional services in diverse settings (Davidson, 1990). Although training requirements vary, most health care professionals—regardless of specialty—are trained to work exclusively in the health care field. Many of the collaborative efforts that social workers make with other professionals may be colored by the fact that these professionals are trained in a narrower field of practice. The training the social worker receives, and the varied job expectations of this professional, help the social worker to provide the diverse forms of helping that is needed in the health care field. It can, however, be confusing to other According to this perspective, the relationship among the client's illness, the health care provider, and the efforts of the social worker need to span the continuum of care (Berkman, 1996). Professionals who do not understand exactly what it is that social workers do—or professionals who put less emphasis on accepting psychosocial interventions as an essential part of medical intervention must be educated (Ben-Sira & Szyf, 1992). Striving to obtain a clear definition of what the health care social worker does can help lay the groundwork for acceptance as part of the team by the other professionals.

A recent study on case management found that although social workers may be trained in a broader area than health care alone, the roles and services they provide in the health care field are often similar to those of other helping professionals (Netting & Williams, 1996). The similarities in professional training and purpose among health care professionals make struggles and competition for a unique service delivery niche more difficult (Richardson, 1988). For example, social work has generally been viewed as the discipline that spans all areas of the health care continuum. Today, nursing is active in advocating for an expanded role for nurses similar to that which was once believed the domain of social work. Nurses are advocating for involvement in every aspect of patient care from primary, secondary, and tertiary services to mental health issues (Carson, 1996).

There are several forms of collaborative practice in which social workers in health care settings engage. The first is a type of *case-by-case collaboration*. Carlton (1984) describes this as practitioners from different disciplines coming together to share and participate in a mode of service delivery emphasizing an individualized intervention plan designed to assist the client, family, or community in need. Generally, this form of collaboration is considered the oldest and most common that may be conducted on a formal or an informal basis.

A second form of collaboration between health care professionals is *consultation*. The NASW defines consultation as the provision of expert advice that can either be accepted or rejected by the consultee (The NASW National Council on Practice of Clinical Social Work (NASW), 1994). Caplan (1970) defines consultation as a process of interaction between two professional persons, where one is viewed as an expert who is called on to help the other regarding current work problems. Basically, the consultant is considered an expert in the area, and the consultee seeks the expert's advice. However, although the consultee seeks the clinical advice of the consultant, he or she is not obligated to follow it or incorporate any of the ideas shared into the treatment context (Carlton, 1984; National Council on Practice of Clinical Social Work (NASW), 1994). This identifies one of the major differences between professional supervision and consultation. A supervisor could be sued for the mistakes a supervisee makes, but it would be difficult to sue a consultant for this because the professional consultee decides whether to follow the consultant's input or not.

A third form of collaborative effort is the provision of *education* (Carlton, 1984). In this form of collaboration, the social worker offers his or her expertise to train other health care providers. When engaging in education to non-social work professionals, three fundamental kinds of knowledge need to be possessed by the social work educator. The first is knowledge of the discipline of social work itself, being able to understand and incorporate the values and apply the skills inherent in the area of health care social work practice. Second, social work educators need to be aware of the professional standards to which those being educated must subscribe. Understanding the ethics and values of the profession will help the social worker to better address and anticipate service-delivery needs. Lastly, social workers need to know how to educate and how to impart information to others effectively. They need to be skilled in different methods of teaching and aware of different learning styles.

The last type of collaborative effort is the *team approach* in which the multidisciplinary and the interdisciplinary team concepts play important roles. In these collaborative team efforts, it appears evident that other disciplines are now moving into new areas and performing many of the tasks that used to be considered the domain of the health care social worker. Social workers need to remain active in this area. In today's practice environment, collaborative team efforts among health care professionals to serve the client better are expected. Collaboration of services is a product of our current health care system that does not appear to be waning.

One important factor that helps in the marketability and service utility of social workers is that they are cost-effective. Even though many of the other health care professionals can do a similar job to the health care social worker, the social worker can still do it with the least cost to the agency or the client (Dziegielewski, 1996; Netting & Williams, 1996). This makes social workers viable and cost-effective attractive team members.

MULTIDISCIPLINARY TEAMS

The term *multidisciplinary* can best be explained by dividing it into its two roots, multi and discipline. Simply stated, multi means many or multiple professionals. Discipline means the field of study in which a professional engages. When these two terms are put together, it therefore refers to "representatives of more than one discipline directing their efforts toward a common problem" (Carlton, 1984, p. 126). "The multidisciplinary team (MT) is composed of a mix of health and social welfare professionals, with each discipline in most part working on an independent or a referral basis" (Siple, 1994, p. 50).

Generally, the multidisciplinary team is composed of several different health and social welfare professionals. These professionals can include physicians, nurses, social workers, physical therapists, and so on. Each of these professionals generally works independently to solve the problems of the individual. Afterward, these opinions and separate approaches are brought together to provide a comprehensive method of service delivery for the client. The role of each professional on the team is usually clearly defined, and each team member knows the role and duties that he or she is expected to contribute. Many times, communication between the professionals is stressed, and goals are expected to be consistent across the disciplines, with each contributing to the overall welfare of the client.

INTERDISCIPLINARY TEAMS

In today's health care environment a transition appears to have occurred, deemphasizing the multidisciplinary team concept of the past while encouraging the continued development of interdisciplinary teams. "The interdisciplinary team (IT) also consists of a variety of health care professionals, but in this model different skills and expertise are brought together to provide more effective, better coordinated, and improved quality of services for patients" (Siple, 1994, p. 50). In health care service, "when clients are different, services are similar, and the size of the service delivery organization is inadequate to justify a great deal of specialization, the primary need is for expertise in dealing with client differences" (Duncan, Ginter, & Swayne, 1992, p. 341). This makes the interdisciplinary team both convenient and cost-effective to health care administrators.

Anticipating the continued emphasis that will be placed on this team approach, Carlton (1984) used the term *interdisciplinary* interchangeably with *collaboration*. Carlton believed that collaboration in the true sense of its definition meant "two or more practitioners from two or more fields of learning and activity, who fill distinct roles, perform specialized tasks, and work in an interdependent relationship toward the achievement of a common purpose" (p. 129). This is the same definition that can be applied to the interdisciplinary team.

The interdisciplinary team, like the multidisciplinary team, consists of a variety of health care professionals. The major difference between the multidisciplinary approach and the interdisciplinary one is that the latter takes on a much more holistic approach to health care practice. Interdisciplinary professionals work together throughout the process of service provision (Abramson, 2002). Generally, all members of the team develop a plan of action collectively. In service provision, the skills and techniques that each professional provides can and often do overlap. A combining of effort similar to the multidisciplinary team is achieved; however, interdependence throughout the referral, assessment, treatment, and planning process is stressed. This is different from the multidisciplinary team, where assessments and evaluations are often completed in isolation and later shared. In the interdisciplinary team process, each professional team member is encouraged to contribute, design, and implement the group goals for the health care service to be provided.

For successful interdisciplinary practice, the following factors should always be considered: (1) recognize the values and ethics of the profession; (2) take into account the individual and the environment; and (3) recognize and understand the interdependency of practice and the contributions and expertise of colleagues that support the helping process. These elements are relevant to both multidisciplinary or interdisciplinary teams, regardless of the model employed.

TODAY'S HEALTH CARE SOCIAL WORKER

Name: Lea Patterson-Lust, LMSW
List State of Practice: Alabama
Professional Job Title: Director of Social Work Services

Duties in a typical day:
I am employed at a regional medical center as the director of social work services. Although I am the director, this title is somewhat of

a misnomer since I am the only person in my department. However, as department director I do oversee and act as a direct service provider, providing 100% of all the social work service needs for this 115-bed inpatient facility, with its full complement of outpatient services as well. It is my responsibility to make sure that all the Joint Commission on Accreditation of Health Care Organizations (JCAHO) standards are met for social services. I wear a beeper 24 hours a day, seven days a week, and I am often on call over the weekends for all social service emergencies.

My duties are varied as a health care social worker, but primarily I am responsible for adoption assistance, discharge planning, advance directives, court-ordered placements (i.e., involuntary commitments, nursing home placement), domestic violence, child abuse and neglect, elder abuse and neglect, and inpatient services (working with uninsured or underinsured).

What do you like most about your position?
Providing direct services to patients and working with other professionals as part of a team.

What do you like least about your position?
What I like the least is the hospital bureaucracy. Also, the unrealistic expectations held by other medical professionals in regard to what the service system can provide.

What "words of wisdom" do you have for the new health care social worker considering work in a similar position?
It is important to remember when working in an acute care setting that social work is generally perceived as a non-revenue-producing service. With all the decreases in health care reimbursement, social work services often feel the brunt end of such cuts. Social workers often are expected to meet the psychosocial needs of clients in crisis, including those who have very complex problems. Although this is a critical service, because it is often not directly linked to reimbursement, it is often not valued.

QUALITY IMPROVEMENT TEAMS

In today's health care environment, health care organizations are faced with conflicting demands. The public demands that organizations and the health care professionals who serve them be innovative, that they deliver high-quality care, and that they do this while containing costs. Often quality of care and cost containment can conflict, if not mutually exclusive (Duncan, Ginter, & Swayne, 1992; Gibelman, 2002). This challenges health care organizations and the professionals who serve them to develop new and innovative ways of balancing these two factors.

Although we typically think of hospitals as the settings where measuring quality of care and establishing quality assessment teams are most important, they are not the only health care delivery organizations that are affected by these processes (Schwab, 1995). The need for quality assurance, sometimes referred to as quality improvement, transcends all health service delivery organizations and includes managed care organizations, clinics in medically underserved areas and rural locations, administrative and headquarter operations, nursing homes, hospices, and group homes. Social workers and other health care professionals will most assuredly serve in some way as the programs and services they deliver are evaluated. All medical, health, mental health, rehabilitation, disease prevention, and health promotion programs need to be monitored.

Quality improvement processes are evaluated in almost all programs and services offered in the area of health care delivery. To assist programs to meet these societal and economic demands, many health care organizations are now implementing *continuous improvement* (CI) teams. These teams are formed to solve specific problems. They take knowledge and insight from several different areas, including statistics, operation management, organizational theory, strategic planning, information management, and service delivery (Batalden, Mohr, Strosberg, & Baker, 1995). Team membership and actual function may vary based on the health care service delivered; however, those chosen to participate in the team must have some *stake* in the service that is being delivered. This means that the participants can benefit from timely and cost-effective solutions to the problem. In the past, one reason for failure was trying to implement quality improvement at the upper level of health care management rather than with the workers who are the most involved (Schalowitz, 1995). To address this weakness, organizations are encouraged to create teams that consist of both management and practice professionals.

Hart, Coady, and Halvorson (1995) continued to emphasize the implementation of a team concept, and they described the professionals that should participate on the teams. The first member of the team, and surely the most important, is the *team leader*. Traditionally, social workers have not been overtly active in this process, although their involvement has been inevitable. Although not referred to by Hart, Coady, and Halvorson (1995), it is as the team leader that the health care social worker can best be used—assuming that this role will allow him or her to become an active and leading member in the workings of the quality improvement team.

In general, it is expected that team leaders be active in leadership and involved in all areas of service delivery. They must also be skilled in the political, social, and cultural environment to anticipate and initiate changes that need to be made. "The call for universal health care coverage with dramatic expansion of resource use becomes a significant challenge to health care leadership. Their [leaders'] ability to proactively lead this effort and to simultaneously engage the delivery system in change is a significant challenge" (Hart, Coady, & Halvorson, 1995, p. 61), and a challenge that social workers have always embraced. The diverse activities of the health care social worker makes him or her an excellent candidate for this leadership role.

To prepare for assuming this role, health care social workers need to be educated in continuous quality improvement (CQI) methods. The skills they possess, with the general knowledge base from which they operate, make them excellent choices for leadership in this area. Although it is beyond the scope of this book to explain the entire quality improvement process, its importance in the teaching and preparation of social workers who choose to practice in the health care arena should not be underestimated. For more information, explanation, and application of continuous quality improvement, the reader is referred to the *Journal of Health Administration Education* (1995, volume 13, number 1), which dedicates the entire issue to the provision and implementation strategy for quality improvement in the health care setting.

To facilitate preparation of health care professionals as team leaders, professional schools need to include this role in their curricula. Recognition of a leader's knowledge and skill, which is not traditionally found in many health administration programs, is essential (Batalden, Mohr, Strosberg, & Baker, 1995; Gelmon, Baker, 1994; Hart, Coady, & Halvorson, 1995). Schools of social work need to adapt leadership as part of training, particularly for those who choose to specialize in the area of health. Whether social workers serve as team leaders or merely as team members, they will undoubtedly be expected to participate in these teams. To participate actively and productively, professional education in this area will be essential.

Once the team leader has been selected, the members of the team must all work together for the common good of the clients. The team's first major task is to develop health care guidelines, which often provide the basis for CQI. The guidelines must address issues of appropriateness, effectiveness, efficiency, and efficacy of the service delivery. In the development of these guidelines, input from the physician is essential. This input requires that physicians be encouraged to think beyond their own role and embrace the total system of service delivery (Hart, Coady, & Halvorson, 1995).

The formulation of guidelines may create the greatest challenge that the physician will face, since he or she must learn to recognize the system influences that interact and permeate the health care arena. Physicians generally receive limited training on the influence of the environment. Many times they are not encouraged to supplement this training in practice, because patient care rewards are generally linked to the concrete service(s) they provide. Because of constant time restraints, it is not uncommon for physicians to depend on other members of the health care delivery team to address the issues that go beyond direct patient care. Although this acceptance seems to be easier when relating to primary care physicians, it can be problematic for all physicians as members of the health care delivery team. In working with the physician, the social work team leader needs to prepare for this problem by sharing with the physician his or her knowledge of environmental and practice systems that can influence guidelines for quality practice.

Another essential member of the quality improvement team is the nurse. Nurses are important members for inclusion on the team because they can be excellent resources as leaders or facilitators in the process. Nurses can assist in making suggestions for improving the process of patient care. It is also important to note that in our changing health care environment, there may be some medical services that are now delivered solely by the nurse. This can make the nurse a solo or entirely responsible medical practitioner regarding some of the patient care services provided. As independent practitioners, nurses' input in establishing guidelines is essential.

A third member for inclusion of the quality improvement team is the administrator or middle-level manager. This person can provide valuable input because he or she is knowledgeable about the daily processes and administrative concerns involved in service delivery. Managers can help to predict problems that will occur within a system and can suggest practical solutions for dealing with service changes from an administrative perspective. Traditionally, on quality improvement teams, it has been the administrator or the middle-level manager who has often assumed the primary leadership role. The advantage of using the social worker as a team leader in addition to or as replacement for the middle manager is the sensitivity that the social worker brings through knowledge of practice issues. The health care social worker can blend practice insight with administrative considerations, while integrating the needs of clients and their families.

Optional team members for inclusion in the quality improvement team can include board members or consumers of the service as well as administrative support personnel, such as receptionists or other front-line contact workers. If a health planning board exists, including one of more of these individuals as participants can be helpful. Members of these boards often are clients who use the service or live in the area where the service is being provided. This participation will allow board members to become empowered through education and understanding while participating in the basics of implementation. If board members are not available or no board exists, inviting individual clients to serve can be invaluable. Meeting the needs of the client is the ultimate objective, and client participation gives input into service delivery designed to address his or her needs. Including the receptionist and other front-line workers can also be helpful. Given their often daily contact with clients, these individuals are in good positions to evaluate front-line needs and desires (Hart, Coady, & Halvorson, 1995).

In summary, the quality improvement process, no matter what form it takes in the future, is here to stay. In the future, continued education and training in this area will probably be the responsibility of the managed care organizations or the service providers themselves. If social workers are taught how to implement, educate, and lead the movement in this form of quality assurance, they will be able to increase employment desirability as well as ensure and improve the measures that lead to continued client health and wellness.

Social workers have a real advantage as team leaders because they are not limited, unlike so many health care executives who cannot engage in direct practice. Social workers cannot only understand and anticipate trends in the turbulent environment, but they can also use their practice expertise to recognize and advocate for system changes that can lead to greater client empowerment and advocacy.

CHAPTER SUMMARY AND FUTURE DIRECTIONS

In current social work health care practice, the behavioral biopsychosocial approach continues to integrate the biomedical, psychosocial, and behavioral outcomes in measuring service necessity, utility, and effectiveness. This integrated approach provides health care social workers with a theory base that can be used to simplify what could otherwise be a complicated process. Today the emphasis is on linking these behaviorally based biopsychosocial issues with medical outcomes data (Rock, 2002). Most of the other health-related disciplines also subscribe to this approach, making the social worker a leader in understanding and interpreting the "psycho" and "social" factors in a client's condition. Because of competition from other allied health professionals, health care social workers, now more than ever, need to emphasize and rely on the strengths of the practice profession, which include remaining active in the planning process for the client.

Teamwork and collaborative efforts to assist clients are the present as well as the future of health care social work. Many professionals truly do not understand the differences between the multidisciplinary and the interdisciplinary team approaches. Interdisciplinary team approaches encourage overlap of roles and integration of services. Social workers need to embrace these changes and allow themselves, as the other professionals are doing, to become more active in areas of service that are not considered traditional. In the provision of health care service there is overlap, blurred definitions, and diffuse boundary distinctions. This is not happening by accident—the interdisciplinary team concept is requiring it. Social workers by their nature can be flexible and should not fear assisting in all areas of the client continuum of care. It is only by being assertive and reaching for more that social workers can help the profession and the clients served. By increasing the marketability of their profession, social workers can also ensure that the services they have traditionally provided to clients will not go unpracticed.

To expand the role of social work, the quality review process should be considered. The quality review process is part of health care delivery that will not go away. Health care social workers can make excellent team leaders and can guide this process, while ensuring quality care services to the clients served. Now is the time for social workers to reach out for new uncharted areas of practice and service delivery. After all, it is clearly efforts such as this that are needed to help secure and maintain the place for social workers at the health care delivery table.

REFERENCES

Abramson, J. S. (2002). Interdisciplinary team practice. In A. R. Roberts & G. J. Greene (Eds.), *Social workers' desk reference* (pp. 44-50). New York: Oxford University Press.

Barker, R. L. (1995). *The social work dictionary* (3rd ed.). Washington, DC: NASW Press.

Batalden, P., Mohr, J., Strosberg, M., & Baker, G. R. (1995). A conceptual framework for learning continual improvement in health administration education programs. *Journal of Health Administration Education, 13,* 67-90.

Ben-Sira, Z., & Szyf, M. (1992). Status inequality in the social worker-nurse collaboration in hospitals. *Social Science Medicine, 34,* 365-374.

Berkman, B. (1996). The emerging health care world: Implications for social work practice and education. *Social Work, 41,* 541-549.

Caplan, G. (1970). *The theory and practice of mental health consultation.* New York: Basic Books.

Carlton, T. O. (1984). *Clinical social work in health care settings: A guide to professional practice with exemplars.* New York: Springer Publishing Co.

Carson, V. B. (1996). Alternate routes for the journey: Practice, roles and settings. In V. B. Carson & E. N. Arnold (Eds.), *Mental health nursing: The nurse-patient journey* (pp. 51-69). Philadelphia: Saunders.

Davidson, K. W. (1990). Role blurring and the hospital social worker's search for a clear domain. *Health and Social Work, 15,* 228-234.

Duncan, W. J., Ginter, P. M., & Swayne, L. E. (1992). *Strategic management of health care organizations.* Boston: PWS-Kent.

Dziegielewski, S. F. (1996). Managed care principles: The need for social work in the health care environment. *Crisis Intervention and Time-Limited Treatment, 3,* 97–110.

Dziegielewski, S. F. (2002). *DSM-IV-TR™ in action.* New York: Wiley.

Engel, G. (1977). The need for a new medical model: A challenge to biomedical science. *Science, 196,* 129–136.

Franklin, C. (2002). Developing effective practice competencies in managed behavioral health care. In A. R. Roberts & G. J. Greene (Eds.), *Social workers' desk reference* (pp. 3-10). New York: Oxford University Press.

Gelmon, S., & Baker, G. R. (1994). *A quality improvement resource teaching guide.* Arlington, VA: Association of University Programs in Health Administration.

Gibelman, M. (2002). Social work in an era of managed care. The biopsychosocial model. In A. R. Roberts & G. J. Greene (Eds.), *Social workers' desk reference* (pp. 17-22). New York: Oxford University Press.

Gilbert, P. (2002). Understanding the biopsychosocial approach: Conceptualization. *Clinical Psychology, 14,* 13-17.

Hart, J., Coady, M. M., & Halvorson, G. (1995). The managed care perspective. *Health Administration Education, 13,* 53–66.

Holliman, D., Dziegielewski, S. F., & Datta, P. (2001). Discharge planning and social work practice. *Journal of Health Care Social Work 32(3),* 1-19.

Kiesler, D. J. (1999). *Beyond the disease model of mental disorders.* New York: Praeger.

Kurtz, R. A., & Chalfant, H. P. (1991). *The sociology of medicine and illness* (2nd ed.). Boston: Allyn & Bacon.

Lawrence, S. A., & Zittel-Palamara, K. (2002). The interplay between biology, genetics, and human behavior. In J. S. Wodarski & S. F. Dziegielewski (Eds.), *Human behavior and the social environment: Integrating theory and evidenced-based practice* (pp. 39-64). New York: Springer Publishing Co.

Lewin, K. (1947). Frontiers in group dynamics. *Human Relations, 1,* 5–41.

McWhinney, I. R. (1989). *A textbook of family medicine.* New York: Oxford University Press.

Meikle, J.C.E. (2002). In defense of the biospychosocial model (letter). *Clinical Psychology, 11,* 3-5.

National Council on Practice of Clinical Social Work (NASW). (1994). *Guidelines for clinical social work supervision.* Washington, DC: NASW.

Netting, F. N., & Williams, F. G. (1996). Case manager–physician collaboration: Implications for professional identity, roles and relationships. *Health and Social Work, 21,* 216-224.

Newman, B. M., & Newman, P. R. (2003). *Development through life: A psychosocial approach.* Belmont, CA: Wadswoth.

Rankin, E. A. (1996). Patient and family education. In V. B. Carson & E. N. Arnold (Eds.), *Mental health nursing: The nurse-patient journey* (pp. 503–516). Philadelphia: Saunders.

Regensburg, J. (1978). *Toward education of the health professions.* New York: Harper & Row.

Richardson, M. (1988). Mental health services: Growth and development of a system. In S. J. Williams & P. R. Torrens (Eds.), *Introduction to health services* (3rd ed., pp. 255–277). Albany, NY: Delmar.

Rock, B. D. (2002). Social work in health care for the 21st century: The biopsychosocial model. In A. R. Roberts & G. J. Greene (Eds.), *Social workers' desk reference* (pp. 10-15). New York: Oxford University Press.

Schalowitz, J. I. (1995). Total quality management at Motorola: A successful blueprint for manufacturing and service organizations. *Health Administration Education, 13,* 15–24.

Schlesinger, E. G. (1985). *Health care social work practice: Concepts and strategies.* St. Louis, MO: Times Mirror/Mosby.

Schwab, P. M. (1995). A federal affair in quality management: A case study. *Health Administration Education, 13,* 129–142.

Shortell, S. M., & Kalunzy, A. D. (1994). Forward. In S. M. Shortell & A. D. Kalunzy (Eds.), *Health care management: Organizational behavior and design* (3rd ed., p. XI). Albany, NY: Delmar.

Shulman, L. (2002). Developing successful therapeutic relationships. In A. R. Roberts & G. J. Greene (Eds.), *Social workers' desk reference* (pp. 375-378). New York: Oxford University Press.

Siple, J. (1994). Drug therapy and the interdisciplinary team: A clinical pharmacist's perspective. *Generations Quarterly, 18,* 49–55.

Sperry, L. (1988). Biopsychosocial therapy: An integrative approach for tailoring treatment. *Individual Psychology, 44,* 225–235.

Spraycar, M. (Ed.). (1995). *PDR: Medical dictionary* (1st ed.). Montvale, NJ: Medical Economics.

Wise, T. N. (1997). Psychiatric diagnoses in primary care: The biopsychosocial perspective. In H. Leigh (Ed.), *Biopsychosocial approaches in primary care: State of the art and challenges for the 21st century* (pp. 9-27). New York: Plenum.

GLOSSARY

Biopsychosocial approach: In this approach to health care practice, the "bio" refers to the biological and medical aspects of an individual's health and well-being; the "psycho" involves the individual aspects of the client, such as individual feelings of self-worth and self-esteem;

and the "social" considers the larger picture and relates to the social environment that surrounds and influences the client.

Biopsychosocial model of practice: When all three areas (the bio, psycho, and social) are identified, assessed, and addressed, a biopsychosocial model of practice intervention is implemented. This approach to practice is viewed primarily as the basis for social work practice in the health care area.

Biopsychosocial–spiritual perspective: This perspective is a modification of the biopsychosocial perspective that includes recognition and influences of client spiritual needs.

Case-by-case collaboration: This is when practitioners from different disciplines come together to share and participate in a mode of service delivery or an individualized intervention plan designed to assist the client, family, or community in need.

Collaboration: This term is often used interchangeably with interdisciplinary. In its most general sense, it means different yet related disciplines working together for the ultimate benefit of the clients served.

Consultation: In this form of collaboration, expert advice that can either be accepted or rejected by the consultee is given.

Continuous quality improvement: A specific method and plan for ensuring that quality care is obtained. The foundation of this method originally comes from a managerial perspective other than health care.

Depersonalization: The essence of the biomedical approach to practice rests in the fact that the professional possesses some type of special esoteric knowledge and skill that can be given to the client. With the advent of increased education, consumers are becoming more knowledgeable and are questioning the special knowledge that professionals have traditionally been considered to possess.

Education: In collaborative education the social worker offers his or her expertise to train other health care providers.

Empowerment: The process of helping clients and their families or significant others to meet their interpersonal, social, socioeconomic, and political goals.

Interdisciplinary teams: Consist of a variety of health care professionals who are brought together to provide effective, better coordinated, and improved quality of services for clients.

Multidisciplinary teams: Are composed of a mix of health and social welfare professionals, with each discipline primarily working on an independent or a referral basis.

Quality assurance: The process or guidelines that a service delivery organization sets to ensure that services measure up to the standards set.

Quality improvement: See definition for *quality assurance*.

Stake: A vested interest in serving as part of the quality assurance team.

Team approach: This type of collaborative effort links professionals from different health care disciplines together to achieve enhanced client outcomes.

Team leader: The individual who is responsible for the coordination, education, and enhanced functioning of the quality assessment team.

QUESTIONS FOR FURTHER STUDY

1. What are the major weaknesses of using a biopsychosocial approach to practice?
2. What are some of the strengths of using the biopsychosocial approach to practice?
3. What forms of collaborative effort should health care social workers participate in, and how could these roles be expanded?
4. Interdisciplinary teamwork seems to be the current trend in health care practice.   Do you believe it will continue, and why?
5. What new roles would you recommend that health care social workers assume as part of the health care delivery team, and how would these roles benefit the profession and the client?

WEBSITES

Behavioral Social Work and Healthcare Settings
Online journal articles from *Social Work in Health Care*.
http://www.haworthpressinc.com/store/TOC.pdf

British Nursing Index
Electronic medical information source for health care and social
    work.
http://www.ais.salford.ac.uk/publica/notes/bni.pdf

Cornell News
Articles about social work in managed care and new developments.
http://www.news.cornell.edu/releases/March 97/social.work.ssl.html

Health Care and Social Work
For everyone involved in one or both fields.
Address: http://www.careandhealth.com

Outcome Measures for Social Work in Health Care
Information and articles on the above topic.
http://www.aascipsw.org/outcome.html

Society for Social Work Administration in Health Care
An association for social workers in administration of health care.
http://www.ala.orglacr4resmar98.html

CHAPTER 6

Practice Strategy: Considerations and Methods for Health Care Social Workers

A revolution in health care delivery is under way. The use of time-limited brief therapeutic approaches can help social workers to be viewed as more competent, effective, and efficient. Time-limited brief treatments remain an integral part of our past and our present, and lastly, can create the basis for our survival in the future.

—Dziegielewski

INFLUENCE OF MANAGED BEHAVIORAL HEALTH CARE

In the field of social work, there is much disagreement over what is considered the best theoretical or methodological basis for current practice (Schram & Mandell, 1997). This is also true of health care social work practice. Furthermore, in this area of social work the pressure is even greater because so many health care social workers simply do not do traditional social work counseling (Dziegielewski & Leon, 2001). To complicate methodological intervention strategy further, health care social workers are often forced to go beyond the traditional bounds of their practice wisdom. For these social workers, selecting the best practice strategy must also be firmly based within the reality of the environment. For the health care social worker who must select a method of intervention, it is not uncommon to feel influenced and subsequently trapped within a system that is driven by social, political, cultural, and economic factors. With the widespread movement of managed behavioral health care, there are many factors in the environment that not only influence current health care practice—they dictate it.

Health care social workers generally work for and are obligated to behavioral health care agencies. The entire health care system is being reorganized by this concept, and the bottom line is to reduce health care costs (Fiesta, 1995; Franklin, 2002). *Fee for service* is decreasing and insurance systems are requiring more partial- or full-risk *capitation* (Rock, 2002). As in the 1990s, managed care remains an alternative or the replacement of fee for service (Burner, Waldo, & McKusick, 1992). This means that managed care organizations must compete to secure service contracts. In the attempt to secure contracts for service, budget restrictions are implemented. Financial incentives are created that encourage the provision of limited service, thereby limiting the number of inpatient or outpatient days (Chambliss, 2000). What this means for health care professionals who accept these contracts is that they will receive a probable decrease in earnings. For example, many physicians in 1995 reported having at least one managed care contract (83%), and those with the largest penetration of managed care reported greater declines in their practice earnings (Meckler, 1996).

This trend of declining income potential for physicians can have direct implications for social work professionals. Two primary reasons for this decline are (a) less money available for health care; and (b) the continued push toward further health care cost reduction. For most managed care organizations, the key strategy for reducing costs is limiting unnecessary health service use. This is generally accomplished by altering the treatment process and services in various ways. These cost-reduction and cost-shifting policies have caused the process of providing health care service to change dramatically over the years. To complicate the selection of a service method further, the provision of counseling, treatment, and discharge planning needs to be set within reimbursement parameters. In today's environment, it is not uncommon for these plans to be guided by the amount of insurance a client has (Fiesta, 1995).

In conjunction with cost-saving strategy, the guidelines and practices developed through quality improvement programs can also be used as preestablished criteria for service delivery (Heeschen, 2000). These preestablished criteria for practice delivery can limit health care social workers in the treatment plans they are able to create or the types of case management strategies they are allowed to employ.

It is believed that the biggest test for health care social workers engaged in practice of any type today (therapeutic or concrete service delivery) will be to link the service to reimbursement patterns. Once this link is made, social workers can only stand to benefit. This will help the health care social worker to justify time spent in the provision of time-limited therapy for increasing client overall health and wellness.

ESTABLISHING THE TIME-LIMITED SERVICE STRUCTURE

Selecting the most appropriate intervention method in today's health care environment requires that a multitude of factors be considered in the selection process. In addition to these numerous factors, there is general support for "traditional methods of time-limited intervention," "lack of a formal space for counseling," and the "time constraints" health care social workers must face in trying to offer services. Many times members of the health care delivery team do not recognize the importance of the social worker as part of the nurse/social worker team (Bristow & Herrick, 2002). Unfortunately, other professionals on the team often believe that the social worker should concentrate on providing more concrete services (Cowles & Lefcowitz, 1992; Holliman, Dziegielewski, & Datta, 2001; Holliman, Dziegielewski & Teare, in press). This view remains debatable, however, since the other professionals continue to recognize the importance of the psychosocial needs of the clients served (Dziegielewski, 1997a; Gross, Rabinowitz, Feldman, & Boerma, 1996).

Unfortunately, in the health area, there is one issue that must be considered in selecting a practice structure—it is the concentration on balancing quality of care and cost-effectiveness. As reinforced throughout the book, when there is a battle between them, it is generally cost-effectiveness that wins. Therefore, health care social workers are expected to provide what they believe is the most beneficial and ethical practice possible, while being pressured to complete it as quickly and efficiently as possible. There is no simple answer. The health care setting, as well as managed care contracts, capitation policies, and direct insurance reimbursement, clearly can affect the choice of health care counseling strategy to be used.

A further complication when selecting a structure for practice intervention is that defending a type of intervention "as in the best interest of the client" may not truly reflect the client's wishes. Traditionally, Americans have been resistant to allowing any interference by political and social factors in service provision. Today, however, because of the promise of lower premiums and lower health care expenditures, this interference has occurred (Burner, Waldo, & McKusick, 1992). It is not uncommon for clients to be more interested in receiving a service that is time limited or reimbursable, regardless of the expected benefit that they may gain from an alternative, possibly longer-term treatment strategy.

TIME-LIMITED SERVICE AND BEHAVIORAL MANAGED CARE PRINCIPLES

Today, time-limited brief practice methods remain in a state of transition, which simply reflects the turbulence in today's general health care environment (Dziegielewski, 1996, 2002; Dziegielewski & Leon, 2001). In choosing a method of practice, health care social workers, like other professionals, are being forced to deal with numerous issues (e.g., limited reimbursement patterns, declining health care admissions, capitation, etc.). Struggling to resolve these issues, as discussed previously, has become necessary because of the inception of prospective payment systems, managed care plans, and other changes in the provision and funding of health care (Johnson & Berger, 1990; Ross, 1993; Simon, Showers, Blumenfield, Holden, & Wu, 1995).

The turbulence in the current health care environment requires health care social workers to struggle with picking a practice structure that is not only efficacious and efficient but one that can also enhance effectiveness in the briefest amount of time. In today's practice environment, practice strategy must encompass two things: maintaining quality of care and joining quality of care with an emphasis on cost containment (Dziegielewski, 1997b). It is no secret, however, that many social workers believe that whether openly stated or not the emphasis is on ensuring cost containment (Dziegielewski, 1996, 2002). Stated simply, in selecting a form of time-limited intervention strategy, health care social workers must remember the importance of remaining viable "dollar generators," or they will feel the brunt of initial dollar savings attempts.

INTERMITTENT THERAPY: APPLICATION OF A TIME-LIMITED STRUCTURE

In the health care setting, as in other practice settings, it is not uncommon for clients to expect that intervention will be brief. In addition to the limitations set by insurance reimbursement patterns, many clients simply do not have the time, desire, or money for longer-term interventions (especially the poor). It has become obvious that the amorphous clinical judgment and vague attempts at making clients "feel better" will no longer be allowed (Araoz & Carrese, 1996; Dziegielewski, Shields, & Thyer, 1998). In the medical setting, as in so many other areas of counseling practice, the days of insurance-covered long-term therapy encounters have ended (Dziegielewski, 2002).

In today's health care practice environment, reality dictates that the duration of most therapeutic sessions, regardless of the intervention used or the orientation of the therapist, remain relatively brief. In social work practice, most of these therapeutic encounters generally range from 6 to 8 sessions (Wells & Phelps, 1990); however, Fanger (1995) noted as many as 20 sessions. Generally speaking, the least number of sessions is 1, and the greatest number is 20. There are some areas in the health care setting where this can apply, but generally client contacts are generally much shorter, with 1- and 2-meeting encounters being the norm rather than the exception. Actually, if polled, many health care social workers would agree that brief or short-term therapy in the traditional sense has become a product of the past. What is used today in this high-pressure environment is more adequately termed *intermittent therapy*, where every session is considered complete and treated as if it is the only session that may occur.

It is essential to realize this short time duration in health care practice and the fact that this may be the only session the social worker is able to provide. Without this framework for practice reality, a lack of planning can result in numerous unexpected and unplanned terminations for the client (Dziegielewski, 2002; Wells, 1994) as well as feelings of failure and decreased job satisfaction for the social worker.

In time-limited intervention strategies, two types of practice delivery formats have emerged: traditional brief intervention and intermittent brief intervention. To capitalize on professional time and the need for "face-to-face" contact, a combination of both formats may also be used. In the traditional format, clients begin and terminate intervention in a close-ended therapeutic environment (Dziegielewski, 1997b).

Intermittent formats, which were rarely used in the past, appear to be gaining in popularity—particularly in the practice of health care social work. This increased acceptance may be viewed as a further response to the limitations instituted by managed care policies. In health care, an intervention plan carried out in one session and monitored periodically over time can be attractive for funding sources. An intermittent format for therapy usually employs fewer sessions; however, sessions can be spread out over a longer period. For health care social workers, use of an intermittent format can provide a "new twist" on intervention.

In summary, for a model to be considered a viable time-limited approach it must include mutually negotiated concrete and realistic goals, a plan for measuring effectiveness, and a specific time frame for conducting and completing the service.

DEVELOPMENT OF TIME-LIMITED GOALS AND OBJECTIVES

No matter what method of time-limited service provision a health care social worker selects, establishing clear goals and objectives is essential. To establish a plan of intervention that is generally of an interdisciplinary nature, behavioral goals and behavioral objectives are required as part of the intervention strategy. Simply stated, a goal constitutes what you and the client want to accomplish; the behavioral objectives state exactly what the client plans to do to address the identified goal(s) (Dziegielewski & Powers, 2000; Roberts & Dziegielewski, 1995). It is important to note, however, that many social work professionals do not make the fine distinction between goals and objectives and use the terms interchangeably.

Cormier and Cormier (1991) stress the importance of clearly defined goals in direct practice. Goals provide direction and structure for the professional practice intervention. This is particularly important when dealing with an individual in the medical setting where clear goals and objectives are part of the client's overall treatment plan. Many times it is this treatment plan that influences accreditation, certification, or reimbursement levels.

Goals also permit the practitioner to establish whether she or he has the skills or desire to work with the client (Cormier & Cormier, 1991). It is important in time-limited service provision to be sure that the individual will be able to secure the services that are needed and, in turn, to ensure that the therapist is able to help the client focus in on change efforts that will allow a healthier homeostatic balance to emerge. The goals and behavioral objectives chosen also help to outline the needed intervention and the particular practice strategies and techniques that will be needed. Finally, goal setting is a crucial element in measuring the effectiveness of service provision because it can provide the standards against which progress is measured (Brower & Nurius, 1993).

Brower and Nurius (1993) suggest two key characteristics that need to be present when designing effective intervention goals. First, goals need to be specific, clear, verifiable, and measurable. This remains consistent with the client's overall plan, where the established goals need to be as concrete and behavior specific as possible. The objectives, therefore, should be designed to further quantify the goals. For example, if an individual were suffering from a grief reaction regarding the sudden illness of a loved one, the social worker would want the goals and objectives to be specifically related to the restoration of equilibrium.

A second major point made by Brower and Nurius (1993) is that the established goals must be mutually agreed on by both the helping professional and the client. This may seem difficult in time-limited service provision, where the health care social worker is pressed for time. However, the role of the therapist, regardless of the method of intervention,should always be one of facilitation in which the client is helped to achieve what he or she has deemed essential to regain an enhanced homeostatic balance (Roberts & Dziegielewski, 1995). The client must also help determine whether the goals and objectives sought are consistent with his or her own culture and values. It is up to the therapist to help the client structure and establish the intervention strategy; however, mutuality is central to the development of goals and objectives.

In implementing the method of intervention, the social worker ensures that the problem that needs to be dealt with is addressed. Goals and objectives should always be stated positively and realistically so that motivation for completion will be increased (Brower & Nurius, 1993). It is also essential, in establishing the effectiveness of what is being done, that the goals (particularly the objectives) be stated in as concrete and functional terms as possible.

TODAY'S HEALTH CARE SOCIAL WORKER

Name: L. Daisy Skinner, MSW, LCSW
List State of Practice:
Professional Job Title: Nephrology Social Worker

Duties in a typical day:
The typical day of a nephrology social worker begins with the pressing problems with patients on the first shift (treatments between 5:00 a.m. and 9:00 a.m.). These issues include having no transportation that morning, utilities being shut off due to nonpayment of bills, the need for medical equipment (walker, wheelchair, etc.), and/or personal issues. The information is given to the nurse or patient care technicians and they refer it to me.

What do you like most about your current position?
People who have end-stage renal disease have a myriad of medical problems that range from diabetes to hypertension (both the leading causes of kidney failure) to cancer and amputations. That said, what I enjoy most about this job is the ability to work with physicians, nurses, and patients to join the psychological with the physical pieces in a way that benefits the patients to their maximum potential. It is critical to guide and provide supportive counseling to the patient through the complicated transplantation process. Working with families to help patients through the medical maze as well as helping to address end-of-life issues with them are the most rewarding aspects to this multifaceted job.

What do you like least about your position?
Arranging for and fielding problems with daily transportation through the countywide transportation system for the disabled and elderly.

What "words of wisdom" do you have for the new health care social worker who is considering working in a similar position?

Breathe! And use humor. Breathe because the problems are numerous and varied, and you must be able to "switch gears" instantly. Humor because even though life is difficult for these patients, a laugh goes a long way. You must be a self-starter and have life's experiences to draw upon. Ask for or arrange a help-network with other nephrology social workers (they are your biggest supporters). Read past case notes, which provide a plethora of information. Above all, when the going gets rough, remember your reason for being there in the first place: You're making a difference for these patients.

FACTORS IN TIME-LIMITED SERVICE PROVISION

Establishing a model for the phases of service provision can be an arduous task. These phases of intervention are generally related to traditional forms of time-limited intervention where there is a predetermined beginning and end. Unfortunately, this is not usually the case for the health care social worker, where intermittent and single-session formats have become a practice reality. Although the traditional forms of brief intervention (with clear plans that are monitored periodically) are attractive to funding sources, they may be impractical to implement. This is particularly problematic when concrete indicators, such as discharge planning, education, and after-care provision, are the primary objectives expected at the completion of service.

In the health care setting, a great deal of intervention is done on an "as-needed basis," so it is important to be flexible in anticipating and experiencing the intervention phases. In time-limited service provision, the phases of intervention may cross several encounters, where at others time they may be condensed into one. Regardless, objectives that lead to the desired outcome must be addressed at each phase of the service provided (Wells, 1994).

Generally, in the *initial phase* of service provision, a hopeful environment is created in which the client begins to feel confident that his or her problem can and will be addressed. It is important that the social worker communicates and starts to build rapport. Many times health care social workers may actually initiate service provision in a hallway or at a client's bedside. No matter where the process starts, it is important that the client feels safe, comfortable, and free to talk about his or her situation. In the hurried rush of the health care social worker's day, it is all too easy to neglect this essential ingredient, which is basic to the start of a successful interventive encounter.

The social worker must further help the client to break down problems into concrete terms, which, once identified, establish the groundwork for the development of concrete goals and objectives (Dziegielewski & Leon, 2001; Roberts & Dziegielewski, 1995; Wells, 1994). Generally, an initial contract is formulated. It does not matter if this is written or verbal, but a clear understanding of what will transpire is essential. It is important that early in the intervention process the social worker starts to think about assessment and assistance to obtain client behavior change. Diagnosis and assessment will be covered in greater depth in chapter 8; however, initiation of a well-rounded and comprehensive assessment at this initial phase is considered essential (Dziegielewski, 2002). Measurement of initial individual, group, or social functioning needs to be established. If measurement scales are not implemented to serve as a baseline, an initial ranking to compare client functioning at the beginning and end of intervention is suggested.

Lastly, an agreed-on time frame for service provision needs to be established (Walter & Peller, 2000). Clients need to know what they can expect from the health care social worker and how much time will actually be devoted to them in addressing their problem. In the initial phase, the measurement of effectiveness will be finalized. It is here that the health care social worker must decide and plan for implementation of how she or he will measure the effectiveness of the intervention strategy.

The *main phase of intervention* is generally based on the model and format chosen in the initial phase. This is the most active of the stages because this is when concrete problem solving actually occurs. Activities that can assist in this stage regardless of the model chosen include planning each session in advance, summarizing of each session, and maintaining flexibility if renegotiation needs to occur in regard to the problem-solving process.

For the health care social worker, planning each session in advance requires commitment of time outside of the formal session. Usually this time is not reimbursable to the social worker or the health care agency. Therefore, both the client and the social worker must be willing to commit this time to planning outside of the traditional session. For the health care social worker, this is particularly important when preparing health and wellness counseling. Generally, there is limited time to do this and not only must the social worker be prepared to discuss the topic, but he or she must have written materials that will assist in making the most of the service time available.

Another essential area where advanced planning is essential concerns the medical aspects of the client's condition. Many times clients suffer from medical problems that complicate the psychosocial aspects they are experiencing. Social workers need to know enough about the "bio" in the behaviorally based biopsychosocial aspects of practice to assist the client in addressing these needs. Also, the issue of medication influence within the counseling environment should not be ignored (Dziegielewski & Leon, 2001). Many times clients are taking medications. The social worker needs to know how these medications can affect them. Medications can influence actions toward family members or significant others as well as impact other social relationships. The increased use of medications for all types of health and mental health problems has a pronounced effect on the practice of health care social work. For a more detailed description of the social worker–client relationship with regard to medication use the reader is referred to the text by Dziegielewski and Leon (2001).

No matter how many sessions are being implemented, the technique of *summarization* should be incorporated into each session (Dziegielewski, 1997b). When each formal encounter begins, the client actually states the agreed-upon objectives that are to be addressed. This will allow both client and social worker to quickly focus on the task at hand. Summarization should also be practiced at the end of each session. This will allow the client to recapitulate what she or he believes has transpired in the session, and how it relates to the stated objectives. Clients should use their own words to summarize what has transpired. In acknowledging and summarizing the content and objectives of the session,(a) the client takes responsibility for his or her own actions; (b) repetition allows the session accomplishments to be highlighted and reinforced; (c) the client and the social worker ascertain that they are working together on the same objectives; and (d) the therapeutic environment remains flexible and open for renegotiation of contracted objectives.

Lastly, the middle phase of intervention will close with consideration for arrangement of future follow-up (Wells, 1994). Resnick and Dziegielewski (1996) completed a study of social workers in the health care area, and one of the conclusions they drew was that health care social workers wanted feedback as to how their clients were doing. They found that receiving this feedback increased overall levels of job satisfaction. It is important at this stage in the intervention process to ensure that proper attention is given to the measurement of feedback and follow-up, particularly if an unplanned termination results. This is important to prepare for, since frequently in the health care environment quick and unplanned terminations occur (Resnick & Dziegielewski, 1996).

In the *final phase* of intervention, a follow-up contact is established. Here the social worker is either to meet the client in person for intermittent sessions or to arrange for telephone communication to review and evaluate current client progress and status (Wells, 1994). A time lapse of no more than 4 months is recommended (Dziegielewski, 1997b). The social worker should prepare in advance for this meeting to continue and reaffirm previous measurement strategies.

TIME-MITED SERVICE PROVISION VERSUS TRADITIONAL PSYCHOTHERAPY

Most psychotherapists, particularly those who support psychoanalytic therapy, believe that managed care policies are biased against them (Alperin, 1994). They believe that making changes in a person takes time and that rushing into changes could lead to further complications in future health and wellness. They urge social workers to realize this danger and advocate strongly for the continuance of psychotherapy before it becomes an extinct mode of practice delivery in today's "big business" practice environment (Alperin, 1994).

The problems of conducting traditional forms of psychotherapy are not unique to the health care environment. For years, the applicability and effectiveness of time-limited methods of practice have been well established (Bloom, 1992; Dziegielewski, Shields & Thyer, 1998; Dziegielewski & Powers, 2000; Epstein, 1994; Ligon, 2002; Mancoske, Standifer, & Cauley, 1994; Wells, 1994). It is easy to see how time-limited interventions have gained in popularity, particularly in the health care setting. They are based on the overall objective of bringing about positive changes in a client's current lifestyle with as little face-to-face contact as possible (Fanger, 1995). It is this emphasis on effectiveness and applicability leading to increased positive change that has helped to make time-limited brief interventions popular. In the health care area, time-limited approaches are the most requested forms of practice in use today.

The major difference between traditional psychotherapy and time-limited approaches is that the foundation for each is different. This difference requires social workers to reexamine some basic premises that have been taught regarding long-term therapeutic models used in a more traditional format. According to Dziegielewski (1997b), seven factors can be identified that highlight the difference between these two methods.

First is the primary difference in the way the client is viewed. Traditional psychotherapy approaches linked individual problems to personal pathology. This is not the case from a time-limited perspective, which sees the client as basically healthy with an interest in increasing personal or social changes (Budman & Gurman, 1988; Roberts & Dziegielewski, 1995).

Second, time-limited approaches may be most helpful when administered during critical periods in a person's life (Roberts & Dziegielewski, 1995). This is a basic difference from traditional psychotherapies, which are seen as necessary and ongoing over a much longer period. Third, in time-limited interventions, the goals and objectives of the formal encounter are always mutually defined by both the client and the social worker (Wells, 1994). This can be different from the traditional psychotherapies, in which goals were first recognized and defined by a therapist and later shared with the client (Budman & Gurman, 1988).

Fourth, time-limited interventions require that goals and objectives be concretely defined and extend beyond the walls of the actual formal encounter (Epstein, 1994).Often, homework or *bibliotherapeutic* (outside reading) interventions are included as a standard part of the practice strategy. In the medical setting, it is also not uncommon for medicines to be considered a part of the treatment regime. The term *biobibliotherapy* refers to the use of a medical intervention, such as medicine, outside reading materials, and brief intervention techniques.

This is different than traditional psychotherapy, in which memories of what happened outside of the session are actually the focus of intervention. In the traditional psychotherapy approaches, issues are generally addressed during the sessions only—not generally outside of them (Budman & Gurman, 1988). This is because the presence of a therapist is seen as a powerful catalyst necessary for change. The client needs this direction to make the therapeutic changes required.

The fifth difference between the time-limited approaches and the traditional psychotherapeutic methods is one of the hardest for social workers that were educated in traditional psychotherapeutic methodology to accept. Simply stated, in time-limited service provision, regardless of the model or method, little emphasis is placed on insight. Neither recognizing nor addressing "insight-oriented change" is considered essential. This is different from traditional psychotherapy, in which development of problem-oriented insight is considered necessary before any type of meaningful change can occur.

Sixth, in time-limited approaches, the therapist is seen as active and directive. Here the social worker goes beyond just active listening and assumes a consultative role with the client (Wells, 1994), which results in the development of concrete goals and problem-solving techniques. This is different from traditional psychotherapeutic approaches, in which emphasis was placed on a more nebulous "inner representation of satisfaction."

Lastly is the issue of termination. In the brief time-limited setting, termination is discussed early in the process (Wells, 1994). Many times discussion for setting a specific time frame for intervention can happen in the first session; termination issues are discussed continually throughout the intervention process. Many times in traditional psychotherapy, termination is not determined in advance; therefore, it is not considered an essential part of the process of therapy.

WHEN THERE SIMPLY IS "NO TIME" FOR THERAPEUTIC INTERVENTION

Social work professionals complain that in the health care setting there is often no time for time-limited brief interventions as discussed previously. It is important to note, however, that this practice reality should not discontinue attempts at conducting it. This lack of time does not mean that if it were available the client would not benefit.

When it is impossible, however, the health care worker still needs to set appropriate objectives (Rock, 2002). Also, it is essential to remember that any service offered today in the health care area is not generally process driven; rather, it is outcomes based. For social workers, the focus needs to be placed on the *outcome* that is desired. One easy way to remember where to put the emphasis in measuring outcome (no matter how little time is available) is to be sure to measure *what comes out at the end*, which is the actual outcome that needs to be identified.

No matter what method of intervention used, you must be prepared to collect outcomes data. Regardless of the clinical health care setting, if you routinely collect and identify the outcomes related to your service provision, you will be able to clearly justify the service that was provided. Always remember that the best place to begin in setting and determining outcomes is "where the client is." What does the client say about the problem? The easiest way to develop specific outcome measures is to use and focus on "behavioral" identifiers. First, the behavior pattern can be established regarding problem gathering, subsequent frequency, and intensity and duration. Questions that can be asked include the following:

- Can you briefly define the problem that needs to be addressed?
- What events in your life make this problem happen?
- What specific things help the problem to reoccur?
- How do others react when the problem occurs?
- Can you tell me how the problem affects your life?
- How do others directly contribute to the problem?

Once this has been completed, you can help the client to redefine and reexamine the problem behavior. In this way, the client is encouraged to focus on specific problem-related talk and strategy. All service provision needs to incorporate this "attention focus limitation." Once the problem has been defined, the social worker needs to urge the client to explore and identify solutions to solve the problem. In general, does the client believe he or she can control the problem, and if so, what types of things have been tried in the past? What new or modified strategies could be tried in the future?

PRACTICE METHODS USED IN TIME-LIMITED SERVICE PROVISION

In this section of the chapter, several methods usually linked to the provision of clinical health care social work services will be briefly summarized: interpersonal psychotherapeutic/psychodynamic approaches, strategic or solution-oriented methods, cognitive-behavioral approaches, crisis intervention, and an introduction to health, education, and wellness counseling. Regardless of what model is being discussed, measurement of behavior change will always be emphasized. In today's health care environment—for reimbursement and marketability purposes—this emphasis is considered essential. It is not uncommon to hear the new terms *managed behavioral health care* or the methods of *behavioral health care management*. These are terms social workers in health care need to cement into their practice vocabulary as they introduce and later define the methods of intervention that they will select for service provision (Franklin, 2002).

In the practice of health care social work, there is a rich history of the use of psychodynamic approaches to practice. It is believed that these models, with a focus on history and past issues, can lend credence to current problem-solving efforts. In many of these current models of practice, the unconscious is considered immediately accessible and changeable (Ecker & Hulley, 1996). Interpersonal psychotherapy (IPT) is one such approach that highlights the psychodynamic aspects of therapeutic practice. IPT is a popular approach in the medical area, where learning to identify personal problems and the concrete means to address them is considered essential. In the solution-focused therapies, a solution (or course of action) is identified, and specific attempts are made to attain it. In the cognitive-behavioral approaches, understanding the complex relationship between socialization and reinforcement as it affects thoughts and behaviors in the current environment is stressed. This results in a clear emphasis on specific goals and objectives that can measure practice effectiveness. Crisis intervention highlights the use of crisis to enhance therapeutic effect. Interpretation of this traditional framework into a single-session intervention is highlighted. The last model is newer (in application) to the field of social work; however, its importance for continued "therapeutic" survival remains clear. In this form of time-limited therapy, social workers focus on providing health counseling and education based on the principle of creating and maintaining wellness. In general, health care social workers have not traditionally viewed health counseling as a viable method of therapeutic social work practice. Refuting this assumption, and recognizing the need for its inclusion, a model for empirically incorporating it into practice is described later in this book.

INTERPERSONAL PSYCHOTHERAPY

IPT is becoming one of the most popular forms of short-term psychotherapeutic therapy used in medical setting today for reducing symptoms and dealing with interpersonal problems. Originally, IPT was formulated as a time-limited outpatient treatment for depressed clients (Rounsaville, O'Malley, Foley, & Weissman, 1988). Numerous studies supporting its effectiveness have been reviewed throughout the years (Friedlander, 1993; Klerman et al., 1994). IPT has also been used to successfully treat substance problems, such as cocaine abuse (Rounsaville, Gawin, & Kebler, 1985).

From a "biopsychosocial" perspective, this form of therapy has gained credibility and recognition among several of the related health care disciplines—particularly in medical settings that employ physicians and nurses as core members of the client care team. In this model, therapists are seen as active, supportive, and contributing factors in therapeutic gain (Fimerson, 1996; Rounsaville et al., 1988). IPT is recommended for professionals such as MDs, PhDs, MSWs, or RNs (Rounsaville et al., 1988), and has been used with individuals, couples, and families (Friedlander, 1993). It is effective in treatment of depression with special populations, such as the elderly (Miller et al., 1994; Sholomskas, Chevron, Prusoff, & Berry, 1983).

Currently, IPT is highlighted as a viable short-term acute treatment to directly address symptom removal and prevention of relapse. In addition, it is also viewed as helpful for clients who have difficulty relating to significant others, careers, social roles, or life transitions (Karasu et al., 1993). IPT treatment generally addresses a client's present situation, and focus on the "here and now" is generally assumed (Rounsaville et al, 1988). The focus on recent interpersonal events is stressed, with a clear effort to link the stressful event to the client's current mood.

In treatment, assessment that includes a diagnostic evaluation and psychiatric history is gathered. Particular attention is paid to changes in relationships proximal to the onset of symptoms. The client's interpersonal situation is highlighted. The focus of intervention is on interpersonal problem areas, such as grief, role disputes, role transitions, or deficits.

Once the goals and objectives have been established, a treatment strategy is applied. This treatment strategy is directly related to the identified interpersonal problem. For example, if there is a role conflict between a client and his or her family member regarding limitations of a particular medical condition, treatment will begin with clarifying the nature of the dispute. Discussion of the medical condition will result, with an explanation of usual limitations that may be beyond the control of the client. Limitations that are causing the greatest problem will be identified, and options to resolve the dispute are considered. If resolution does not appear possible, strategies or alternatives to replace it are contemplated. In some cases, application manuals can be acquired and followed that give specific treatment approaches regarding certain interpersonal problem areas (Rounsaville et al., 1988).

In using IPT as a treatment model, attention needs to be given to the varied and diverse types of training that each member of the interdisciplinary team has received. When using different health care professionals with differing backgrounds and education levels, the use of treatment manuals may be of benefit to highlight psychosocial areas of intervention. The use of manuals continues to gain in popularity because of the current pressure to use specific goals and objectives (Rounsaville et al., 1988).

Lastly, when using IPT, the social worker seeks to incorporate change strategy into the therapeutic environment. Generalization of what was learned in the clinical appointments is related to situations or symptoms that may arise in the future. It is important to note, however, that the therapist cannot expect to solve all the issues involved in an interpersonal conflict. Therefore, at the end of treatment, it is possible that some concerns might not be resolved. These issues will be left up to the client to continue to address.

In summary, when using this method of intervention, the role of the health care social worker is essential in helping the client to identify treatment issues of concern and to provide the groundwork for how they can be addressed. Many times, this includes helping the client to learn how to recognize the need for continued intervention. This is especially important when problems seem greater than what the client is capable of handling at the time. The social worker is influential in helping the client to feel comfortable about seeking additional treatment when needed. This help-seeking behavior is an important step in establishing and maintaining a basis for continued health and wellness.

The application of this method of practice in the different health care social work settings is variable. Because of the "medical model" and the fact that "therapeutic treatment" is planned and coordinated throughout the sessions, it may be best suited for an inpatient or therapeutic case management setting. Today, this method continues to be used primarily in inpatient and structured rehabilitative settings, which generally involve the work of a coordinated interdisciplinary team. The use of manuals and specifically outlined steps to structure the intervention process has made it a viable practice methodology for managed care and other service reimbursement considerations.

Solution-Focused Intervention Strategy

In a solution-focused intervention strategy, it is assumed that clients are basically healthy individuals. All clients possess the skills they need to address their problems and remain capable of change (De Shazer, 1985). In this approach to health care practice, specific problem solving is not the focus; rather, it is an exploration that is designed to find, identify, and consider "alternative solutions" for implementation. There does not need to be a causal link between the antecedent and the actual problem; this connection is not needed to establish a link between the problem and the solution (O'Hanlon & Weiner-Davis, 1989).

In this model of intervention, the social worker is active in helping the client to find and identify strengths in his or her current functional patterns of behavior. A dialogue of "change talk" is created rather than "problem talk" (Walter & Peller, 1992). In "change talk," the problem is viewed positively with patterns of change highlighted that appear successful for the client. Positive aspects and exceptions to the problem are explored, allowing for alternative views of the problem to develop. Once the small changes have been highlighted, the client becomes empowered to elicit larger ones (O'Hanlon & Weiner-Davis, 1989; Walter & Peller, 1992).

The key ingredients in a solution-based approach to time-limited health care practice appear to be (a) focusing on what the client sees as the problem; (b) letting the client establish what is the desired outcome; (c) beginning to analyze and develop solutions focusing on the individual strengths the client can contribute; (d) developing and implementing a plan of action; and (e) assisting with termination and follow-up issues if needed (Dziegielewski, 1997b).

Simply stated, in "solution-focused" interventions, the emphasis is placed on constructing probable solutions to a problem. The idea is that it is easier to construct solutions than it is to attempt to change problem behaviors. By not spending a great deal of time on the cause of the problem, the emphasis on the intervention is switched away from the past toward present or future survival. There is often more than one solution, and it becomes the role of the health care social worker and the client together to help construct alternative and possible scenarios of assistance. Basically, the duty of the practitioner with this type of intervention strategy is to create an interactive process that formulates solution-focused questions from the language or meaning reflected in the client's answers (De Jong, 2002). For example:

- What would have to occur to make the problem more tolerable for you?
- What specific changes would you need to achieve to make you feel more comfortable with the problem?
- What can you do to make these changes occur?
- If you woke up tomorrow and the problem was solved, what would be different?
- In what ways would it be different?

In the managed health care environment, this method continues to gain in popularity. For more specifics on how to apply this model, see De Jong (2002) and De Jong and Berg (2002). One reason for this attention rests in the kind of measurement that is highlighted as part of the intervention. Often, "scaling questions" that involve specific aspects of a client's life that can be translated into numbers and reflect progress are used. For example, if a client is depressed about his or her medical condition, a self-reported level of scaling this depression is used. A scale can be devised that reflects the way the client perceives the depression. Current mood could be rated from 0 as feeling "free" from depression, 3 or 4 as in the middle, and 7 as feeling "completely" depressed. Once completed, the identified solutions are tied to the ratings and can be tracked over time.

COGNITIVE-BEHAVIORAL INTERVENTION APPROACHES

In the early 1970s, the importance of applied behavioral analysis and the influence of reinforcement on human behavior were explored (Skinner, 1953). However, many theorists believed that behavior alone was not enough, and that human beings acted or reacted based on an analysis of the situation and the thought patterns that motivated them. Here the thought process, including how cognitive processes and structures influence individual emotions, was highlighted (Roberts & Dziegielewski, 1995). The roots of cognitive therapy are often linked to the work of Arron Beck (Beck, 1991). Beck and his colleagues postulated the use of this form of intervention in addressing numerous mental health problems across many different population groups (Beck, Emery, & Greenberg, 1985; Beck & Freeman, 1990; Beck, Rush, Shaw, & Emery, 1979; Beck, Wright, Newman, & Leise, 1993). Cognitive-behavioral therapy (CBT) is considered a number of related theories that focus on recognizing the importance of cognitions in the psychological process (Vonk & Early, 2002).

When working from a cognitive-behavioral perspective, one develops a *schema* (Beck & Weishaar, 2000; Beck & Freeman, 1990). The schema that develops is referred to as the cognitive structure that organizes experience and behavior (Beck & Freeman, 1990). Schemas involve the way individuals view certain aspects of their lives, including relationship aspects such as adequacy and the ability for others to love them. Once these schemas have been formulated as part of normal development, the individual will be exposed to critical incidents that he or she will interpret and react to (Roberts & Dziegielewski, 1995). The literature supports the fact that individuals develop different styles or patterns of information processing based on their life experiences. Therefore, CBT allows for individual interpretation (Dobson & Dozois, 2001). These schemas may influence an individual's reactions, resulting in cognitive distortion when interpreting a current situation or event (Beck et al., 1979).

Cognitive-behavioral therapies focus on the present and seek to replace distorted thoughts or unwanted behaviors with clearly established goals (Fanger, 1995; McMullin, 2000). In the cognitive behavioral approach, the setting of goals and objectives is crucial for measuring the effectiveness of the intervention (Brower & Nurius, 1993). In cognitive-behavioral intervention, goals should always be stated positively and realistically so that motivation for completion will be increased (Dziegielewski & Powers, 2000). Also, to facilitate the measurement of effectiveness, objectives must be stated in concrete and functional terms. In setting the appropriate objectives, the focus is not necessarily on process but rather on the outcome that is desired (Roberts & Dziegielewski, 1995). The adaption of cognitive and behavioral principles in the time-limited framework creates a viable climate for change.

A cognitive-behavioral approach can be helpful to the health care social worker who must deal with clients who are suffering from medical problems. Medical problems often happen quickly, and individuals may be frustrated by their inability to perform in areas in which they previously were proficient. When faced with a medical situation, clients may develop negative schemas or ways of dealing with the situation that can clearly cause conflicts in their physical, interpersonal, and social relationships. Specific techniques, such as identifying irrational beliefs and using cognitive restructuring, behavioral role rehearsal, and systematic desensitization, can help the client to adjust and accommodate to the new life status. When a client experiences a physical change in capability, the urgency to respond can be stronger than that of a psychological problem. Physical or biomedical changes can force a client into immediate lifestyle changes. Many of these behavior changes may be drastic (movement disability) or psychologically challenging (quitting smoking).

Cognitive and behavioral techniques can help the client to not only recognize the need for change, but to create a plan that will produce the behavior change needed for continued health and functioning. In the managed care setting, the basic ideas from this method of health care service delivery remain essential. Often, whether this method is used directly or not, the ideas and principles that it explicates are incorporated into service delivery. Cognitive-behavioral relationships fit ideally into the behavioral health care delivery services of today.

CRISIS INTERVENTION

Because of a growing awareness of the need for principles and techniques of time-limited clinical intervention that deal with survivors of crisis, crisis intervention has come to be accepted as a viable modality for health care social work practice. Crisis intervention addresses acute problem situations and can help the individual discover an adaptive means of coping with a particular life stage, tragic occurrence, or problem that generates a crisis situation (Laube, 2002). Today, crisis intervention is used in a wide range of primary and secondary settings and with many different individuals, families, communities, and groups. Health care settings where crisis intervention techniques are often employed include hospitals (especially hospital emergency rooms), public health agencies, hospice services, home health care agencies, and almost all other agencies that employ health care social workers. In addition, crisis intervention has been found to be successful in the health area with survivors of rape, domestic violence, mental illness, and numerous other medical or life-threatening illnesses.

A major characteristic of crisis intervention is the short duration of the therapeutic experience. Brief time-limited intervention is important because the state of crisis is by its nature self-limiting (Roberts, 1996, 2000). Time-limited intervention is intended to accomplish a set of therapeutic objectives with a sharply limited time frame, and its effectiveness appears to be indistinguishable from that of long-term treatment (Reid & Fortune, 2002). According to Parad, Hoard, and Lab (1990) and Roberts (1995), minimum therapeutic intervention during the brief crisis period can often produce a maximum therapeutic effect. These authors suggest the use of supportive social resources and focused intervention techniques to facilitate therapeutic effectiveness (Parad et al., 1990). Crisis intervention is a dynamic form of intervention that focuses on a wide range of phenomena that affect individual, family, or group equilibrium.

Generally, the term *crisis* is defined as a temporary state of upset and disequilibrium, characterized chiefly by an individual's inability to cope with a particular situation. During this crisis period, customary methods of coping and problem solving do not work. According to Gilliland and James (2001), a crisis is a perception of an event or situation as an intolerable difficulty that exceeds the resources and the coping mechanisms of the individual. This is further supported by Roberts (2000), who stated that a person in a crisis state has experienced a hazardous or threatening event; is in a vulnerable state; has failed to cope and lessen the stress through customary coping methods;

and therefore, enters into a state of disequilibrium. It is important to note, however, that any definition of the term *crisis* must remain somewhat subjective because what precipitates a crisis state in one individual might not generate such a response in another (Roberts & Dziegielewski, 1995; Roberts, 1996, 2000).

With the techniques used in crisis intervention, the crisis situation can eventually be reformulated within the context of growth. Ultimately, the client is expected to reach a healthy resolution by which he or she can emerge with greater strength, self-trust, and sense of freedom than before the crisis event occurred (Roberts, 1996, 2000). In crisis intervention, the social worker practices with the assumption that acute crisis events can be identified, controlled, and lessened. Successful resolution is therefore achieved when social workers apply crisis intervention techniques to help clients successfully resolve the emotional crisis. The health care social worker is essential in helping the client reach a healthier resolution of the problem. Most health care practitioners agree that assisting an individual in a state of crisis can provide an important opportunity for achieving client-oriented health behavior change.

Stages of Crisis Intervention

Generally, in the application of crisis intervention, a psychosocial assessment is implemented to identify the triggering or precipitating event or particular problem that started the chain of events leading to an acute crisis state. In behavioral health, emergency medicine, and surgical recovery, the application of Roberts's seven-stage crisis intervention model is imperative (Roberts, 1996, 2000). The first stage refers to assessing the nature and extent of the life-threatening illness or psychiatric emergency that is overwhelming the client at the time. The second stage involves helping the person in crisis to prioritize his or her concerns. The first and second stages of intervention often lead to what is referred to as the middle phase. In this middle phase, the crisis intervention approach should focus on encouraging the person to talk to the counselor about the event; understand and conceptualize the meaning of the event; and integrate the cognitive, affective, and behavioral components of the crisis. The third stage of intervention consists of helping the person in crisis to problem-solve and find effective coping methods.

In the middle phase of intervention, social workers are encouraged to view a psychological crisis as both danger and opportunity. Generally, when an individual is in this crisis phase, he or she is open to the future and has heightened motivation to try new coping methods. It is important to remember that the outcome of a crisis is either a change for the better or a change for the worse. Although uncomfortable, this active crisis state provides an important turning point and energy for the change effort. The client's individual personal resources, problem-solving skills, adaptability to withstand sudden intensely stressful life events, and social support networks need to be assessed.

In the final phase of intervention, whether the client is seen in person or counseled on the telephone (as a hotline caller), the client needs to be prepared to deal with recurring problems stemming from the original crisis event. For example, violent crime victims in the aftermath of gunshot wounds may experience flashbacks or intrusive thoughts about the victimization. This makes it essential to prepare the client for common reactions that may occur. Another example is the person who has recently been diagnosed as HIV positive, who may receive mixed messages from those she or he encounters. In the final session, it would be useful to help the client decide on the best person to turn to for support in dealing with delayed or post-traumatic reactions if they should develop, even if at the present time they are not being experienced. The working through of the actual traumatic event and integrating of the self are considered the primary goals in the middle phase. In the final phase of intervention, emphasis is placed on the ability of an individual to adapt or restore himself or herself to a balanced state—preferably one that exhibits restored or enhanced levels of confidence and coping.

In the application of crisis intervention, it is important to note that psychological trauma can be understood as an "affliction of the powerless" (Herman, 1992, p. 33). Threat to life and bodily integrity overwhelms normal adaptive capabilities, producing extensive symptomatology. Adopting a pathological view of symptomatology is not helpful; it is more beneficial when clients can comprehend their symptoms as signs of strength. Symptoms that are understood as coping techniques developed by the survivor to adapt to a toxic environment can enhance self-esteem (Roberts & Dziegielewski, 1995).

APPLICATIONS: ROBERTS' SEVEN-STAGE CRISIS INTERVENTION MODEL

Effective intervention with survivors of trauma precipitated by a crisis requires a careful assessment of individual, family, and environmental factors. A crisis by definition is short term and overwhelming. According to Roberts (2000), a crisis is an emotionally distressing change. The crisis can cause a disruption of an individual's normal and stable state in which the usual methods of coping and problem solving do not work.

Roberts (1995, 2000) describes seven stages of working through a crisis: (a) assessing lethality and safety needs; (b) establishing rapport and communication; (c) identifying the major problems; (d) dealing with feelings and providing support; (e) exploring possible alternatives; (f) formulating an action plan; and (g) providing follow-up. Roberts' seven-stage model applies to a broad range of crises addressed by health care providers and has been recommended as the framework for time-limited cognitive treatment throughout the book.

To enhance the application of this crisis intervention the following assumptions are made: (a) all strategy will follow a "here-and-now" orientation; (b) the intervention period will be time limited (typically 6 to 12 sessions); (c) the adult survivor's behavior is viewed as an understandable (rather than a pathological) reaction to stress; (d) the mental health worker will assume an active and directive role; and (e) the intervention strategy will strive to increase the survivor's remobilization and return to the previous level of functioning (Resnick & Dziegielewski, 1996).

STAGE 1
Assessing Lethality
There are many hazardous events that can initiate a traumatic response. Listed subsequently are some of the hazardous events or circumstances that can be linked to the recognition or reliving of traumatic events. These events can trigger anxious responses from clients so that they seek help, even if the traumatic event is not immediately identified as the crisis issue. They include (a) growing public awareness of the prevalence of the traumatic event or similar

traumatic events; (b) the acknowledgment by a loved one or some-one that the client respects that he or she has also been a victim; (c) a seemingly unrelated act of violence being committed to the client or someone he or she loves, such as rape or sexual assault; (d) the changing of family or relationship support issues; and (e) the sights, sounds, or smells that trigger events from the client's past (these can be highly specific to individuals and the trauma experienced).

With the number of suicides on the rise, intervention requires careful assessment of suicidal ideation and the potential for initial and subsequent hospitalization or medication. Questions to elicit pervasive symptomatology should be asked (e.g., depression, suicid-al ideation, anxiety, eating disorders, somatic complaints, sleep dis-orders, sexual dysfunction, instances of promiscuity, substance abuse, psychological numbing, self-mutilation, flashbacks, and panic attacks). Based on the age and the circumstances of the trauma experienced, the client's living situation should be assessed to ensure that the client is not still in danger and that an adequate support system does exist. Several structured and goal oriented sessions may be needed to help the client move past the traumatic event. Generating an understanding that what happened in regard to the traumatic event may have been beyond his or her control.

In these initial sessions of therapy (sessions 1–3) the goal of the therapeutic intervention is recognizing the hazardous event and ac-knowledging what has actually happened. For some reason (based on the triggering catalyst) the survivor of trauma is currently being subjected to periods of stress that disturb his or her sense of equilib-rium. (It is assumed that the individual wants to maintain homeo-static balance and that physically and emotionally the body will seek to regain equilibrium.) As stated earlier, the survivor may not present with the actual crisis event, and the mental health counse-lor may have to help the survivor get to the root of the problem (i.e., the real reason for the visit). During these initial sessions the survi-vor becomes aware and acknowledges the fact that the trauma has occurred; and once this happens, the survivor enters into a vulner-able state. The impact of this event disturbs the survivor, and tradi-tional problem solving and coping methods are attempted. When these do not work, tension and anxiety continue to rise, and the individual becomes unable to function effectively. In the initial sessions the assessment of both past and present coping behaviors is important; however, the focus of intervention clearly must remain in the "here and now." The mental health worker must attempt to stay away from past issues or unresolved issues unless they relate directly to the handling of the traumatic event.

STAGE 2
Establishing Rapport and Communication
Many times, survivors of trauma may feel as though family and friends have abandoned them, or that they are being punished for something they did or did not do. These unrealistic interpretations may result in feelings of overwhelming guilt. It is possible that the capacity for trust has been damaged, and this may be reflected in negative self-image and poor self-esteem. A low self-image and poor self-esteem may increase the individual's fear of further victimization. Many times, survivors of trauma question their own vulnerability and know that revictimization remains a possibility. This makes the role of the counselor in establishing rapport with the client essential.

Whenever possible, the mental health professional should progress slowly and try to let the survivor set the pace of treatment. Let the client lead, because he or she may have a history of being coerced; and forcing confrontation on issues may not be helpful. Allowing the client to set the pace creates a trusting atmosphere, which gives the message "the event has ended, you have survived and you will not be hurt here." Survivors often need to be reminded that their symptoms are a healthy response to an unhealthy environment (Resnick & Dziegielewski, 1996). They need to recognize that they have survived heinous circumstances and continue to live and cope. Trauma victims may require a positive future orientation, with an understanding that they can overcome current problems and arrive at a happy, satisfactory tomorrow (Dolan, 1991). Hope that change can occur is crucial to the survivor's well being.

Perhaps more than anything else, throughout each of the sessions, these clients need unconditional support, positive regard, and concern. These factors are especially crucial to the working relationship because a history of lack of support, "blaming," and breach of loyalty are common. The therapeutic relationship is seen as a vehicle for continued growth, development of coping skills, and the ability to move beyond the abuse (Briere, 1992).

STAGE 3
Identifying the Major Problems
Once the major problems relevant to the particular event are identified and addressed, support should still be given. Group participation has been effective, as well as the use of journal writing, relaxation techniques, physical exercise, and development of an understanding that the victim needs to be good to himself or herself.

In these next few sessions (sessions 3–6) the mental health worker needs to assume an active role. First the major problems to be dealt with and addressed must be identified. The mental health worker must study how they have affected the survivor's behavior. Education in regard to the effects and consequences of this type of trauma will be discussed. Here the precipitating factor, especially if the event was in the past, must be clearly identified. Complete acknowledgment of the event can push the person into a state of active crisis marked by disequilibrium, disorganization, and immobility (e.g., the last straw). Once the survivor enters full acknowledgment, new energy for problem solving will be generated. This challenge stimulates a moderate degree of anxiety, plus a kindling of hope and expectation. This actual state of disequilibrium can last four to eight weekly sessions or until some type of adaptive or maladaptive solution is found.

STAGE 4
Dealing with Feelings and Providing Support
The energy generated from the survivor's personal feelings, experiences, and perceptions steers the therapeutic process (Vonk & Early, 2002). It is critical that the social workers demonstrate empathy and an anchored understanding of the survivor's world. These symptoms are seen as functional, and as a means of avoiding abuse and pain. Even severe symptoms such as dissociative reactions should be viewed as a constructive method of removing oneself from a harmful situation and exploring alternative coping mechanisms. Survivors' experiences should be normalized so that they can recognize that they are not at fault. Reframing symptoms is a coping technique that can be helpful. In this stage (sessions 6–8), the

survivor begins to reintegrate and gradually becomes ready to reach a new state of equilibrium. Each particular crisis situation (i.e., type and duration of incest, rape, etc.) may follow a sequence of stages, which can generally be predicted and mapped out. One positive result from generating the crisis state in stage three is that in treatment, after reaching active crisis, survivors seem particularly amenable to help.

Once the crisis situation has been obtained, distorted ideas and perceptions regarding what has happened need to be corrected and information updated so that the client can better understand what he or she has experienced. Victims eventually need to confront their pain and anger so that they can develop better strategies for coping. Increased awareness helps the survivor to face and experience contradicting emotions (anger/love, fear/rage, dampening emotion/intensifying emotion) without the conditioned response of escape (Briere, 1992). Throughout this process, there must be recognition of the client's continued courage in facing and dealing with these issues.

STAGE 5
Exploring Possible Alternatives
Moving forward requires traveling through a mourning process (generally in sessions 8-10). Sadness and grief at the loss need to be experienced. Grief expressions surrounding betrayal and lack of protection permit the victim to open to an entire spectrum of feelings that have been numbed. Now accepting, letting go, and making peace with the past begins.

STAGE 6
Formulating an Action Plan
Here the mental health worker must be active in helping the survivor to establish how the goals of the therapeutic intervention will be completed. Practice, modeling, and other techniques, such as behavioral rehearsal, role play, the process of writing down of one's feeling, and an action plan, become essential in addressing intervention planning. The survivor has come to the realization that he or she is not at fault or to blame. The doubt and shame of what his or her role was and what part he or she played become more clear and self-fault less pronounced. The survivor begins to acknowledge that he or she did not have the power to help himself or herself, or to

change things. Oftentimes, however, these realizations are coupled with anger at the helplessness a client feels to control what has happened to him or her. The role of the mental health professional becomes essential here in helping the client to look at the long-range consequences of acting on his or her anger, and in planning an appropriate course of action. The main goal of these last few sessions (sessions 10–12) is to help the individual reintegrate the information learned and process it into a homeostatic balance that allows him or her to function adequately once again. Referrals for additional therapy should be considered and discussed at this time (i.e., additional individual therapy, group therapy, couples therapy, family therapy).

STAGE 7
Providing Follow-up Measures
This area is important for intervention in general, but one that is almost always forgotten. In the successful therapeutic exchange significant changes have been made for the survivor in regard to his or her previous level of functioning and coping. Measures to determine whether these results have remained consistent are essential. Often follow-up can be as simple as a telephone call to discuss how things are going. Follow-up within one month of termination of the sessions is important.

Other measures of follow-up are available but require more advanced planning. A pretest/posttest design can be added to the design by simply using a standardized scale at the beginning of treatment and at the end. Scales to measure depression, trauma, and so on are readily available. See Corcoran and Fischer (2000) or Hudson (1992) for potential measurement scales that can be used in the behavioral sciences.

Finally, it is important to realize that at follow-up many survivors may realize that they want additional therapeutic help. After they have adapted to the crisis and have learned to function and cope, they may find that they want more. After all, returning the survivor to a previous state of equilibrium is the primary purpose for the application of this brief crisis intervention therapy. If this happens, the health worker should be prepared to help the client become aware of the options for continued therapy and emotional growth by giving the appropriate referrals. Referrals for group therapy with

> other survivors of similar trauma, individual growth-directed thera-
> py, couples therapy that is to include a significant other, or family
> therapy should be considered.

In the health care setting, crisis intervention can be severely limited by resources and agency role and function. Often the health care social worker simply does not have the time to follow through with the formal intervention described here. In these cases, recognition of the problem, assessment of immediate danger, and referral with subsequent follow-up is most important. Because many individuals present in hospital emergency rooms as well as before surgery in acute crisis, it is important when feasible for social workers to apply Roberts's seven-stage sequential practice model of crisis intervention. Practice models can serve as a guideline to help the health care social worker act quickly and confidently. Health care social workers may be the first helping professional these individuals meet that is willing to spend time with them. Many times, simply normalizing or giving clients permission to feel as they do is critical to starting the return to healthy homeostatic balance.

Assessing client danger to self or others is also essential. Individuals in crisis are experiencing feelings and emotions that they are not able to resolve by the usual methods of coping. This means that "unusual" or "permanent" solutions may be selected to handle what could be viewed as a temporary setback. The role of the health care social worker is essential in assessing of the situation and helping to provide service to combat the stress, whether that be done directly through intervention or indirectly through planned and actively assisted referral.

INTRODUCTION TO HEALTH AND WELLNESS EDUCATION AND COUNSELING

Through the document *Healthy People 2000* (U. S. DHHS, 1990), health promotion has been incorporated into the nation's health delivery agenda. However, despite the emphasis placed in this area, health promotion remains fragmented. Often, its implementation is characterized by "poor communication between the many disciplines contributing to this area and little interaction between the research and the practitioner communities" (O'Donnell, 1994, p. ix).

Many times in the medical field, health care social workers are called on to participate in a type of counseling that is not considered traditional. This type of counseling can include many different techniques; however, at a minimum, it must be time limited, must be focused on goal sand objectives and must assist clients to address present and future health and wellness issues. More and more health care social workers are being called on to provide this type of "health counseling" or "health education," yet rarely is it openly discussed and accepted as a method of providing social work practice.

In today's current health care environment, many believe that counseling to maintain health and wellness is essential. Openly acknowledging this method as part of health care social work practice can assist social workers in identifying with this commonly provided service. Social workers are in a unique position to participate in health counseling and prevention services. The overall practice of social work is health oriented, both conceptually and philosophically. The social worker can serve as a link between the person and a system of support, and can assist in maintaining health, detecting illness early, or preventing deterioration of existing problems (Skidmore, Thackeray, & Farley, 1997). The chapter in this book entitled "New Horizons: Health and Wellness Counseling" is dedicated to the introduction and specific application of this form of intervention.

CHAPTER SUMMARY AND FUTURE DIRECTIONS

The infected populations that suffer from acquired immunodeficiency syndrome (AIDS) are shifting, and the number of infections is continuing to grow (Centers for Disease Control, 1998; Giddens, Ka'opua & Tomaszewski, 2002). According to Armas (2002), reporting for the Associated Press, the latest U.S. Census Bureau information for 2001 stated that about 1.4 million people were without health insurance last year as a result of increased unemployment as businesses were forced to scale back benefits. In addition, 41 million people, or 14.6 % of U.S. residents, lacked health coverage for all of 2001. These are just some of the problems that health care social workers must face. Thus it is no surprise that the recognition and provision of counseling services have declined. If general health benefits are being cut at such drastic rates, counseling services will clearly be pushed aside, since they are not considered a necessary part of the health care benefit package. To complicate this situation further, too many social workers in the field are quick to say we do not do counseling anymore. With the desperate need for this type of intervention in the health care setting, commentaries such as this should be avoided. Health care social workers should not allow administrative pressure to provide only reimbursable services in their practice strategy. The bottom line is that clients need and continue to want supportive counseling in the health care setting. It is true that as the number of people suffering from anxiety and depressive disorders, self-destructive acts, and life-threatening illnesses has steadily risen, so has the need for counselors, social workers, and psychologists (Dziegielewski, 2002). To receive and continue to qualify for reimbursement for such services, social workers need to remain aware and active in the social and political climate that surrounds the health care practice arena.

Generally, social and political changes do not happen quickly. In the meantime, health care social workers are encouraged to engage in time-limited methods. These time-limited methods of practice offer promise for meeting urgent biopsychosocial and crisis-related needs of clients in distress. Regardless of what intervention method is selected, an building strength and helping the client to identify his or her own resources are important. All methods of practice need to help clients reframe their thinking patterns and use their strengths.

Because of the turbulence and insecurity in our current health care environment, clients need the help and assistance that can only be given by competent professional social workers. Consequently, professional social workers need to be knowledgeable of the methods, tools, and techniques that are currently being used to provide this service.

For health care social workers, clearly stated objectives are most important. It is these objectives and the outcome result (not the practice method that is used) that are considered the "bread and butter" in the billing process. Stated simply, the goal is the overall task that the health care social worker wants to establish; however, it is the clearly stated outcome-based concrete objective that will help to ensure reimbursement and facilitate the measurement of service effectiveness. Never forget that the resultant objective must clearly be related to the outcome measure. This means that regardless of what time-limited method you use in the process, it will only be considered important to funding sources when it brings about changes in outcome (i.e., the end result).

REFERENCES

Alperin, R. M. (1994). Managed care versus psychoanalytic psychotherapy: Conflicting ideologies. *Clinical Social Work Journal, 22,* 137–148.

Araoz, D. L., & Carrese, M. A. (1996). *Solution-oriented brief therapy for adjustment disorders: A guide for providers under managed care.* New York: Brunner/Manzel.

Armas, G. C. (September 30, 2002). More people lose health insurance: The Census Bureau blamed the trend on the recession. *Orlando Sentinel,* Monday, Associated Press, A9.

Beck, A. T. (1991). Cognitive therapy: A 30-year retrospective. *American Psychologist, 46,* 368–375.

Beck, A. T., & Emery, G., with Greenberg, R. L. (1985). *Anxiety disorders and phobias: A cognitive perspective.* New York: Basic Books.

Beck, A. T., & Freeman, A. (1990). *Cognitive therapy of personality disorders.* New York: Guilford Press.

Beck, A. T., Rush, A. J., Shaw, B. F., & Emery, G. (1979). *Cognitive therapy of depression.* New York: Guilford Press.

Beck, A. T., & Weishaar, M. E. (2000). Cognitive therapy. In R. J. Corisini & D. Wedding (Eds.), *Current psychotherapies* (6th ed., pp. 241-272). Itasca, IL: F.E. Peacock.

Beck, A. T., Wright, F. D., Newman, C. F., & Leise, B. S. (1993). *Cognitive therapy of substance abuse.* New York: Guilford Press.

Bloom, B. L. (1992). *Planned short-term psychotherapy: A clinical handbook.* Boston: Allyn & Bacon.

Briere, J. N. (1992). *Child abuse trauma: Theory and treatment of the lasting effects.* Newbury Park, CA: Sage.

Bristo, D. P., & Herrick, C. A. (2002). Emergency department case management: The dyad team of the nurse case manager and social worker. *Lippincott's Case Management, 7,* 121-128.

Brower, A. M., & Nurius, P. S. (1993). *Social cognitions and individual change: Current theory and counseling guidelines.* Newbury Park, CA: Sage.

Budman, S., & Gurman, A. (1988). *Theory and practice of brief therapy.* New York: Guilford Press.

Burner, S. T., Waldo, D. R., & McKusick, D. R. (1992). National health expenditure projections through 2030. *Health Care Financing Review, 14,* 1–29.

Centers for Disease Control. (1998). *Trends in HIV and AIDS epidemic.* Atlanta, GA: Author.

Chambliss, C. H. (2000). Psychotherapy and managed care. New York: Allyn & Bacon

Corcoran, K., & Fischer, J. (2000). *Measures for clinical practice* (3rd ed.). New York: Free Press.

Cormier, W. H., & Cormier, L. S. (1991). *Interviewing strategies for helpers* (3rd ed.). Pacific Grove, CA: Brooks Cole.

Cowles, L. A., & Lefcowitz, M. J. (1992). Interdisciplinary expectations of medical social workers in the hospital setting. *Health and Social Work, 17,* 58–65.

De Jong, P. (2002). Solution-focused therapy. In A. R. Roberts & G. J. Greene (Eds.), *Social workers' desk reference* (pp. 112-116). New York: Oxford University Press.

De Jong, P., & Berg, I. K. (2002). *Interviewing for solutions* (2nd ed.). Pacific Grove, CA: Brooks Cole.

De Shazer, S. (1985). *Keys to solution in brief therapy.* New York: W. W. Norton & Co.

Dobson, K. S., & Dozoi, D. J. (2001). Historical and philosophical bases of the cognitive behavioral therapies. In K. S. Dobson (Ed)., *Handbook of cognitive behavioral therapies* (2nd ed., pp. 3-39). New York: Guilford Press.

Dolan, Y. M. (1991). *Resolving sexual abuse.* New York: Norton.

Dziegielewski, S. F. (1996). Managed care principles: The need for social work in the health care environment. *Crisis Intervention and Time-Limited Treatment, 3,* 97–110.

Dziegielewski, S. F. (1997a). Should clinical social workers seek psychotropic medication prescription privileges?: Yes. In B. A. Thyer (Ed.), *Controversial issues in social work practice* (pp. 152–165). Boston: Allyn & Bacon.

Dziegielewski, S. F. (1997b). Time limited brief therapy: The state of practice. *Crisis Intervention and Time Limited Treatment, 3,* 217–218.

Dziegielewski, S. F. (2002). *DSM-IV-TR™ in action.* New York: Wiley.

Dziegielewski, S. F., & Leon, A. M. (2001). *Psychopharmacology and social work practice.* New York: Springer.

Dziegielewski, S. F., & Leon, A. M. (2001). Time-limited case recording: Effective documentation in a changing environment. *Journal of Brief Therapy, 1*(1), 51–66.

Dziegielewski, S. F., & Powers, G. T. (2000). Procedures for evaluating time-limited crisis intervention. In A. R. Roberts (Ed.), *Crisis intervention handbook (2nd ed.).* New York: Oxford University.

Dziegielewski, S. F., Shields, J., & Thyer, B. A. (1998). Short-term treatment: Models and methods. In J. Williams & K. Ell (Eds.), *Advances in mental health research: Implications for practice.* Washington, DC: NASW Press.

Ecker, B., & Hulley, L. (1996). *Depth-oriented brief therapy: How to be brief when you were trained to be deep—and vice versa.* San Francisco: Jossey-Bass.

Epstein, L. (1994). Brief task-centered practice. In R. Edwards (Ed.), *Encyclopedia of social work: 19th edition* (pp. 313-323). Washington, DC: NASW Press.

Fanger, M. T. (1995). Brief therapies. In R. Edwards (Ed.), *Encyclopedia of social work* (19th ed., pp. 323-334). Washington, DC: NASW Press.

Fiesta, J. (1995). Managed care: Whose liability? *Nursing Management, 26,* 31–32.

Fimerson, S. S. (1996). Individual therapy. In V. B. Carson & E. N. Nolan (Eds.), *Mental health nursing: The nurse patient journey* (pp. 367–384). Philadelphia: Saunders.

Franklin, C. (2002). Developing effective practice competencies in managed behavioral health care. In A. R. Roberts & G. J. Greene (Eds.), *Social workers' desk reference* (pp. 3-10). New York: Oxford University.

Friedlander, M. L. (1993). Does complementarity promote or hinder client change in brief therapy? A review of the evidence from two theoretical perspectives. *Counseling Psychologist, 21,* 457–486.

Giddens, B., Ka'opua, L. S., & Tomaszewski, E. P. (2002). HIV/AIDS case management. In A. R. Roberts & G. J. Greene (Eds.), *Social workers' desk reference* (pp. 506-510). New York: Oxford University Press.

Gilliland, B., & James, R. (2001). *Crisis intervention strategies.* Pacific Grove, CA: Brooks/ Cole.

Gross, R., Rabinowitz, J., Feldman, D., & Boerma, W. (1996). Primary health care physicians' treatment of psychosocial problems: Implications for social work. *Health and Social Work, 21,* 89–94.

Heeschen, S. J. (2000). Making the most of quality indicator information. *Geriatric Nursing, 21(4),* 206-209.

Herman, J. L. (1992). *Trauma and recovery.* New York: Basic Books.

Holliman, D., Dziegielewski, S. F., & Datta, P. (2001). Discharge planning and social work practice. *Journal of Health Care Social Work. 32(3),* 1-19.

Holliman, D., Dziegielewski, S. F., & Teare, R. (in press). Differences and similarities between social work and nurse discharge planners. *Health and Social Work.*

Hudson, W. (1992). *The WALMYR Assessment scales scoring manual.* Tempe, AZ: WALMYR Publishing.

Johnson, R. S., & Berger, C. S. (1990). The challenge of change: Enhancing social work services at a time of cutback. *Health and Social Work, 15,* 181–190.

Karasu, T. B., Docherty, J. P., Gelenberg, A., Kuper, D. J., Merriam, A. E., & Shadoan, R. (1993). Practice guidelines for major depressive disorder in adults. *American Journal of Psychiatry, 150(Suppl),* 1–26.

Klerman, G. L., Weissman, M. M., Markowitz, J. C., Glick, I., Wilner, P. J., Mason, B., & Shear, M. K. (1994). Medication in psychotherapy. In A. E. Bergin & S. B. Garfield (Eds.), *Handbook of psychotherapy and behavior change* (4th ed., pp. 734–782). New York: Wiley.

Laube, J. (2002). Crisis groups. In A. R. Roberts & G. J. Greene (Eds), *Social workers' desk reference* (pp. 428-432). New York: Oxford University.

Ligon, J. (2002). Fundamentals of brief treatment. In A. R. Roberts & G. J. Greene (Eds.) *Social workers' desk reference* (pp. 96-100). New York: Oxford University.

Mancoske, R., Standifer, D., & Cauley, C. (1994). The effectiveness of brief counseling services for battered women. *Research on Social Work Practice, 4*, 53–63.

McMullin, R. E. (2000). *The new handbook of cognitive therapy techniques.* New York: W. W. Norton.

Meckler, L. (1996, September 3). Managed care brings decrease in doctor's pay. *Tuscaloosa News*, pp. 1A, 4A.

Miller, M. D., Frank, E., Cornes, C., Imber, S., Anderson, B., Ehrenpreis, L., Malloy, J., Silberman, R., Wolfson, L., Zaltman, J., & Reynolds, C. F. (1994). Applying interpersonal psychotherapy to bereavement-related depression following loss of a spouse in late life. *Journal of Psychotherapy Practice and Research, 3*, 149–162.

O'Donnell, M. P. (1994). Preface. In M. P. O'Donnell & J. S. Harris (Eds.), *Health promotion in the work place* (pp. ix–xvi). Albany, NY: Delmar.

O'Hanlon, W. H., & Weiner-Davis, M. (1989). *In search of solutions: A new direction in psychotherapy.* New York: Norton.

Parad, H., Hoard, L., Lab, J., et al. (1990). *Crisis intervention: The practitioner's source book for brief therapy.* Milwaukee, WI: Family Service America.

Reid, W. J., & Fortune, A. E. (2002). The task-centered model. In A. R. Roberts & G. J. Greene (Eds.), *Social workers' desk reference* (pp. 101-104). New York: Oxford University Press.

Resnick, C., & Dziegielewski, S. F. (1996). The relationship between therapeutic termination and job satisfaction among medical social workers. *Social Work in Health Care, 23*, 17–35.

Roberts, A. R. (1995). *Crisis intervention and time-limited cognitive treatment* (pp. 3–27). Thousand Oaks, CA: Sage.

Roberts, A. R. (1996). Epidemiology and definitions of acute crisis in American society. In A. R. Roberts (Ed.), *Crisis management and brief treatment: Theory, technique, and applications* (pp. 16–34). Chicago: Nelson Hall.

Roberts, A. R. (2000). *Crisis intervention handbook: Assessment, treatment and research* (2nd ed.). New York: Oxford University Press.

Roberts, A. R., & Dziegielewski, S. F. (1995). Foundation skills and applications of crisis intervention and cognitive therapy. In A. R. Roberts (Ed.), *Crisis intervention and time-limited cognitive treatment* (pp. 3–27). Thousand Oaks, CA: Sage.

Rock, B. D. (2002). Social work in health care in the 21st century: The biopsychosocial model. In A. R. Roberts & G. J. Greene (Eds.), *Social workers' desk reference* (pp. 10-15). New York: Oxford University Press.

Ross, J. (1993). Redefining hospital social work: An embattled professional domain [Editorial]. *Health and Social Work, 18*, 243–247.

Rounsaville, B. J., Gawin, F., & Kebler, H. (1985). Interpersonal psychotherapy adapted for ambulatory cocaine abusers. *American Journal of Drug and Alcohol Abuse, 11*, 171–191.

Rounsaville, B. J., O'Malley, S., Foley, S., & Weissman, M. M. (1988). Role of manual-guided training in the conduct and efficacy of interpersonal psychotherapy for depression. *Journal of Consulting and Clinical Psychology, 56,* 681–688.

Schram, B., & Mandell, B. R. (1997). *Human services: Policy and practice* (3rd ed.). Boston: Allyn & Bacon.

Sholomskas, A. J., Chevron, E. S., Prusoff, B. A., & Berry, C. (1983). Short-term interpersonal therapy (IPT) with the depressed elderly: Case reports and discussion. *American Journal of Psychotherapy, 38,* 552–566.

Simon, E. P., Showers, N., Blumenfield, S., Holden, G., & Wu, X. (1995). Delivery of home care services after discharge: What really happens. *Health and Social Work, 20,* 6–14.

Skidmore, R. A., Thackeray, M. G., & Farley, O. W. (1997). *Introduction to social work* (7th ed.). Boston: Allyn & Bacon.

Skinner, B. F. (1953). *Science and human behavior.* New York: MacMillian.

U.S. Department of Health and Human Services. (1990). *Healthy people 2000: National health promotion disease and prevention objectives.* DHHS Publication No. (PHS). 91-50212. Washington, DC: U.S.Government Printing Office.

Vonk, M. E., & Early, T. J. (2002). Cognitive-behavioral therapy. In A. R. Roberts & G. J. Greene (Eds.), *Social workers' desk reference* (pp. 116-120). New York: Oxford University Press.

Walter, J. L., & Peller, J. E. (1992). *Becoming solution-focused in brief therapy.* New York: Brunner/Mazel.

Walter, J. L., & Peller, J. E. (2000). *Recreating brief therapy: Preferences and possibilities.* New York: Norton.

Wells, R. A. (1994). *Planned short-term treatment* (2nd ed.). New York: Free Press.

Wells, R. A., & Phelps, P. A. (1990). The brief psychotherapies: A selective overview. In R. A. Wells & V. J. Giannetti (Eds.), *Handbook of the brief psychotherapies* (pp. 3–26). New York: Plenum.

GLOSSARY

Bibliotherapeutic intervention: The assignment of reading materials to the client, generally completed as therapeutic "homework" to expand the formal limits of the counseling session.

Biobibliotherapy: The client is usually prescribed medication to supplement treatment, and is also given reading materials to be completed as therapeutic "homework" to expand the formal limits of the counseling session.

Capitation: Under this provision, providers are paid a certain amount to provide a fixed amount of care for a certain period.

Cognitive-behavioral therapy: This method of practice uses a combination of selected techniques incorporating the theories of behaviorism, social learning theory, and cognition theories to understand and address a client's behavior.

Crisis: Generally, the term *crisis* is defined as a temporary state of upset and disequilibrium that is characterized by an individual's inability to cope with a particular situation.

Crisis intervention: A therapeutic practice used to help clients in crisis regain a sense of healthy equilibrium.

Fee for service: Defined simply, it is the amount of money paid for the service that is delivered.

Goal: A statement of the overall process a client wants to achieve.

Intermittent therapy: A type of intervention strategyin which every session is considered complete and treated as if it is the only session that may occur. Acknowledgment of this format allows for planned intervention and closure with each therapeutic encounter.

Interpersonal therapy: A form of time-limited treatment used in the medical setting. Generally, an assessment is made that includes a diagnostic evaluation and psychiatric history. The focus of treatment is on interpersonal problem areas, such as grief, role disputes, role transitions, or deficits.

Managed behavioral health care: In this type of health care coverage, services are based, determined, and/or assessed on the basis of clear and specific outcome criteria.

Objectives: Specific statements that tell specifically how the goal will be accomplished.

Outcomes: These are the consequences of a situation; simply stated, attention is focused on what comes out at the end of the intervention process.

Psychotherapy: A form of therapy that involves understanding the "inner processes" of the individual regarding his or her personal situation.

Schema: This is considered a pattern of thinking that is referred to as the cognitive structure that organizes an individual's experience and behavior.

Summarization: The process of describing what has occurred in a situation, highlighting the goals and objectives that have been met in the session. This process should always be completed at the beginning and end of every time-limited session.

QUESTIONS FOR FURTHER STUDY

1. What can health care social workers do to stress the value of the counseling services they provide?
2. What can social workers do to increase the reimbursement potential of the counseling services they provide?
3. Which form of time-limited service provision seems most appropriate to use in the hospital setting and why?
4. Which form(s) of counseling seem to be most beneficial in the public health setting and why?
5. What things can social workers do to support the inclusion of counseling as part of the services provided in the managed care system?

WEBSITES

The Centers for Disease Control and Prevention (CDC)
Provides health news, publications, software, data, and statistics.
http://www.cdc.gov/

Health Care Financing Administration
HCFA provides health insurance for 74 million Americans and
    regulates all laboratory testing (except research) in the U.S.
http://www.hcfa.gov/

Psychotherapy Finances and Managed Care Strategies
News related to financing for psychotherapy and managed care.
http://www.199.190.86.8/

SOSIG
British site for the Social Work in Health Care journal.
http://www.sosig.ac.uk/social_welfare/social_work/

Yahoo Social Science/Social Work
A website for social workers with links, articles, and forums.
http://www.dir.yahoo.com/Social_Science/Social_Work

CHAPTER 7

Documentation and Record Keeping in the Health Care Setting

In this era of intermittent and time-limited therapeutic encounters, human service workers are expected to have correct and complete client documentation. Client records must clearly reflect assessment and treatment progress while demonstrating worker efficiency, effectiveness, and accountability. Without organized and complete client records, helping professionals cannot accurately document the services that they provide (Kagle, 2002). Furthermore, inaccurate records may result in clients losing their insurance coverage from third party payers.

Kagle (1993) stated that one of the major problems for social workers is the lack of training in documentation; this lack of training can make it difficult for them to meet record-keeping requirements for a growing number of clients. Furthermore, Kagle (2002) believes that many social workers simply do not recognize the actual purpose that a record serves. Therefore, when a trial-and-error approach is used to document services, the worker may be uncertain about the nature, duration, and outcomes of the therapeutic encounter. Nevertheless, many workers believe that investing time in ensuring that they have complete and accurate records results in less quality time to spend with clients. In fact, many human service workers feel that a minimal amount of time should be allowed for documentation because they do not consider this activity a part of the therapeutic process (Moreland & Racke, 1991; Rock & Congress, 1999; Wilson, 1980). This results in a strong desire by many human service workers to postpone or defer documentation to a later time. In addition, when a human service worker is not properly trained about the best way to document client progress and services, anxiety can be expected to rise.

Since there are no national policies regarding documentation guidelines for many mental health conditions, professionals in the field often struggle with what to do (APA Online, 2001). Whether a human services worker is involved in indirect practice (focusing on policy, planning, administration, and community organization) or direct practice (involving assessment, intervention, prevention, and alleviation of negative situations) with individuals, couples, families, or groups, the development of good documentation skills remains essential for quality intervention. Limited resources and specific program guidelines make it increasingly imperative that human services professionals be responsive to growing expectations of accountability and improved program effectiveness. Furthermore, most human service agencies expect their new employees to know how to document client progress and how to identify what information should be included in the files (Gelman, Pollack, & Weiner, 1999; Moreland & Racke, 1991; Wilson, 1980). Most human service professionals agree that good record keeping is essential for effective practice. According to Dust (1996), "with accurate records, a clinician can examine the past and prepare for the future" (p. 50).

RECORD KEEPING AND JUSTIFICATION OF SERVICE

Health care social workers need to be knowledgeable of the different types of professional record keeping that are completed in the health care area. Professional record keeping can serve many purposes. First, record keeping can help health care social workers maintain the basic written information that is needed in the practice environment. To qualify for reimbursement, most third-party payers require that counselors record specific assessment, goals, objectives, and the actual treatment process that will be employed in the helping environment (Okum, 1997; Kagle, 2002). In health care, the social worker's records must be brief and concise (Dziegielewski, 2002). Furthermore, in this society where litigation is common, adequate documentation must reflect the legal and ethical concerns in the helping relationship (Dziegielewski & Leon, 2001b). It is important for the health care social worker to always remember that "some day the health care social worker will die but not the medical record you charted in—it will live on." What is meant by this is simple; social workers may discharge a client from service or go to work at another agency, but their responsibility to the client never ends. A written synopsis that describes the treatment a client receives will always create an essential piece of information if a situation arises where the social worker or medical record is ever subpoenaed into court.

A second reason for maintaining accurate records in the health care environment is related to the concept of evidence-based practice. In evidence-based practice, maintaining objective and impartial records can assist in understanding, establishing, and justifying the intervention process that has been initiated. Record keeping in the evidence-based practice setting can be used for numerous purposes, including providing information on the rate of progress; providing information on nonprogress and retrogression; molding or shaping the intervention program; highlighting if changes in the current program are needed; determining whether the program is moving too quickly; determining whether the client can complete the tasks and behavioral requirements assigned; determining whether it is essential to move back to an earlier stage of intervention; evaluating factors that are impeding progress; establishing the extent to which problems have been stabilized; determining whether the terminal goal has been reached; assessing the efficiency and effectiveness of the service delivered (Fischer, 1978); and, lastly, justifying that the services provided were delivered in the most cost-effective way possible (Dziegielewski & Leon, 2001b).

Lastly, the importance of the written record in today's health care practice environment cannot be overstated—particularly in the area of service accountability and reimbursement. Managed care organizations and other external reviewing bodies tasked with monitoring service can hold health care social work providers responsible for quality of care issues, length of service provision, level of care provided, use of ancillary and other therapeutic services, referral patterns and use, cost-restraining interventions, appropriateness or suitability of service, compliance to a standard set of provision criteria, the use of outcome criteria, and so on. Therefore, the health care service record is audited to determine whether professionals have applied the most affordable services prudently dedicated to quality service provision.

TYPES OF RECORD KEEPING

Throughout the history of health care social work, some type of medical record or recording process has been required. In the beginning, most records were in the form of *ledgers* and *narrative records*. This early form of record keeping merely provided the facts regarding the client's situation (Timms, 1972). When public health services were delivered, they were documented, but little clinical interpretation generally occurred. This did change, and in the second half of the nineteenth century, a more sophisticated approach was used. This new approach went beyond simply listing the problems to "making a case" for a client's needs and resources (Sheffield, 1920).

In 1920 Sheffield wrote a book titled *The Social Case History: Its Construction and Content*. In this method of recording, she highlighted what the facts meant and how they could be applied to relieve suffering. Sheffield, like Mary Richmond, believed that accountability meant improving social conditions (public health) as well as delivering effective services and enhancing practitioner skills.

PROCESS RECORDING

Another type of record keeping that influenced health care social work was *process recording*. This form of recording became popular in the 1920s, and its introduction was influenced heavily by the field of sociology. It was expected to facilitate research and practice by allowing a client to reveal the self by using his or her own dialogue (Burgess, 1928). Often this type of recording format was used (a) to gather information for the development of social work practice theory and (b) to monitor service evaluation. However, it did not take long for this method of case recording to lose favor. Many social workers thought it was too long, detailed, and cumbersome to use in the practice setting.

Today, process recording is generally not used in the health care practice setting. However, it is used in hospital training programs, in cases involving the courts and legal issues, and in other educational settings. For the most part, process recording remains a type of case-based documentation primarily used to assist beginning-level social workers and other health care providers to learn counseling and practice strategy. In training, it is not uncommon for students to be asked to create a detailed chronological format that includes a face sheet, goals, contracts or agreements and client interpretations, as well as telephone and in-person contacts with all involved in the service that was provided.

DIAGNOSTIC RECORDING

A fourth type of early case-based recording that was often used in health and mental health settings was *diagnostic recording*. Hamilton (1936, 1946) grounded this type of case recording in psychosocial theory. Diagnostic recording was based on process recording in that the exploration of social causes was expanded to include those issues of a psychosocial nature. A trained diagnostician completed this assessment and interpretation. It was the use of diagnostic recording that is said to have cemented the relationships among practice, the practitioner, supervision, and the record (Kagle, 1995). The format for this type of recording often varied in length and content and had little unifying structure. This form of record keeping quickly lost favor in the medical setting because it became too hard to find important information and often the information simply was not there to find at all, since what was to be recorded was at the discretion of the recorder.

AUDIOTAPING AND VIDEO RECORDING

Audiotaping and *video recording* are methods of case-based recording currently used in the medical setting; however, this type of recording is almost always limited to training programs and is primarily used for educational purposes only. For example, to train primary care physicians, nurses, and so on, particularly in the area of family dynamics. Often the interdisciplinary team reviews sessions and makes suggestions for improving service delivery. Generally, audiotaping and video recording are not used as the sole method of recording service delivery. In health care practice today, this method of recording alone is considered deficient and is never used without supplementation.

TIME-SERIES RECORDING

In evidence-based practice, *time-series recording* offers an efficient and effective way to establish whether an intervention is successful and to display this difference graphically. Generally, this form of recording is most commonly associated with behavioral interventions and single-subject designs. It is highlighted in the term *scientist-practitioner.* Bloom, Fischer, & Orme (1999) encourage the use of this type of design to document and measure specific client problem behaviors. This method of recording can be helpful in providing information to meet goals and objectives.

In this method, data are collected and displayed visually on a graph. The information gathered is later analyzed statistically or visually. One major weakness of this form of record keeping is that it requires expertise in the design and setup of the recording. One of the major limitations for the use of time-series recording in the health care setting appears to be lack of knowledge about this format. Many health care supervisors and other medical professionals are not familiar with single-subject designs and the methods of recording generally practiced in this context. Therefore, they do not encouragethe use of time-series recording. A second factor for the lack of popularity is the charting procedure. This form of record keeping is generally limited to documenting only certain aspects of the client's problem or situation. This makes it essential for health care social workers to not only know the basics of this approach to recording but to be willing to teach it to others on the interdisciplinary team.

In time-series recording, the *single-subject research design* is used. In this design, the individual is studied throughout the treatment process. Use of this type of design can help the health care social worker answer the question "Is what I am doing working?" The attractiveness of this design in the health care setting is that it can be used with individual clients, a couple, a family, or a group. It is beyond the scope of this chapter to go into depth in this area, but for further information on the single-subject design, the reader is referred to a workbook written by Westerfelt and Dietz (1997) entitled *Planning and Conducting Agency-Based Research* that assists the health care worker through the research process while presenting different research designs used in the practice setting.

COMPUTERIZED AND STANDARDIZED RECORDS

The *computerized* or *standardized record* is gaining in popularity in the area of health care delivery. In the 1980s, agencies, hospitals, and other health care facilities began to recognize the benefits of computer technology in record keeping. Today, almost all health care agencies keep standardized and computerized administrative files. The most common use of computers involves word processing, making computers invaluable tools for writing assessments, progress notes, correspondence, and reports (Gingerich, 2002). Although this is changing, in many facilities more personal and problem-oriented notes are still generally maintained outside of the computer. The primary reason for this separation is the difficulty with protecting client confidentiality within the computerized record. To protect the confidentiality of the client, information and computer access must be guarded. Guarded access is important to restrict information to only select professionals with a need to know. This type of record keeping is expanding, especially in regard to outcome measures and symptom checklists, as a diagnostic tool and for graphing or analysis of data (Gingerich, 2002). In terms of the future, it appears likely that eventually total client record keeping will be within an automated system.

PERSON-OR FAMILY-ORIENTED RECORDING

The *person-*or *family-oriented* record is a new type of record keeping found in the health care setting. Generally, it is seen most in a community-oriented practice model for health care delivery. A database, treatment plan, assessment, progress notes, and progress review are included; however, special attention is given to the uniqueness of the client and his or her family. Particularly in the family-oriented record, a concentration on wellness is highlighted because information on everyone in the household may be viewed at the same time. The entire family is kept in one file. Similarly, in the client-oriented record, the responsibility for the record rests with the client. All information from numerous providers is kept in one record, and at times the record may be released directly to the client to ensure that continuity in health care treatment is documented. The emphasis in the family-and person-oriented record is measuring individual family or client progress over time and with different providers.

PROBLEM-ORIENTED RECORDING

Among the various types of record keeping formats, many health care facilities use problem-oriented recording (POR) (Dziegielewski, 2002;

Rankin, 1996). Traditionally used in health care or medical settings, this type of recording was originally formulated to encourage multidisciplinary and interdisciplinary collaboration and to train medical professionals (Weed, 1969). As members of either multidisciplinary or interdisciplinary teams, helping professionals find that problem-oriented case documentation enables them to maintain documentation uniformity while remaining active within a team approach to care.

For the health care social worker POR emphasizes accountability through brief and concise documentation of client problems, services, or interventions as well as client responses. Although there are numerous formats for problem-oriented case recording, always keep comments brief, concrete, measurable, and concise. Many professionals feel strongly that problem-oriented recording is compatible with the increase in client caseloads, rapid assessments, and time-limited treatment. By maintaining brief but informative notes, health care professionals are able to provide significant summaries of intervention progress. Generally, the health care social worker cannot select the type of problem-oriented recording that will be utilized as this choice is based on agency, clinic, hospital, or practice's function, need, and accountability. Clear and concise documentation reflects the pressure indicative of evidence-based practice. This makes it critical for the health care social worker to be familiar with the basic types of problem-oriented recording and with how to utilize this format within the case record.

One thing that all problem-oriented recording formats share is that all start with a problem list that is clearly linked to the behaviorally based biopsychosocial intervention (Frager, 2000). This problem-focused documentation helps the health care social worker focus directly on the presenting problems and coping styles that the client is exhibiting, thereby helping to limit abstractions and vague clinical judgments. Therefore, this type of documentation should include an inventory reflective of current active problems that are periodically updated. When a problem is resolved, it is crossed off the list with the date of resolution clearly designated. The active problems a client is experiencing are considered the basic building blocks for case recording within the problem-oriented record.

Although numerous formats for the actual progress note documentation can be selected, the SOAP is considered the most commonly used. See Table 7.1 for SOAP, SOAPIE, and SOAPIER recording formats.

TABLE 7.1   SOAP, SOAPIE, and SOAPIER Recording Formats

Subjective, Objective, Assessment, Plan (SOAP)

Subjective, Objective, Assessment, Plan, Implementation, Evaluation (SOAPIE)

Subjective, Objective, Assessment, Plan, Implementation, Evaluation, Response (SOAPIER)

S = subjective data relevant to the client's request for service; client and practitioner impressions of the problem

O = objective data such as observable and measurable criteria related to the problem. If client statements are used, put the statement in quotes

A = assessment information of the underlying problems; diagnostic impression

P = plan that outlines current intervention strategy and specific referrals for other needed services

I = implementation considerations of the service to be provided

E = evaluation of service provision

R = client's response to the diagnostic process, treatment planning, and intervention efforts

The Subjective-Objective-Assessment-Plan (SOAP) is the most common form of POR and became popular in the 1970s. In this format, the health care social worker utilizes the "S" (subjective) to record the data relevant to the client's request for service and the things the client says and feels about the problem. In this section the health care professional can use his or her clinical judgment in documenting what appears to be happening with the client. Some professionals prefer to document this information in terms of major themes or general topics addressed, rather than making specific statements about what the practitioner thinks is happening. Generally, in this section intimate personal content or details of fantasies and process interactions should not be included. When charting in this section of the SOAP note, the health care social worker should always consider whether this statement could be open to misinterpretation. If the statement is vulnerable to misinterpretation or it resembles a personal rather than professional reaction to what is said, it should not be included.

The "O" (objective) includes observable and measurable criteria related to the problem. These are symptoms, behaviors, and client-focused problems observed directly by the social worker during the assessment and intervention process. In addition, some agencies, clinics, and practices have started to include client statements in this section as well. If a client statement is to be utilized as objective data, however, exact quotes must be used. For example, if in the session the client states that he will not harm himself, the practitioner must document exactly what the client has said and use quotation marks. Under the objective section of the summary note it is also possible to include the results from standardized assessment instruments designed to measure psychological or social functioning.

The "A" (assessment) includes the therapist's assessment of the underlying problems, which in the mental health setting might include a DSM-IV-TR multiaxial system. Since application of this framework is beyond the scope of this chapter, please see Dziegielewski (2002) for more specific applications. In "P" (plan), the practitioner records how treatment objectives will be carried out, areas for future interventions, and specific referrals to other services needed by the client.

With today's increased emphasis on time-limited intervention efforts and accountability, two new areas have been added to the original SOAP format (Dziegielewski & Leon, 2001b). This extension, referred to as SOAPIE, identifies the first additional term as "I," which stands for the implementation considerations of the service to be provided. Here the health care social worker explains exactly how, when, and who will implement the service. In the last section of the SOAPIE format, an "E" is designated to represent service provision evaluation (Dziegielewski, 2002). It is here that all health care professionals are expected to identify specific actions related to direct evaluation of progress achieved after any interventions are provided. When treatment is considered successful, specific outcome-based objectives established early in the treatment process are documented as progressing or checked off when attained. In some agencies a modified version of the SOAPIE has been introduced and is referred to as SOAPIER. In this latest version, the "R" outlines the client's response to the intervention provided.

A second popular problem-oriented recording format used in many health and mental health care facilities today is the DAP (data, assessment, and plan) format. The DAP encourages the social worker to identify only the most salient elements of a practitioner's client contact. Using the "D" (data), the social worker is expected to record objective client data, statements related to the presenting problem, and the focus of the therapeutic contact. The "A" is used to record the diagnostic assessment intervention from the multiaxial format, the client's reactions to the service and intervention, and the social worker's assessment of the client's overall progress toward the treatment goals and objectives. Specific information on all tasks, actions, or plans related to the presenting problem and to be carried out by either the client or the helping professional is recorded under "P" (plan). Also recorded under "P" (plan) is information on issues related to the presenting problem to be explored at the next session and the specific date and time of the next appointment (Dziegielewski, 2002). Again, like the SOAP, the DAP format has undergone some changes. For example, some counseling professionals who generally apply the DAP are now being asked to modify this form of record keeping to add an additional section. This changes the DAP into the DAPE and adds a section where documentation under the "E" reflects what type of educational and evaluative services have been conducted. See Table 7.2.

Two other forms of problem-based case recording formats often used in health and mental health settings are the PIRP (Problem, Intervention, Response, and Plan) and the APIE (Assessed information, Problems addressed, Interventions provided, and Evaluation). A structure similar to the SOAP and DAP structures is employed (see Table 7.3). All four of these popular formats of problem-oriented case recording have been praised for supporting increased problem identification and standardizing what and how client behaviors and coping styles are reported, thus providing a greater understanding of health and mental health problems and the various methods of managing them. This type of problem-oriented record allows all helping professionals to quickly familiarize themselves with a client's overall situation (Starfield, 1992). For health care social workers, utilizing a problem-focused perspective must go beyond merely recording information that is limited to the client's problems. When the focus is limited to gathering only this information, important strengths and resources that clients bring to the therapeutic interview may not be validated. Furthermore, partialization of client problems creates the potential risk that other significant aspects of a client's functioning will be overlooked in treatment planning and subsequent practice strategy. Therefore, problem-oriented forms of case recording need to extend beyond the immediate problem, regardless of whether managed care companies require it (Dziegielewski, 2002; Rudolph, 2000).

TABLE 7.2   DAPE Recording Format

Data, Assessment, Plan (DAP)
Data, Assessment, Plan, Education (DAPE)

D = data that are gathered to provide information about the identified problem

A = assessment of the client in regard to his or her current problem or situation

P = plan for intervention and what will be completed to help the client achieve increased health status or functioning

E = professional education that is provided by the mental health practitioner to ensure that problem mediation has taken place or evaluation information to ensure practice accountability

DOCUMENTATION, TREATMENT PLANNING, AND PRACTICE STRATEGY

Throughout history, health care social workers have relied on some form of record keeping to clearly document information on client situations and problems. Although the formats used by professionals have changed, documentation for maintaining case continuity has remained a professional priority (Dziegielewski, 2002). In its most basic form, case recording provides the helping professional with a "map" that indicates where the client and practitioner have traveled in their treatment journey (Dziegielewski & Leon, 2001b). And, because experience is dynamic and words are static the intervention process goes beyond what written words can describe (Lauver & Harvey, 1997). Therefore, the exact words used must be chosen carefully, which makes case documentation an evolving process. Case documentation must also be geared toward maintaining high-quality service as well as toward preserving continuity of service when different mental health professionals are involved (Welfel, 1998). In addition, well-documented diagnostic assessments and interventions can protect the health care social worker in high-risk cases, making him or her less likely to be judged negligent in the legal setting (Bernstein & Hartsell, 1998; Welfel, 1998).

Understanding the relationship between client problems, interventions used, and client progress enables the social worker to assess the interventions provided and make necessary changes in the intervention

TABLE 7.3 PIRP and APIE Recording formats

Problem, Intervention, Response, Plan (PIRP)

P = presenting problem(s) or the problem(s) to be addressed
I = intervention to be conducted by the mental health practitioner
R = response to the intervention by the client
P = plan to address the problems experienced by the client

Assessed information, Problems addressed, Interventions provided,
Evaluation (APIE)

A = documentation of assessed information in regard to the client problem
P = explanation of the problem that is being addressed
I = intervention description and plan
E = evaluation of the problem once the intervention is completed

process. Sheafor, Horesjsi, & Horesjsi (1997) stated that the purpose of documentation and accurate record keeping in helping professions is multifaceted. Therefore, good record keeping must (1) provide an accurate and standardized account of the information gathered; (2) support this information with introspective and retrospective data collection; (3) provide the information needed for good practice standards that include relevant ethical, legal, billing, and agency requirements; and (4) provide clearly stated information that will withstand scrutiny by external reviewers such as accreditation bodies, ombudsmen, lawyers, insurance companies, and quality assurance/improvement and control personnel.

For the health care social worker, accurate case documentation is necessary or most third-party payers will not reimburse for the start or continuation of services. Therefore, the link between clinical indicators and clinical interventions in the health care setting cannot be overemphasized. This emphasis on accountability and reimbursement is mandated by managed care organizations and other external reviewing bodies that monitor client services (Dziegielewski & Holliman, 2001). All social workers are expected to justify and document client eligibility for service, appropriateness for continuation of services, length of treatment, level of care, interventions provided, and the use of outcome criteria (Holliman, Dziegielewski, & Datta, 2001; Lowery, 1996).

Utilizing a holistic framework that stresses the client's behavioral and biopsychosocial factors allows health care social workers to play an important role in the efficient delivery of interdisciplinary psychological and social services. As part of an interdisciplinary team, practitioners can also assist other team members to document effectively while collaborating with other interdisciplinary team members on client progress and problems (Abramson, 2002). Providing accurate, up-to-date, and informative records is vital to the coordinated planning efforts of the entire team.

With the advent of behaviorally based managed care, however, high caseloads and shorter lengths of stay have caused health care social workers to adapt a style of documentation that is brief yet informative (Dziegielewski, 1997, Holliman, Dziegielewski, & Datta, 2001). The challenge then is to summarize important client information into meaningful yet concise notes and treatment plans. Given the litigious nature of our society, informative records that demonstrate treatment interventions and reflect legal and ethical values and concerns become important documents that can be recalled long after the therapeutic intervention has ended (Bernstein & Hartsell, 1998). The pressure for accurate documentation rests in the growing emphasis and on using evidence-based professional practice and justification for the course of intervention.

When utilizing evidence-based practice, clear documentation as reflected in the case record can be used for numerous purposes. Furthermore, regardless of the helping discipline or practice setting, standard rules for efficient and effective documentation should be implemented. The social worker should always:

- Clearly document problem behaviors and coping styles.
- Clearly outline behavioral symptoms, because this will provide the basis for subsequent goals and interventions.
- The intervention plan must clearly reflect progress indicators and time frames that are reflective and supportive of the identified problem.
- Case notes and intervention plan must clearly document and show response to interventions.
- Case notes are used to assess goal accomplishment and to evaluate the efficiency, treatment, and whenever possible the cost-effectiveness of the service delivered.

MEASURING GOALS AND OBJECTIVES

In the health care setting, the time-limited and/or unstructured nature of the setting clearly presents challenges for the social worker trying to measure the effectiveness of his or her interventions. Basically, no matter what evaluative effort is employed, it must be initiated early and brought to closure fairly quickly. In addition, in establishing effectiveness, this experience should not be seen as being intrusive in the helping process. Consequently, the purposes of both the intervention and the evaluation should be compatible and mutually supportive. The first task for the health care social worker is to help the client not only to participate in the development of the change efforts but also to express these efforts in specific time limited goals and objectives. Goals permit the practitioner to establish whether he or she has the skills and/or desire to work with the client (Cormier & Cormier, 1991).

Brower and Nurius (1993) suggest two key characteristics of goals that need to be present when designing effective intervention. First, goals need to be specific, clear, verifiable, and measurable, as well as concrete and behavior-specific as possible. The objectives should be designed to further quantify the goals. Second, whenever possible, both the social worker and the client should mutually agree upon all goals and objectives. Clients must also contribute in order to determine whether the goals and objectives sought are consistent with their own culture and values. It is up to the social worker to help the client structure and establish the intervention strategy; however, mutuality is central to the development of goals and objectives.

In social work we have long realized the importance of goal setting in facilitating the intervention process. With the advent of managed behavioral health care, however, an increased emphasis has been placed on the means of ensuring that a specific goal and the subsequent objectives have been accomplished. Therefore, for evidence-based practice to be meaningful, social workers must establish a climate where goals, and the specific objectives to meet them, are viewed as realistic, obtainable, and measurable. This suggests that no one methodological approach is likely to be appropriate for all types of client problems or health care settings. The evidence-based challenge is to fit the method to the problem, and not vice versa. This requires a thoughtful selection of research strategies, the various threads of which can be creatively woven throughout the broader fabric of the overall intervention plan (Dziegielewski & Powers, 2000).

USING MEASUREMENT INSTRUMENTS AS OUTCOME INDICATORS

Once the goals and objectives have been established, the difficult task of evaluating the clinical intervention in standardized or evidence-based terms must be addressed. This task is simplified when problems are addressed directly by the goals and objectives rather than characterized in somewhat vague and nebulous language. With the emphasis on treatment efficacy and accountability in today's practice environment, it is essential that mental health practitioners learn to include objective measures that help to evaluate the interventions used within the health care setting. Included in these measures are standardized scales, surveys, and RAIs (rapid assessment instruments). These tools provide evidence-based data that identify the changes occurring over the course of the intervention (Corcoran & Boyer-Quick, 2002). It is extremely important that health care social workers become familiar with and integrate measurement instruments in their practice and in their documentation to determine if treatment interventions have impacted baseline behaviors and problems (Dziegielewski, 1997). Gathering pre-and postdata on a client's problem enables both the practitioner and the client to examine whether progress has occurred and provides regulatory agencies with tangible objective evidence of client progress. By using a holistic framework that stresses the client's behaviorally based biopsychosocial factors, health care social workers play an important role in the efficient delivery of interdisciplinary health services.

One evaluation model that has historically gained and continues to receive widespread attention and use is Goal Attainment Scaling (GAS) (Lambert & Hill, 1994). This type of scaling appears to be adaptable to a wide range of situations and was originally introduced by Kiresuk and Sherman (1968) as a way of measuring programmatic outcomes for community mental health services. GAS employs a client-specific technique designed to provide outcome information regarding the attainment of individualized clinical and social goals. The GAS requires that a number of individually tailored intervention goals/objectives be specified in relation to a set of graded scale points ranging from the least to the most favorable outcomes considered likely. Although at first it may seem somewhat dated, the GAS remains consistent with today's behaviorally based, outcome-focused practice environment because it is constructed with a specific time frame in mind. With this type of measure any number of goals may be specified for a particular client, and any subject area may be included as an appropriate goal. Even the same goal can be defined in more than one way. For example, the goal of alleviating depression could be scaled in relation to self-reports or in relation to specific cutoff points on a standardized instrument such as the Beck Depression Inventory (Beck, 1967). It is essential, however, that all goals be defined in terms of a graded series of verifiable expectations in ways that are relevant to the idiosyncrasies of the particular case.

In summary, the GAS is given as an example of how goal and objective attainment can be specified as a means toward establishing evidence-based practice (Hart, 1978). Basically, systems such as the GAS can provide a systematic yet flexible practice evaluation model that can help bridge the methodological gap between clinical and administrative interests.

For health care social workers, understanding and concretely defining terms such as *stress, anxiety,* and *depression* and how these conditions can relate to the medical condition a client is experiencing cannot be overestimated. Understanding a client's health condition requires a full assessment of his or her biopsychosocial functioning. Although commonplace in our professional jargon, such terms tend to carry rather subjective connotations, and as a result can be difficult to measure. Therefore, establishing and monitoring a method for measuring effectiveness of the intervention process becomes a practice necessity. The first step in measuring practice effectiveness, as stated earlier, generally begins with being able to show how mutually negotiated goals and objectives have been met. Change must be documented through some type of concrete measurement with clear clinical indicators indicative of client progress. Once goals and objectives have been clarified, establishing baselines through the use of concrete and/or standardized measurement instruments begins (Lewis & Roberts, 2002). Therefore, it is often the task of the health care social worker to select, implement, and evaluate the appropriate measurement instruments.

Most professionals agree that standardized scales (that have been assessed for reliability and validity) are generally recommended.

In recent years social workers have begun to rely more heavily on the use of these types of standardized instruments in an effort to achieve greater accuracy and objectivity in measuring some of the more commonly encountered clinical problems. The most notable development in this regard has been the emergence of numerous brief pencil-and-paper assessment devices known as rapid assessment instruments (RAIs). As standardized measures, RAIs share a number of characteristics. They are brief, relatively easy to administer, score, and interpret, and they require very little knowledge of testing procedures on the part of the clinician. For the most part, they are self-report measures that can be completed by the client, usually within 15 minutes. They are independent of any particular theoretical orientation, and as such can be used with a variety of interventive methods. Since they provide a systematic overview of the client's problem, they often tend to stimulate discussion related to the information elicited by the instrument itself. The score that is generated provides an operational index of the frequency, duration, or intensity of the problem. Most RAIs can be used as repeated measures and thus are adaptable to the methodological requirements of both research design and goal assessment. In addition to providing a standardized means by which change can be monitored over time with a single client, RAIs can also be used to make equivalent comparisons across clients experiencing a common problem (e.g., marital conflict).

One of the major advantages of RAIs is the availability of information concerning reliability and validity. *Reliability* refers to the stability of a measure. In other words, do the questions that constitute the instrument mean the same thing to the individual answering them at different times, and would different individuals interpret those same questions in a similar manner? Unless an instrument yields consistent data, it is impossible for it to be valid. But even highly reliable instruments are of little value unless their validity can also be demonstrated. Validity speaks to the general question of whether an instrument does in fact measure what it purports to measure.

There are several different approaches to establishing validity (Chen, 1997; Cone, 1998; Schutte & Malouff, 1995), each of which is designed to provide information regarding how much confidence we can have in the instrument as an accurate indicator of the problem under consideration. While levels of reliability and validity vary greatly among available instruments, it is very helpful to the social worker to know in advance the extent to which these issues have been addressed. Information concerning reliability and validity, as well as other factors related to the standardization process (e.g., the procedures for administering, scoring, and interpreting the instrument), can help the professional make informed judgments concerning the appropriateness of any given instrument.

The key to selecting the best instrument for the intervention is knowing where and how to access the relevant information concerning potentially useful measures. Fortunately, there are a number of excellent sources available to the clinician to help facilitate this process. One such compilation of standardized measures is *Measures for Clinical Practice* by Corcoran and Fischer (2000), and another is by Schutte and Malouff (1995), *Sourcebook of Adult Assessment Strategies*. These books can serve as valuable resources of rapid assessment instruments specifically selected for review because they measure the kinds of problems most commonly encountered in clinical social work practice. Fischer and Corcoran have done an excellent job, not only in identifying and evaluating a viable cross-section of useful clinically grounded instruments, but also in discussing a number is issues critical to their use. Further, Schutte and Malouff (1995) provide a list of mental health-related measures for adults and what areas they can best assist in. In addition to introducing to the basic principles of measurement, these books discuss various types of measurement tools, including the advantages and disadvantages of RAIs. Corcoran and Fischer (2000) also provide some useful guidelines for locating, selecting, evaluating, and administering prospective measures. In this text the instruments are provided in two volumes in relation to their appropriateness for use with one of three target populations: adults, children, or couples and families. They are also cross-indexed by problem area, which makes the selection process very easy. The availability of these, as well as of numerous other similar references related to special interest areas, greatly enhances the social work professional's options with respect to monitoring and evaluation practice.

In summary, to further enhance the measurement of practice effectiveness many social workers are feeling pressured to incorporate additional forms of measurement in the treatment plan (Dziegielewski,

1997). The pressure to incorporate individual, family and social rankings is becoming more common. This requires that specific measurement scores that establish functioning levels for the clients served be clearly measured and documented. To provide this additional measurement, more and more professionals are turning to the DSM-IV-TR and providing Axis V (Generalized Assessment of Functioning (GAF) rating scores for each client served. When utilizing the GAF functioning ratings are assigned as clients enter therapy and again upon discharge (Dziegielewski, 2002). The GAF scale allows for assignment of a number that represents a client's behaviors. On the GAF behaviors are ranked from zero to 100, with the higher numbersbeing considered more indicative of higher levels of functioning and coping. In rating the highest level of functioning a client has maintained over the past year and comparing it to the current level of functioning, the social worker can make helpful comparisons to quantify the client problems and changes resulting within the counseling relationship. This allows for a comparison of scores to show increased client functioning. See the DSM-IV-TR, published by the American Psychiatric Association (2000) for scale rankings for the above. Also, in the DSM-IV "Criteria Sets and Axes Provided for that might be particularly helpful to social work professionals. The first of these optional scales is the relational functioning scale termed the Global Assessment of Relational Functioning (GARF). This index is used to address family or other ongoing relationship status on a hypothetical continuum from competent to dysfunctional (American Psychiatric Association, 2000). The second index is the Social and Occupational Functioning Assessment Scale (SOFAS). With this scale an "individual's level of social and occupational functioning that is not directly influenced by overall severity of the individual's psychological symptoms" can be addressed (American PsychiatricAssociation, 2000). The complementary nature of these scales in identifying and assessing client problems is evident in the fact that all three scales, the GARF, GAF, and SOFAS, use the same rating system. The ranking scale for each remains from zero to 100, with the lower numbers being representative of the more severe problems. The use of all three of these tools is encouraged because they can help social workers to employ concrete measurements from a more multifaceted perspective. All three involve the clinical documentation of increased levels of functioning from the individual (GAF), family (GARF), and social (SOFAS) perspective.

TREATMENT AND INTERVENTION PLANNING

Once the problem behaviors have been identified, this information can be utilized to start a treatment or intervention plan. When working with the client, it is important that each treatment plan be individualized. Treatment plans have gained in importance in the health care setting. One reason for this popularity is that most programs require reimbursement and this makes following the requirements and standards of organizations such as the Joint Commission for the Accreditation of Healthcare Organizations (JCAHO) very important (Maruish, 2002). This means that the plans must reflect the general as well as the unique symptoms and needs the client is experiencing. A formal intervention plan will help determine the structure and provide focus for any type of health intervention. Furthermore, a clearly established treatment plan can help deter any litigation by either the client or a concerned family member (Bernstein & Hartsell, 1998). When the treatment plan clearly delineates the intervention plan, families and friends of the client may feel more at ease and may actually agree to participate and assist in any behavioral interventions.

In developing the intervention plan, Maruish (2002) identifies several assumptions that are always considered in the health care environment:

- The client is experiencing behavioral health problems.
- The client is motivated to work on the problems.
- Treatment goals are tied to identified problems.
- Treatment goals are achievable, collaboratively developed, and prioritized.
- Progress indicators are noted and tracked.

In formulating the plan, several critical steps need to be identified (Jongsma & Peterson, 1999). First, problem behaviors that are interfering with functioning must be noted. It is considered essential that the client and his or her family participate and assist in this process of identifying the issues, problem behaviors, and coping styles that are either causing or contributing to the client's discomfort. Of all of the problem behaviors a client may be experiencing, the ones that should receive the most attention are those behaviors that impair independent living skills or cause difficulties in completing tasks of daily living. Once identified, these behaviors need to be linked to the intervention process. The identification of specific problem behaviors or coping styles can provide an opportunity to facilitate educational and communicative interventions that can further enhance communication between the client and family members. Involving the family and support system in treatment plan formulation and application can be especially helpful and productive since at times individuals experiencing mental confusion and distortions of reality may exhibit bizarre and unpredictable symptoms. If support systems are not included in the intervention planning process and the client's symptoms worsen, the client-family system environment may become characterized by increased tension, frustration, fear, blame, and helplessness. To avoid support systems from withdrawing from the client and thereby decreasing the support available to the client, family members and key support system members need to either be involved or at a minimum be made aware of the treatment plan goals and objectives that will be utilized if the client consents to their involvement.

Second, not only do family and friends need to be aware of the treatment plan initiatives, but they also need to be encouraged to share valuable input and support to ensure intervention progress and success. Family education and supportive interventions for family and significant others can be listed as part of the treatment plan for an individual client. It is beyond the scope of this chapter to discuss the multiple interventions available to the family members of the mentally ill individual; however, interested readers are encouraged to refer to Walsh (2000), which provides an excellent strategy for working with families of a relative who suffers from mental illness.

Next, in order to assist in treatment plan development, it is critical to state the identified problem behaviors in terms of behaviorally based outcomes (Dziegielewski, 2002). In completing this process, the assessment data that lead to the diagnostic impression, as well as the specific problems often experienced by the client, need to be outlined. Once identified, the clients' problems are then prioritized so that goals, objectives, and action tasks may be developed. The goals of intervention, which constitute the basis for the plan of intervention, must then be clearly outlined and applied. These goals must be broken down into specific objective statements that reflect target behaviors to be changed and ways to measure the client's progress on each objective. As subcomponents to the objectives, action tasks must be included that clearly delineate the steps to be taken by the client and the helping professional to ensure successful completion of each objective. For example, if the problem behavior is ambivalent feelings that impair general task completion, the main goal may be to help the client decrease feelings of ambivalence. It is therefore important to document a behavioral objective that clearly articulates a behavioral definition of ambivalence, ways that the ambivalence will be decreased, and the mechanisms used to determine if the behavior has been changed. The therapeutic intervention involves helping the client develop specific and concrete tasks that are geared toward decreasing this behavior and consequently meeting the objective. The outcome measure simply becomes establishing whether the task was completed. It is important to note that no treatment plan is designed to be all-inclusive; rather it is designed to provide the guidelines for effective documentation of the assessment and intervention process. Furthermore, the treatment plan must be individualized for the client, outlining the specific problem behaviors and how each of these behaviors can be addressed.

MEASURING CHANGE IN THE HEALTH CARE SETTING

It remains obvious that the helping relationship is a complex one that cannot be measured completely through the use of standardized scales or assessment measures. To facilitate measurement of effectiveness, specific concrete goals and objectives must incorporate a number of direct behavioral observation techniques, self-anchored rating scales and client logs. Together these methods can provide a range of qualitative and quantitative measures for initiating evidence-based practice.

For the health care social worker, evidence-based practice interventions can lead to greater efficiency and effectiveness. For many social workers this requirement to concretely identify all problem behaviors in clear terms or indicators has led to frustration because social workers are expected to operationalize the change-behaviors as part of the assessment process (Dziegielewski, 1996, 2002). In addition, the link between the actual practice components and the strategies needed to assess them can be elusive. For example, in the case plan a problem statement along with behaviorally based goals and objectives must be clearly identified. The client's capacity for self-determination must be recognized as well as the accountability issues that remain germane to the profession, the agency, and the requirements and conditions relevant to service reimbursement.

MAINTAINING CLINICAL RECORDS

Since records can be maintained in more than one medium, such as written case files, audio-or videotaped material, and computer-generated notes, special attention needs to be given to ensuring confidentiality and ethical release of client information. Probably the greatest protection a health care social worker has in terms of risk management for all types of records is accurate, clear, and concise clinical records (Reamer, 2001). This means that an unbroken chain of custody between the social worker and/or the multidisciplinary/interdisciplinary team and the record must always be maintained. Since health care providers will ultimately be held responsible for producing a clinical record in case of litigation, this policy cannot be overemphasized. Furthermore, documentation in the health care record should always be clearly sequenced and easy to follow. If a mistake occurs, never change a summary note or intervention plan without acknowledging it. When changes need to be made to the clinical case record, the intervention plan, or any other types of case recording clearly indicate that a change is being made by drawing one thin line through the mistake and dating and initialing it. For these and other directions, see Table 7.4. Records that are legible and cogent limit open interpretation of the services provided. In addition, the health care practitioner will always be required to keep clinical case records (including written records and computerized backup files) safeguarded in locked and fireproof cabinets. Most health care facilities use archiving types of storage systems such as microfiche or microfilm to preserve records and maximize space.

As the use of computer-generated notes continues to become more common different forms of problem-oriented case recording will be linked directly into computerized databases (Starfield, 1992; Gingerich, 2002). In terms of convenience, this can mean immediate access to fiscal and billing information as well as client intervention strategy, documentation, and treatment planning. When working with computerized records, Bernstein & Hartsell (1998) suggest the following: (1) when recording client information on a hard drive or disk, be sure

TABLE 7.4   Documentation Reminders

Because accurate and ethical documentationeinsures continuity of care and ethica, and legal aspects of practice, and also provides direction for the focus of intervention, every record must have the following essential information:

- Date and time of entry
- Interview notes that clearly describe the presenting problem
- Evidenced-based format for recording of behaviors
- An intervention plan that clearly establishes overall goals, objectives, and intervention tasks

In addition:

- Always use ink that does not run (ball point pens are best)
- Never use pencil or white-out to erase mistakes
- Draw a line through an error, marking it "error" and initialing the error;
- Print and sign social worker's name, title, and credentials with each entry
- Document all information in the case record as if you might some day have to defend it in a court of law

Criteria modified from Dziegielewski (2002).

storage is in a safe and secure place; (2) be sure to secure any passwords from detection; (3) if you are treating a celebrity or a famous individual, use a fictitious name and be sure to keep the "key" to the actual name in a protected place; (4) always maintain a backup system and keep it secure; (5) be sure that everyone who will have access to the client's case file reads and signs an established protocol concerning sanctity, privacy, and confidentiality of the records; and (6) take the potential of computer theft or crash seriously and establish a policy that will safeguard what will need to happen if this should occur. The convenience of records and information now being easily transmitted electronically produces one major concern. Since clinical case records are so easy to access and are portable, there is a genuine problem of possible unauthorized access of the recorded information. This means that if a health care social worker is dealing with personal and confidential information, every precaution should be taken to safeguard the information. In addition, since medical records are kept for the benefit of the client, access to the record by the client is generally allowed. When engaging in any type of disclosure or transfer issues to either the client or third parties, however, a written consent from the client is expected (Lauver & Harvey, 1997).

ETHICAL AND LEGAL CONSIDERATIONS IN RECORD KEEPING

Malpractice is negligence in the exercise of one's profession (Schroeder, 1995). Schroeder (1995) warns that one way to protect professionals against malpractice is to encourage them to keep careful records that clearly and accurately reflect the service that was rendered. Social workers in health care, like all social workers, have to be careful to protect the client's right to privacy and confidentiality. Many times, these records involve personal information that can be damaging to the client served, especially when records are subpoenaed into a court of law. Although often state and federal workers may be exempt from responsibility and may carry qualified immunity against judgment (Schroeder, 1995), other professionals may not be so lucky. This is particularly problematic for social workers, who work in home health care agencies and so on. All social workers practicing in the health care field should contemplate maintaining their own malpractice insurance. The National Association of Social Workers sponsors a professional liability policy that should be considered. For clarification and more updated information on the malpractice insurance coverage available to health care social workers (e.g., rates, services, and policies), contact with the national office of NASW is recommended. Further, it is important to note that in August 1996 social workers were granted privilege in the federal court system. The effect that this decision may have on record keeping is still to be determined. Again, contact with NASW for updated information regarding ethics and legal implications is highly recommended.

CHAPTER SUMMARY AND FUTURE DIRECTIONS

Managed care presents a type of service delivery never before experienced. Health care social workers are expected to show that the intermittent or time-limited brief services they provide are necessary and effective. This challenge has been a particularly vigorous one for the health care social worker because of the variation and lack of clarity in the types of interventions provided. Health care social workers must be aware of and capable of using the different methods of record keeping often used in the health care setting. Regardless of the specific style or type of record keeping being used, all records need to (a) identify, describe, and assess the client's situation; (b) describe the reason or purpose for the service being provided; (c) describe the goals and objectives to be obtained, listed as behavioral outcome measures; (d) establish the plan for intervention; and (e) evaluate the process and outcome of therapeutic process.

It is the responsibility of the health care social worker to ensure that records are maintained that are both accountable and accurate. These records are essential for effective and efficient communication with other team members. In health care delivery, the medical record is often considered central for treatment coordination; it generally reflects the planning of the entire team. The social worker's written input as a professional part of the health care delivery team is indispensable in the documentation of services rendered.

Every record must have basic information that includes the date and time of entry, interview notes that describe the client and the problem or situation that requires treatment, an assessment and initial treatment plan, and therapeutic objectives and treatment responses. A time frame for intervention must be clearly established, and progress regarding that time frame must be documented. When family interventions are included, the time, date, and who was involved should always be inserted. Also, when discharge services are addressed, such as placement and so on, they need to be formally documented in the record.

The social worker practicing in today's behaviorally based managed care environment must be aware of the direct link between service delivery and good record keeping. The written connection to outcome measurement is essential. The process of assessing pretreatment, posttreatment, and follow-up measures of client progress or change must be clearly demonstrated through this written exchange. When symptom description is made, it must be stated clearly in observable, demonstrable terms that can clearly relate to the measurable treatment intervention presented. The treatment plan should also always include a detailed description of client complaints with the specific interventions used to address them. Health care social workers need to always remember the importance and power that is ascribed to this written document—especially in this time of litigation, limited service delivery access, and the movement to control health care costs.

REFERENCES

Abramson, J. S. (2002). Interdisciplinary team practice. In A. R. Roberts & G. J. Greene (Eds.), *Social workers' desk reference* (pp. 44–50). New York: Oxford University Press.

American Psychiatric Association. (2000). *Diagnostic and statistical manual of mental disorders: Text revision* (4th ed.). Washington, DC: Author.

APA Online. (2001). Documentation. *APA Practice.* http://www.apa.org/practice/meddocum.html.

Beck, A. T. (1967). *Depression: Clinical, experimental and theoretical aspects.* New York: Harper & Row.

Bernstein, B. E, & Hartsell, T. L. (1998). *The portable lawyer for mental health professionals.* New York: Wiley.

Bloom, M., Fischer, J. & Orme, J. (1999). *Evaluating practice: Guidelines for the accountable professional.* Boston: Allyn and Bacon.

Brower, A. M. & Nurius, P. S. (1993). *Social cognitions and individual change: Current theory and counseling guidelines.* Newbury Park, CA: Sage.

Burgess, E. W. (1928). What social case records should contain to be useful for sociological interpretation. *Social Forces, 6,* 539–544.

Chen, S. (1997). *Measurement and analysis in psychosocial research.* Brookfield, VT: Avebury

Cone, J. D. (1998). Psychometric considerations: Concepts, contents and methods. In A. S. Bellack & M. Hersen (Eds.) *Behavioral assessment: A practical handbook* (4th ed.; pp. 22–46), Boston: Allyn and Bacon.

Corcoran, K., & Boyer-Quick, J. (2002). How clinicians can effectively use assessment tools to evidence medical necessity and throughout the treatment process. In A. R. Roberts & G. J. Greene (Eds.), *Social workers' desk reference* (pp. 198–204). New York: Oxford University Press.

Corcoran, K., & Fischer, J. (2000). *Measures for clinical practice: A source book* (4th ed., Vols. 1 and 2). New York: Free Press.

Cormier, W. H., & Cormier, L. S. (1991). *Interviewing strategies for helpers* (3rd ed.). Pacific Grove, CA: Brooks/Cole.

Dust, B. (1996). Training needs. *Training & Development, 50,* 50–51.

Dziegielewski, S. F. (1996). Managed care principles: The need for social work in the health care environment. *Crisis Intervention and Time Limited Therapy, 3*(2), 97–110.

Dziegielewski, S. F. (1997). Time limited brief therapy: The state of practice. *Crisis Intervention and Time Limited Treatment, 3,* 217–228.

Dziegielewski, S. F. (2002). *DSM-IV-TR™ in action.* New York: Wiley.

Dziegielewski, S. F. & Holliman, D. (2001). Managed care and social work: Practice implications in an era of change. *Journal of Sociology and Social Welfare, 28*(2), 125–138.

Dziegielewski, S. F., & Leon, A. (2001a). *Social work practice and psychopharmacology.* New York: Springer Publishing Co.

Dziegielewski, S. F., & Leon, A. (2001b). Time-limited case recording: Effective documentation in a changing environment. *Journal of Brief Therapy, 1*(1), 51–66.

Dziegielewski, S. F., & Powers, G. T. (2000). Procedures for evaluating time-limited crisis intervention. In A. Roberts (Ed.), *Crisis intervention handbook (2nd ed.).* New York: Oxford University Press.

Fischer, J. (1978). *Effective casework practice: An eclectic approach.* New York: McGraw-Hill.

Frager, S. (2000). *Managing managed care.* New York: Wiley.

Gelman, S. R., Pollack, D., & Weiner, A. (1999). Confidentiality of social work records in the computer age. *Social Work, 44,* 243–252.

Gingerich, W. J. (2002). Computer applications for social work practice. In A. R. Roberts & G. J. Greene (Eds.), *Social workers' desk reference* (pp. 23–28). NewYork: Oxford University Press.

Hamilton, G. (1936). *Social case recording.* New York: Columbia University Press.

Hamilton, G. (1946). *Principles of social case recording.* New York: Columbia University Press.

Hart, R. R. (1978). Therapeutic effectiveness of setting and monitoring goals. *Journal of Consulting and Clinical Psychology, 46,* 1242–1245.

Holliman, D. C., Dziegielewski, S. F., & Datta, P. (2001). Discharge planning and social work practice. *Social Work in Health Care, 32*(3), 1–19.

Jongsma, A. E., & Peterson, L. M. (1999). *The complete adult psychotherapy treatment planne.* (2nd ed.) New York: Wiley.

Kagle, J. D. (1993). Record keeping: Directions for the 1990's. *Social Work, 38,* 190–197.

Kagle, J. D. (1995). Recording. In *Encyclopedia of social work* (19th ed., Vol. 2, pp. 2027–2033). Washington, DC: NASW Press.

Kagle, J. D. (2002). Record-keeping. In A. R. Roberts & G. J. Greene (Eds.), *Social workers' desk reference* (pp. 28–32). New York: Oxford University Press.

Kiresuk, T .J., & Sherman, R. E. (1968). Goal attainment scaling: A general method for evaluating comprehensive community mental health programs. *Community Mental Health Journal, 4,* 443–453.

Lambert, M. J., & Hill, C. E. (1994). Assessing psychotherapy outcomes and process, In S. L. Garfield & A. E. Bergin (Eds.), *Handbook of psychotherapy and behavior change* (4th ed., pp. 72–113). New York: Wiley.

Lauver, P., & Harvey, D. R. (1997). *The practical counselor: Elements of effective helping.* Pacific Grove, CA: Brooks/Cole.

Lewis, S. J., & Roberts, A. R. (2002). Crisis assessment tools. In A. R. Roberts & G. J. Greene (Eds.). *Social workers' desk reference* (pp. 208–216). New York: Oxford University Press.

Lowery, M. (1996). Total quality management. In V. B. Carson & E. N. Arnold (Eds.), *Mental health nursing: The nurse-patient journey* (pp. 1173–1192). Philadelphia: Saunders.

Maruish, M. E. (2002). *Essentials of treatment planning.* New York: Wiley.

Moreland, M. E., & Racke, R. D. (1991). Peer review of social work documentation. *Quality Review Bulletin,* 236–239.

Okum, B. F. (1997). *Effective helping: Interviewing and counseling techniques* (5th ed.). Pacific Grove, CA: Brooks/Cole.

Rankin, E. A. (1996). Patient and family education. In V. B. Carson & E. N. Arnold (Eds.), *Mental health nursing: The nurse-patient journey* (pp. 503–516). Philadelphia: Saunders.

Reamer, F. G. (2001). *Tangled relationships: Managing boundary issues in the human services.* New York: Columbia University Press.

Rock, B., & Congress, E. (1999). The new confidentiality for the 21st century in a managed care environment. *Social Work, 44,* 253–262.

Rudolph, C. S. (2000). Educational challenges facing health care social workers in the twenty-first century. *Professional Development, 3*(1), 31–41.

Schroeder, L. O. (1995). *The legal environment of social work* (rev. ed.). Washington, DC: NASW Press.

Schutte, N. S., & Malouff, J. M. (1995). *Sourcebook of adult assessment strategies.* New York: Plenum Press.

Sheffield, A. E. (1920). *The social case history: Its construction and content.* New York: Russell Sage.

Sheafor, B. W., Horejsi, C. R., & Horejsi, G. A. (1997). *Techniques and guidelines for social work practice* (4th ed.). Needham Heights, MA: Allyn & Bacon.

Starfield, B. (1992). *Primary care, concept, evaluation, and policy.* New York: Oxford University Press.

Timms, N. (1972). *Recording in social work.* Boston: Routledge & Kegan Paul.

Walsh, J. (2000). *Clinical case management with persons having a mental illness: A relationship-based perspective.* Belmont, CA: Wadsworth/Thompson Learning.

Weed, L. (1969). *Medical records, medical evaluation, and patient care.* Cleveland: Case Western Reserve University Press.

Welfel, E. R. (1998). *Ethics in counseling and psychotherapy: Standards, research and emerging issues.* Pacific Grove, CA: Brooks/Cole.

Westerfelt, A., & Dietz, T. J. (1997). *Planning and conducting agency-based research.* New York: Longman.

Wilson, S. J. (1980). *Recording guidelines for social workers.* New York: Free Press.

GLOSSARY

Accountability: When managed care and other health care delivery reviewing bodies hold social workers and other health care professionals responsible for the services provided. Important elements for consideration include quality-of-care issues, level of care used, use of ancillary services and resources, appropriate referrals, and other activities that produce cost-effective and efficient service delivery.

APIE: A form of problem-oriented record keeping often used in the medical setting. *A* = assessment, *P* = problem identification, *I* = intervention, and *E* = evaluation.

Appropriateness: The degree of compatibility, suitability, and compliance with standardized sets of criteria for service provision and delivery.

ASAP: Affordable services applied by professionals.

Audiotape recording: This form of record keeping is often used for educational purposes in the medical setting. Generally, if this form of record keeping is used in establishing service provision, it is not used alone, and another form of recording, such as the problem-oriented format, is used to supplement its use.

Audit: A standard "criteria-based" examination and review of written documentation and clinical practice provision.

Care management: Using the client's allowed benefits, a program is established to determine eligibility and direct service provision to achieve maximum functioning.

Computer standardized records: This form of record keeping first became popular in the 1980s and has significantly grown as computer technology continues to grow. A particular concern in the use of this form of record keeping is ensuring client confidentiality.

DAP or *DAPE*: A form of problem-oriented recording that is often used in health and mental health settings. *D* = data, *A* = assessment, and *P* = plan (DAP); or *D* = data, *A* = assessment, *P* = plan, and *E* = education (DAPE).

Diagnostic recording: This form of early social work record keeping was completed by a trained diagnostician. The notes were generally long and not uniform. It is rarely used as a form of record keeping in health care practice setting today.

Family-oriented records: This form of record keeping generally includes the entire household of a client, and all information is generally recorded in the same file. This type of record is considered particularly good for prevention and wellness services because it relates to the entire family. For example, when one individual is in for treatment, the medical personnel can also screen for information relevant to other family members, which is all located in the same record.

Ledgers: An early form of writing in the field of social work that recorded events after they occurred.

Malpractice: Negligence in the practice of one's profession.

Narratives: A form of early social work documentation that simply documented what transpired with a client seeking services.

Outcome criteria: Specific elements relative to evaluating end results in terms of the level of client functioning.

Outcomes management: Feedback related to the outcomes identified to improve service delivery.

Outcomes measurement: The process of assessing pretreatment, posttreatment, and follow-up measures of client change or progress.

Person-oriented record: In this form of record keeping, wellness and prevention are stressed. In addition, the record is generally considered the property of the client, who ensures that different professional services are recorded in one central record. This type of record keeping seems to be most popular in community practice or rural health care delivery settings.

PIRP: A form of problem-oriented recording that is often used in the health and mental health setting. P = problem(s), I = intervention, R = response, and P = plan.

Problem-oriented records: In this form of record keeping, emphasis is placed on limiting documentation to the problem being addressed. This is the most popular form of recording today, with numerous variations in the formats used. Examples of such formats include the SOAP, SOAPIE, PIRP, DAP, DAPE, and so on.

Process recording: An early form of social work recording that was used in the health care environment as a means of verbatim recording of the events that transpired in a session. This form of recording is still used in the medical setting; however, it is only used for educational purposes.

Single-subject research designs: Designs that help a provider establish whether the treatment provided to a client works. Target behaviors are identified and tracked throughout the treatment process.

SOAP and SOAPIE: This is one of the most popular formats for problem-oriented recording. This form is often used in medical and mental health settings. S = subjective, O = objective, A = assessment, and P = plan (SOAP); and S = subjective, O = objective, A = assessment, P = plan, I = intervention used, and E = evaluation (SOAPIE).

Time-series recording: This form of record keeping is continuing to evolve in the medical setting. Generally, target behavior(s) are clearly identified and followed over time.

Videorecording: This form of record keeping is often used in the medical setting for educational purposes. At times, recordings of surgery, procedures, and so on have been made to accompany the written record. This form of record keeping is usually supplemental.

QUESTIONS FOR FURTHER STUDY

1. Do you believe there is a need for cost-benefit information to be included in the client record?
2. How can empirical practice strategy best be reflected in the case-recording format chosen?
3. Why do you believe that problem-oriented records have gained in popularity over the years? With the advent of managed care, do you believe this popularity will decline?

CHAPTER 8

Health and Mental Health Assessment

This chapter introduces the concepts and current application principles that outline the relationship between an individual's physical health and his or her mental health. Too often distinctions are made between health and mental health when these two concepts cannot be separated. To highlight their relationship, assessment and diagnostic impressions will be exemplified to show how these terms are applied in current health care practice. The argument has been made that the health and mental health of a person are always intertwined (Dziegielewski, 2002a). Health care practice strategy is highlighted, with an explanation and emphasis on the person-in-environment (PIE) assessment scheme, and later relating the scheme to the multiaxial system of the *Diagnostic and Statistical Manual of Mental Disorders* (DSM-IV-TR) multi-axial system. In addition, considerations for future exploration and refinement are noted in this chapter.

ASSESSMENT AND DIAGNOSIS: IS THERE A DIFFERENCE?

Over the years, the formulation of an *assessment* leading to a *diagnosis* has been a source of serious debate within the profession. Carlton (1984) believed that the debate essentially stems from the fact that the profession of social work has not always separated these two entities into distinct clinical aspects of practice. This means that the clinical features inherent in either one can and often do overlap. This complicates explication and definition in many health care settings, with the result that both services (diagnosis and assessment) are viewed as interchangeable (Dziegielewski, 2002a). It is this hesitancy and inability to differentiate between these concepts that can create obvious difficulties in practice reality.

When elements within the same process are not considered distinct, the inherent concepts are allowed to blur and overlap. There is no clear difference between *assessment, diagnosis, and the relationship between the mental diagnosis and the physical health condition*. This lack of clarity within definitions and overlapping relationships causes social, personal, and professional interpretation to be varied and nonuniform in definition, practice, or approach.

To highlight the difficulty in differentiating between assessment and diagnosis further, it is important to note that the profession of social work did not develop in isolation. The social work profession and professional practice strategy have been influenced greatly by such disciplines as general medicine, psychiatry, and psychology. Moreover, in order for health care strategy to remain competitive, it is forced to adapt to the dominant culture. Most of the time health care social workers are part of the agency structure and are forced to practice within the organizational budget. Because of the pressures in the environment, it is not uncommon for social workers to feel that they are forced to reduce services to clients, treat only those who are covered by insurance or can pay privately, or terminate clients because the services are too costly (Ethics Meet Managed Care, 1997).

For the health care social worker, *assessment* is "the thinking process by which one reasons from the facts to tentative conclusions regarding their meaning" (Sheafor, Horejsi, & Horejsi, 1997, p. 134). Meyer (1995) believes that in all professions, assessment is viewed as an essential step in starting the therapeutic process "and may be viewed as the hallmark of all professional (as opposed to lay) activity" (Meyer, 1995, p. 260). She believes that assessment is truly the process that controls and directs all aspects of practice, including its nature, direction, and scope (Meyer, 1995).

Given that health care social work is such an eclectic field with many different duties, it is not unusual that the assessment process reflects this diversity. There are numerous health care settings in which social workers provide service. This makes the process of assessment dependent on a multiplicity of factors, including client need, agency function, practice setting, service limitations, and coverage for provision of service. Many times, narrowing the content of the assessment has become necessary because of reduced economic support (Meyer, 1995).

Dziegielewski (2002a) warns that although assessments completed today may appear to have a narrower focus, it is essential that utility, relevance, and salience be maintained. Therefore, for the health care social worker the process of assessment must continually be examined and reexamined carefully to ensure quality of service. If the process of assessment is rushed in the health care setting, observed mental health features may not be clearly related to physical health factors and vice versa. This can lead to important psychosocial factors being deemphasized or overlooked. Health care social workers are tasked with establishing that the practice provided is quality driven, no matter what the administrative and economic pressures may be (Davis & Meier, 2001). To support this idea, social workers remain active in reviewing changes in health care and making recommendations for consumer protection and health care quality (Steps Taken to Watchdog Managed Care, 1997). Therefore, health care social workers are tasked with not only helping to develop a comprehensive strategy to help clients, but to also ensure that quality service is provided (Dziegielewski & Holliman, 2001).

TODAY'S HEALTH CARE SOCIAL WORKER

Name: Lisa "Todd" Graddy, MSW
Title of Current Position: Mental Health Therapist
Where You Practice: Kentucky
Professional Job Title (s):   Mental Health Therapist, Hospice
                                Social Worker, and Lifestyle/
                                Behavioral Management Therapist

Duties in a typical day:
(1) I am a therapist for families of the terminally ill. I perform suicide risk assessments, drug diversion assessments, and grief counseling to those who are involved in the patient's life.
(2) In my position as a wellness/lifestyle therapist, I assess clients for their ability to change their current lifestyle. I use a model to predict success for their ability to change.

What do you like most about your current position?
I like to work with the individual as a whole. I am able to perform a psychosocial assessment that includes both their mental capabili-

ties and their physical limitations. This ability gives me a broader framework for assisting patients and their families.

What do you like least?
What others see as the role of social work and the limits it places on what I can do to help others.

What "words of wisdom" do you have for the new health care social worker who is considering working in a similar position?
Get a variety of education and experience. Try not to specialize in the established areas of medical social work. The medical arena is changing rapidly, and there is much room for medical social workers to expand their expertise and skills in new areas.

What is your favorite health care social worker story?
The chaplain and I look alike. We are the same age and have the same haircut. One time she was working with a terminally ill man who wanted to give his confession. They spent a long time working on this issue together. A few days later I was in the man's home and he leaned over to me and said, "Now I sure feel better about telling you all of that stuff so just make sure that no one else knows about it." I reported this to the chaplain and she asked if I had written up her note for visiting the patient that day since she did not have to go to make her weekly visit, having already been there that day!

CLINICAL ASSESSMENT: A SYSTEMATIC APPROACH

There are many forms of formal assessment that can support and assist in the development of an intervention plan. One system of assessment designed by social workers that has gained recent favor is that of the person-in-environment (PIE) classification system. The PIE was developed through an award given to the California Chapter of the National Association of Social Workers (NASW) by the NASW Program Advancement Fund (Whiting, 1996). Basically, the PIE is built around two major premises: recognition of social considerations and the person-in-environment stance. Both of these premises provide the cornerstones on which all social work practice rests.

According to Karls and Wandrei (1996a), the PIE system calls first for a social work assessment of the client's problems in social functioning.

"Social functioning is the client's ability to accomplish the activities necessary for daily living (for example, obtaining food, shelter and transportation) and to fulfill major social roles as required by the client's subculture or community" (p. vii). The PIE was formulated in response to the need to identify the problems of clients in a way that health professionals could easily understand (Karls & Wandrei, 1996a, 1996b). As a form of classification system for adults, the PIE provides the following:

- A Common language for all social workers in all settings to describe their clients' problems in social functioning
- A common capsulated description of social phenomena that could facilitate intervention or ameliorate problems presented by clients
- A basis for gathering data needed to measure the need for services and to design human service programs to evaluate effectiveness
- A mechanism for clearer communication among social work practitioners and between practitioners, administrators, and researchers
- A basis for clarifying the domain of social work in human service fields (Karls & Wandrei, 1996a)

The PIE system breaks down clients' problems into four distinct categories or "factors." An abbreviated version of these factors is presented here in this text. The first area is termed *Factor I*. Here the social role within each problem is identified and explored. Factor I has five categories. The first, social role, is divided into four subcategories: family roles, the role a person performs within the family (e.g., parent role, spouse role, child role, sibling role, other family role, and significant other role); other interpersonal roles where interpersonal relationships between individuals who are not family members are considered (e.g., lover role, friend role, neighbor role, member role, and other interpersonal role); occupational roles, either paid or unpaid, that a client fills (e.g., worker role—paid economy, worker role—home, worker role—volunteer, student role, and other occupational role); and special life situation roles that clients assume that are time-limited and situation-specific (e.g., consumer role, inpatient/client role, outpatient/client role, probationer/parolee role, prisoner role, immigrant role—undocumented, immigrant role—refugee, and other special life situation role) (Wandrei & Karls, 1996).

The second category to be considered under Factor I is the type of social problem that is being experienced. In the first category, emphasis is placed on identifying the social role that is causing difficulty; in this second category of Factor I, emphasis is placed on the kind of problem experienced. It is believed that there are nine types of interactional difficulties that social workers most often encounter: power, ambivalence, responsibility, dependency, loss, isolation, victimization, and the categories of "mixed" and "other." Because problems often interact and are not mutually exclusive, Wandrei and Karls (1996) recommend using the mixed category, if needed, to describe these types of problems. When the interactional difficulty cannot be related to any of these types, the category of "other" is used.

The third, fourth, and fifth areas or categories under Factor I were designed to help social workers decide if intervention was needed, the severity of the impairment, the level of impairment, and how quickly services needed to be provided. Therefore, the following three indexes were developed: the severity index, the duration index, and the coping index.

In the *severity index*, the prospect of change is measured. Generally, change factors are a necessary and functioning part of life; however, when the change factors get too extensive or rapid, problems can occur in adaptation and adjustment for the client. Wandrei and Karls (1996) proposed six levels for rating severity. In scaling, the higher the number given, the higher the degree of problem noted. The six levels identified by Wandrei and Karls (1996) are (a) no problem, (b) low severity, (c) moderate severity, (d) high severity, (e) very high severity, and (f) catastrophic. In (a), no problem, both client and practitioner perceive the problem as nondisruptive, and no intervention is needed. In (b), low severity, there are some changes noted, but the client sees the problem as nondisruptive. It is important to note, however, that although the client notes no disruption, the practitioner may note some disruption occurring. In this case, intervention is desirable but not necessary. In category (c), moderate severity, intervention would be helpful. Here the problem is viewed as disruptive to the client's level of functioning, but the level of distress does not impair function. In (d), high severity, the client is in a clear state of distress, and early intervention is indicated. In (e), very high severity, the client is in a high state of distress and *immediate* intervention is probably necessary. Here the client is subjected to significant and multiple changes in the environment that must be addressed. Lastly, in (f), catastrophic, immediate intervention is needed because the client's problem is characterized by sudden, negative changes that can have devastating implications.

In the *duration index*, the length of time of the problem has existed is noted. This can also help in assessing the chronicity of the problem and how this length of time may be related to prognosis. The duration index has six levels: (a) more than 5 years, (b) 1 to 5 years, (c) 6 months to 1 year, (d) 1 to 6 months, (e) 2 to 4 weeks, and (f) 2 weeks or fewer.

In the *coping index*, the degree to which a client can handle a problem within his or her internal resources is noted. The coping index is reflective of "the social worker's judgment of the client's ability to solve problems, capacity to act independently, and his or her ego strength, insight and intellectual capacity" (Wandrei & Karls, 1996, p. 33). There are six levels in the coping index: (a) outstanding coping skills, reflecting the client's ability to solve problems and act independently using intellectual capability and insight; (b) above-average coping skills, which is similar to level one, and several coping skills are generally expected from the average individual; (c) adequate coping skills, where the client is able to function adequately in the earlier stated areas; (d) somewhat inadequate coping skills, where the client has a fair problem-solving ability but has major difficulty in addressing and solving current problems; (e) inadequate coping skills, where the client has some skills but is unable to solve current problems and ego strength, insight, or intellectual ability are impaired when applied to the problem-solving process; and (f) no coping skills, where the client shows little or no ability to solve problems or act independently. At this level, ego strength, insight, and intellectual ability are impaired. for a review of PIE Factor I, see Table 8.1)

The second area for consideration in the PIE is *Factor II.* (see Table 8.2). In Factor I, consideration was given to explaining the problem of the client in conjunction with interpersonal relationships. Factor II goes beyond the interpersonal and looks at issues and forces that have to do with social systems. Six social system environmental problem areas are delineated: the economic/basic needs system, the educational/ training system, the judicial/legal system, the health safety and social services system, the voluntary association system, and the affectional support system. Once the areas to be considered have been

TABLE 8.1   PIE Factor I: Structural Breakdown

Type	Definition
Social role	Where each problem is identified (four categories)
Type of problem	Clarifies the interactional difficulty within the social role (nine types)
Severity of the problem	Where the problem is rated for severity based on change factors on a scale from one to six
Duration	Identifies the length and frequency of the problem (six categories)
Coping index	Measures the client's ability to cope with the problem (six levels)

established, the specific type of problem within each social system is identified. Each of the major six categories has numerous subcategories that can further describe it. The last two considerations for Factor II involve assessing a measure for the severity of the problem and recording the duration of the problem (similar to Factor I).

Factor III of the PIE classification system looks specifically at mental health problems. Clinical syndromes as recorded in the DSM-IV classification system on Axis I are recorded on Factor A. This codification system is covered later in this chapter, and special attention should be given to Axis I and its application here. Category B of Factor III deals with personality and developmental disorders. In the DSM-IV classification, most of these (except the developmental disorders) are generally recorded on Axis II and would be listed here. See Table 8.3.

Factor IV of the PIE classification scheme looks at physical health problems. Factor IV, category A, deals with diseases that are generally diagnosed by a physician. Factor IV, category B, looks at other health problems reported by the client and or other individuals (e.g., family, significant others, etc.) that may be important to the assessment process. See Table 8.4.

Using the PIE in the health care setting is similar to its use in mental health; however, greater emphasis needs to be placed on Factor IV (the physical health problems). Adkins (1996) believes that this makes knowledge of the health and medical conditions clients suffer from essential for social work professionals. Establishing Factors I and

II can help social workers get a clear sense of the relationship the problem has to the environment in a friendly and adaptable way.

As with any coding scheme, learning to use the PIE will take time. The book and manual with its practical application guidelines make the PIE a viable and practical method for assessment. However, it is important to stress that the PIE is not an independent classification system. It uses the diagnostic classification system of either the *International Classification of Diseases* (ICD-9) or the *Diagnostic and Statistical Manual* (DSM-IV-TR). This means that health care social workers must also know these two other codification systems. Actually, this may be positive for the health care social worker because it incorporates the methods used within the health care and mental health setting, which most often govern reimbursement patterns. Usage of the PIE gives health care social workers a way to categorize the numerous factors regarding the client's environment that must be considered.

CLINICAL DIAGNOSIS IN THE HEALTH CARE SETTING

Numerous types of diagnostic and assessment measurements are currently available—many of which are structured into unique categories and classification schemes. As stated earlier, it is essential for the health care social worker to be familiar with some of the major formal methods of diagnosis and assessment—especially those used and accepted in health service delivery. Social workers need this information (a) to be able to choose, gather, and report this information systematically; (b) to be aware and assist other interdisciplinary team members in the diagnostic process; (c) to interpret assessment results and help the client understand what the results of the diagnostic assessment mean; and (d) to assist the client to choose empirically sound and ethically wise modes of practice intervention. Because most fields of practice in the health care area subscribe to the medical model, the DSM-IV-TR is examined as a formal diagnostic system.

THE DSM-IV-TR

In practice today few professionals would debate that the most commonly used and accepted sources of diagnostic criteria are the

TABLE 8.2   PIE Factor II: Structural Breakdown

Type	Definition
Environmental systems	Six types of system difficulties usually beyond the individual control of the client
Economic/basic needs system	Refers to the production, distribution, and consumption functions of the economic system (e.g., food, shelter, and employment)
Education/training system	Refers to the ability of the community to meet the goals of the educational system (e.g., access to education, nurture intelligence, provide quality education programs, etc.)
Judicial/legal system	Refers to factors related to the criminal justice system of social control (e.g., lack of adequate prosecution, inadequate defense, and insufficient police services)
Health/safety and social services system	Refers to the factors in the community regarding health, safety, and so on that are beyond the direct control of the client (e.g., absence of support services impairing use of mental health services and the occurrence of a natural disaster)
Voluntary association system	Refers to the ways clients meet needs through the community by participating in social or religious groups, and so on (e.g., lack of client's preference for religious affiliation, etc.)
Affectional support system	Refers to clients who have under-involved or over-involved support systems in the marital family, extended family, friends, acquaintances, and so on
Specific type of problem in each system	Clarifies the system difficulty
Severity of the problem	Where the problem is rated for severity based on change factors on a scale from 1 to 6
Duration	Identifies the length and frequency of the problem (6–point indicator)

TABLE 8.3   PIE Factor III: Structural Breakdown

Type	Definition
Clinical	Refers to DSM-IV Axis I classifications
Personality and developmental disorders	Refers to most of the mental health conditions that are coded on Axis II

TABLE 8.4   PIE Factor IV: Structural Breakdown

Type	Definition
Physical health diagnoses	Refer to diseases that are actually diagnosed by a physician. These are related to Axis III of DSM-IV or the ICD-9.
Other health problems	Refers to conditions that are noted that may impair functioning that are reported by clients and others by a physician

Diagnostic and Statistical Manual for Mental Disorders (Fourth Edition) *Text Revision* (DSM-IV-TR) and the *International Classification of Diseases* (Tenth Edition) (ICD-10). These books are generally considered to reflect the official nomenclature in all mental health and other health-related facilities in the United States. The DSM-IV-TR (2000) is the most current version of the APA's *Diagnostic and Statistical Manual,* and revisions to this edition are expected to be completed in 2005 with the publication of the DSM-V.

Since the DSM has historically been used as an educational tool, it was felt that recent research might be overlooked if a revision was not published prior to DSM-V, which is anticipated to be published in 2005. Surprisingly, however, even with the addition of much new research and information, the DSM-IV (published in 1995), continues to be relatively up to date. Therefore, in formulating the text revision published in 2000, none of the categories, diagnostic codes, or criteria from the DSM-IV were changed. What has changed, however, is that more supplemental information is now provided for many of the current categories (American Psychiatric Association, 2000). In addition, more information is provided on many of the field trials that were introduced in the DSM-IV but were not yet completed or required updated research findings to be applied. Furthermore, special attention was paid to updating the sections in terms of diagnostic findings, cultural information, and other information to clarify the diagnostic categories (American Psychiatric Association, 2000).

Today, the DSM is similar to the ICD in terms of diagnostic codes and the billing categories that result; however, this wasn't always the case. As late as the 1980s, clinical practices often used the ICD for billing but referred to the DSM to clarify diagnostic criteria. It was not uncommon in the past to hear psychiatrists, psychologists, social workers, and mental health technicians "moan and groan" about the lack of clarity and uniformity in both of these texts (Dziegielewski, 2002a). This professional discontent became so pronounced that the message for revamping was received. Therefore, later versions of these texts clearly responded to the professional outcry of dissatisfaction over the disparity between the two texts, and similar criteria wree used in the DSM and the ICD when outlining descriptive classification systems that cross all theoretical orientations. Historically, while most clinicians are knowledgeable about both books, the DSM appears to have gained the greatest popularity and is the resource most often used by psychiatrists, physicians, psychologists, psychiatric nurses, social workers, and other mental health professionals throughout the United States. In terms of licensing and certification of most social workers, a thorough knowledge of the DSM is considered essential for competent clinical practice. Since all professionals working in health and mental health need to be capable of completing what is needed for service, it is not surprising that the majority of mental health professionals support the use of this manual (Corey, 2001).

Nevertheless, some professionals, such as Carlton (1984) questioned the choice of this path. Carlton believed that all health and mental health intervention needed to go beyond the traditional bounds of simply diagnosing a client's mental health condition. From this perspective, social, situational, and environmental factors are considered key ingredients for addressing client problems. Therefore, to remain consistent with the "person-in-situation" stance, utilizing the DSM as the path of least resistance might lead to a largely successful fight—yet would it compromise social work values. Carlton, along with other professionals of his time, feared the battle was being fought on the wrong battlefield and advocated for a more comprehensive system of reimbursement that took into account environmental aspects. Furthermore, research findings have suggested that when engaging in clinical practice many professionals did not use the DSM to direct their interventions at all. Rather, the manual was used primarily to ensure third-party reimbursement, to qualify for agency service, or to avoid placing a diagnostic label. For these reasons, clients were being given diagnoses not based solely on diagnostic criteria, and the diagnostic labels assigned were being connected to unrelated factors such as reimbursement. Therefore, some health and mental health professionals were more likely to pick the most severe diagnoses so that their clients could qualify for agency services or insurance reimbursement. Other mental health professionals engaged in the opposite behavior by assigning clients the least severe diagnoses to avoid stigmatizing and labeling them (Kutchins & Kirk, 1986, 1988, 1993).

Historically, although use of the DSM is clearly evident in mental health practice, some professionals have contested its use. The controversy centers on whether it is being utilized properly. Yet, regardless of the controversy in mental health practice, the continued and increased popularity of the *Diagnostic and Statistical Manual of Mental Disorders* (DSM) makes it the most frequently used publication in the field of mental health. In addition, the connection this diagnostic system makes between the medical condition and the mental health condition cannot be overlooked.

For some professionals such as social workers, however, the controversy over using this system for diagnostic assessments remains. Regardless of the school of thought or specific field of training a mental health practitioner ascribes to, most professionals would agree that there is no single diagnostic system that is completely acceptable by all. Furthermore, it is the opinion of this author that some degree of skepticism regarding of the appropriateness of this manual needs to continue. Since placing a diagnostic label needs to reach beyond ensuring service reimbursement and can have serious consequences for the individual client, knowledge of how to properly use the manual is necessary. In addition, there must be knowledge, concern, and continued professional debate about the appropriateness and utility of certain diagnostic categories, since those with professional experience are well aware of the fertile ground that exists for abuse.

FACTORS SUGGESTIVE OF A MENTAL DISORDER

The following indications are suggestive of a mental disorder:

- Previous psychosocial difficulties not related to a medical or neurodevelopmental disorder
- Chronic unrelated complaints that cannot be linked to a satisfactory medical explanation
- A history of object relations problems such as help-rejecting behavior, codependency, and other relationship problems
- A puzzling lack of concern on the part of the client as to the behaviors he or she is engaging in, including a detached attitude and tendency to minimize or deny the circumstances
- Evidence of secondary gain when the client is reinforced by such behaviors by significant others, family, or other members of the support system
- A history of substance abuse problems (alcohol or medication abuse)
- A family history of similar symptoms and/or mental disorders
- Cognitive or physical complaints that are more severe than what would be expected for someone in a similar situation

A detailed explanation of the DSM's multiaxial system is beyond the scope of this chapter. To learn more about the diagnostic system itself, it is suggested that the reader go to the original source, the *DSM-IV-TR.* For a further description and in-depth application of this information, Dziegielewski (2002a) is suggested. Generally, all clinical syndromes are coded on Axis I (e.g., mood disorders, chizophrenia, dementia, anxiety disorders, substance disorders, disruptive behavior disorders, etc.). In addition, all other codes that are not attributed to a mental disorder but are the focus of intervention are also coded here.

The *DSM-IV-TR* clearly states that Axis I does not denote the severity of the illness (American Psychiatric Association, 2000). It is merely where a disorder is classified, and the diagnostic category has been placed there for convenience. In completing the diagnostic assessment, there needs to be a plan for addressing every axis. The following questions relate to Axis I:

1. What are the major psychiatric symptoms a client is displaying?
2. What is the frequency, intensity, and duration of the symptom?
3. Have environmental factors, such as cultural and social factors, been considered as a possible explanation?

Axis II is used to code personality disorders in adults (but can also include those of children and adolescents) and mental retardation. Generally, disorders on Axis II start in childhood or adolescence and persist in a stable form into adulthood (generally there are not periods of remission). Like Axis I, Axis II also needs to have a plan for addressing the disorders coded on this axis. Questions to be considered include the following:

1. Is the client experiencing any lifelong maladaptive patterns?
2. Do these identified patterns tend to cause difficulty in intimate, social, or work relationships?
3. Based on these patterns, what developmental issues are arrested or currently presenting difficulty?

In the *DSM-IV-TR*, there was only one condition not attributable to a mental illness that was coded on Axis II, rather than Axis I, and that is a condition called "borderline intellectual functioning." This diagnosis was placed on Axis II because it was similar to the other disorders in that the personality traits present are believed to be enduring and pervasive.

On Axis III, physical (medical) conditions that may be relevant to the condition being addressed are listed. This section is particularly important for the health care social worker because often medical and mental health conditions overlap. To facilitate coding on Axis III, an Appendix section in *DSM-IV* lists the proper codes for these conditions. To prepare for use of this category, health care social workers should inquire into the signs and symptoms of these conditions and attempt to understand the relationship of these medical conditions to the assessment and planning process.

To assist the health care social worker, Pollak, Levy, and Breitholtz (1999) suggest several factors that can help a practitioner separate mental health clinical presentations that may have a medical contribution. First, the practitioner should give special attention to clients that present with the first episode of a major disorder. In these clients, particularly when symptoms are severe (e.g., psychotic, catatonic, and nonresponsive), close monitoring of the original presentation, when compared with previous behavior, is essential.

Second, the worker should note if the client's symptoms are acute (just started or relative to a certain situation) or abrupt with rapid changes in mood or behavior. Examples of symptoms that would fall in this area include both cognitive and behavioral symptoms such as marked apathy, decreased drive and initiative, paranoia, lability or mood swings, and poorly controlled impulses.

Third, the practitioner should pay particular attention when the initial onset of a problem or serious symptoms occurs after the age of 40. Although this is not an iron-clad rule, most mental disorders become evident before the age of 40. Thus, onset of symptoms after 40 should be carefully examined to rule out social and situational stressors, cultural implications, and medical causes.

Fourth, the social worker should note symptoms of a mental disorder that occur immediately preceding, during, or after the onset of a major medical illness. It is very possible that the symptoms may be related to the progression of the medical condition or to medication or some other substance (Dziegielewski & Leon, 2001). Polypharmacy can be a real problem for the many individuals who are unaware of the dangers of mixing certain medications and substances that they do not consider medications (i.e., herbal preparations) (Dziegielewski, 2002b).

Fifth, when gathering information for the diagnostic assessment, one should note whether there is an immediate psychosocial stressor or life circumstance that may contribute to the symptoms the client is experiencing. This is especially relevant when the stressors present are so minimal that a clear connection between the stressor and the reaction cannot be made. One very good general rule is to remember that anytime a client presents with extreme symptomoolgy of any kind and no previous history of such behaviors, attention and monitoring for medical causes are essential.

Sixth, the social worker should pay particular attention in the screening process when a client suffers from a variety of different types of *hallucinations*. Basically, a hallucination is the misperception of a stimulus. In psychotic conditions, *auditory hallucinations* are most common. When a client presents with multiple types of hallucinations such as *visual* types (seeing things that are not there), *tactile* types, which pertain to the sense of touch (e.g., bugs crawling on them), *gustatory* types, pertaining to the sense of taste; or *olfactory* types, relating to the sense of smell, this is generally too extreme a hallucination to be purely a mental health condition.

Seventh, the practitioner should note any simple repetitive and purposeless movements of speech (e.g., stuttering or indistinct or unintelligible speech), of the face (e.g., motor tightness or tremors), and of the hands and extremities (e.g., tremor, shaking, and unsteady gait). He or she should also note any experiential phenomena such as derealization, depersonalization, and unexplained gastric or medical complaints and symptoms such as new onset of headache accompanied by physical signs such as nausea and vomiting.

Eighth, one should note signs of cortical brain dysfunction such as aphasia (language disturbance) and apraxia (movement disturbance), agnosia (failure to recognize familiar objects despite intact sensory functioning), and visuo-constructional deficits (problems drawing or reproducing objects and patterns).

Lastly, the social worker should note any signs that may be associated with organ failure, such as jaundice related to hepatic disease or dyspnea (difficulty breathing) associated with cardiac or pulmonary disease. For example, if a client is not getting proper oxygen, he or she may present as very confused and disoriented. When oxygen is regulated, the signs and symptoms would begin to decrease and quickly subside. Although mental health practitioners are not expected to be experts in diagnosing medical disorders, being aware of the medical complications that can influence mental health presentations are necessary to facilitate the most accurate and complete diagnostic assessment possible (Dziegielewski, 2002a).

In closing, the following questions can be used to guide the social worker.

- Has the client had a recent physical exam? If not, suggest that one be ordered.
- Does the client have a summary of a recent history and physical exam that could be reviewed?

• Are there any laboratory findings, test, or diagnostic reports that can assist in establishing a relationship between the mental and physiological consequences that result?

Axis IV is designed to address the severity of the psychosocial stressors that have happened in a client's life over the last year. Here we are reminded of the importance of the environment. If a stressors is considered great when a mental health disorder develops, the prognosis for recovery is better. Axis IV is relevant to the profession of social work because it considers the environment. Generally, both the stressor and the severity were listed on this axis.

Axis V is used to rate the client's psychosocial and occupational functioning in the past year. To complete this task, a scale known as the Generalized Assessment of Functioning (GAF) is used. In DSM-IV-TR, the scale of the GAF has now been extended to 100 points. As before, the lower the number, the lower the level of functioning (1 = minimal functioning; 100 = highest level of functioning). The scale is listed in the DSM-IV-TR, and most professionals are not expected to memorize what each of the numbers means. The GAF continues to assess both symptomology and level of functioning. Generally, the *highest* level of functioning is determined and rated.

With the pressure in the health care field for measurement of competent and professional service, some social workers and other professionals are now turning to the GAF and other forms of measurement to provide rating scores for each client that they see (Dziegielewski, 1997, 2002a). Generally, in the health setting, functional ratings are assigned as clients enter therapy and again upon discharge. This allows for a comparison of scores that can reflect increased client functioning.

Also, in the DSM-IV "Criteria Sets and Axes Provided for Further Study," there are two scales that provide a format for ranking function that might be particularly helpful to social work professionals. The first relational functioning scale is the Global Assessment of Relational Functioning (GARF). This scale is used to address family or other ongoing relationship status on a hypothetical continuum from competent too dysfunctional (American Psychiatric Association, 2000). The second scale is the Social and Occupational Functioning Assessment Scale (SOFAS). With this scale, an "individual's level of social and occupational functioning that is not directly influenced by overall severity of the individual's psychological symptoms" can be addressed (American Psychiatric Association, 1994, p. 760). The use of these tools can help social workers to employ concrete measurements that help establish increased levels of functioning from the individual (GAF), family (GARF), and social (SOFAS) perspectives.

SPECIAL CONSIDERATIONS FOR HEALTH CARE SOCIAL WORKERS

When completing the diagnostic assessment, there are two areas coded on Axis III that are often overlooked and neglected, yet they are critical to a well-rounded comprehensive diagnostic assessment. The first falls under Diseases of the Eye and has to do with *Visual Loss* (coded 369.9) or *Cataracts* (coded 366.9). Visual loss is related to a decrease in vision (sight), yet the apparent loss of vision acuity or visual field is not related directly to substantiating physical signs. This problem may be best addressed with client reassurance (*PDR Medical Dictionary*, 1995). Cataracts are the loss of transparency in the lens of the eye. Both of these conditions result in vision impairment.

For the health care social worker, assessing for problems with vision is critical because decreased or impaired vision may lead individuals to interpret daily events incorrectly. For example, if a client is sitting by a window, he or she could be easily startled by his or her own reflection. The client might even be shocked and frightened, believing that someone is watching him or her. Clients that have trouble with vision could very easily misinterpret what is happening around them. If they do not have their glasses with them or if they have cataracts, their vision may become obstructed, and what is seen is clouded or shadowed in appearance. This lack of vision can be very frustrating for clients, especially when they cannot distinguish the shape in the window as their own. Imagine how frightened these clients might become and how easy it could be for them to become convinced a stranger is watching their every move. For health care social workers, the most salient issue to identify once the vision difficulty is recognized or corrected is whether the problem resolves itself. Regardless, as part of the general assessment special attention should always be given to screening for vision problems that may cause distress to the individual in terms of individual and social functioning.

The second medical area that is often overlooked in the mental health and health assessment process is related to *Hearing Loss* (Coded 389.9). A client with hearing impairment or hearing loss will experience a reduction in the ability to perceive sound that can range from slight impairment to complete deafness (*PDR: Medical Dictionary*, 1995). Many times a client who is having hearing difficulty may not want to admit it. At times, when an individual does not hear what is said, he or she may try to compensate by answering what he or she thought was asked or refusing to respond at all. In addition, many individuals may rely on hearing enhancement devices such as hearing aids, which amplify sound more effectively into the ear. Such hearing aids may not be able to differentiate among selected pieces of information as well as the human ear. Furthermore, as a normal part of aging, high frequency hearing loss can occur. Most noises in a person's environment, such as background noise, are low frequency. Therefore, an individual with high frequency loss may not be able to tune out background noise such as television sets or side conversations. He or she may get very angry over distractions that other people who do not have a similar hearing loss do not perceive.

Special attention should always be given during the diagnostic assessment process to ask very specific questions in regard to hearing and vision problems, since these medical problems can be misinterpreted as signs of a mental health problem. Dziegielewski (2002a) suggests that the social worker ask the following questions:

- Do you have any problems with your hearing or vision?
- How would you rate your current ability to hear and see?
- Can you give examples of specific problems you are having?
- When did you have your last vision or hearing check-up?
- Have you ever worn glasses or contact lenses?

THE ASSESSMENT PROCESS

There are five expectations or factors that need to guide the initiation of clinical assessment in the health care setting.

1. *Clients need to be active and motivated in the intervention process.* As in almost all forms of intervention, the client is expected to be active.

Furthermore, client motivation for participation in intervention planning in the health area is essential. Generally, the issues that the client must face often require serious exertion of energy in attempting to make behavioral change. This means that clients must not only agree to participate in the assessment process but must be willing to embark on the intervention plan that will result in behavioral change.

2. *The problem needs to guide the approach or method of intervention used.* Health care social workers need to be aware of different methods and approaches for clinical intervention; however, the approach should never guide the intervention chosen. Sheafor, Horejsi, and Horejsi (1997) warn against social workers becoming overinvolved and wasting valuable clinical time by trying to match a particular problem to a particular theoretical approach, especially because so much of the problem identification process in assessment is an intellectual activity. The health care social worker should never lose sight of the ultimate purpose of the assessment process. Simply stated, the purpose is to complete an assessment that will help to establish a concrete service or intervention plan to address a client's needs (see Table 8.5).

3. *The influence and effects of values and beliefs should be made apparent in the process.* Each individual, professional or not, is influenced by his or her own values and beliefs. It is these beliefs that create the foundation for who we are. In the practice of health care social work, it is essential that these individual influences do not directly affect the assessment process. Therefore, the individual values, beliefs, and practices that can influence intervention outcomes must be clearly identified from the onset of treatment. For example, an unmarried client at the public health clinic tested positive for being pregnant. The social worker assigned to her case personally believes that abortion is "murder" and cannot in good conscience recommend it as an option to her client. The client, however, is unsure of what to do and wants to explore every possible alternative. The plan that evolves must be based on the client's needs and desires, not the social worker's values.. Therefore, the social worker is advised to tell the client of her prejudice and refer her to someone who can be more objective in exploring abortion as a possible course of action. Clients have a right to make their own decisions, and health care social workers must do everything possible to ensure this right and not allow personal opinion to impair the completion of a proper assessment.

TABLE 8.5   Areas for Consideration in the Diagnostic Assessment

Area	Explanation
Biomedical factors	
General medical condition	Describe the physical illness or disability from which the client is suffering.
Overall health status	Client is to evaluate his or her own self-reported health status and level of functional ability.
Maintenance of continued health and wellness	Measurement of the client's functional ability and interest in preventive interventions.
Psychological factors	
Life stage	Describe the developmental stage in life in which the individual appears to be functioning.
Mental functioning	Describe the client's mental functioning. Complete a mental status measurement. Can the client participate knowledgeably in the intervention experience?
Cognitive functioning	Does the client have the ability to think and reason what is happening to him or her? Is he or she able to participate and make decisions regarding his or her own best interest?
Level of self-awareness	Does the client understand what is happening to him or her?
Is the client capable of and assisting in his or her level of self-care?	Is the client capable of understanding the importance and being educated about health and wellness information? Is the client open to help and services provided by the health care team?
Social factors	
Social/societal help-seeking behavior	Is the client open to outside help? Is the client willing to accept help from those outside the immediate family or the community?

TABLE 8.5 *(continued)*

Occupational participation	How does a client's illness or disability impair or prohibit functioning in the work environment?
	Is the client in a supportive work environment?
Significant other support	Does the significant other understand and show willingness to help and support the needs of the client?
Ethnic or religious affiliation	If the client is a member of a certain cultural or religious group, will this affiliation affect medical intervention and compliance issues?

Functional/situational factors

Financial condition	How does the health condition affect the financial status of the client?
	What income maintenance efforts are being made?
	Do any need to be initiated?
	Does the client have savings or resources from which to draw?
Entitlement	Does the client have health, accident, disability, or life insurance benefits to cover his or her cost of health service?
	Has insurance been recorded and filed for the client to assist with paying of expenses?
	Does client qualify for additional services to assist with illness and recovery?
Transportation	What transportation is available to the client?
	Does the client need assistance or arrangements to facilitate transportation?
Placement	Does the client have a place to return or a plan for continued maintenance when services are terminated?
	Is alternative placement needed?
Continuity of service	If the client is to be transferred to another health service, have the connections been made to link services and service providers appropriately?
	Based on the services provided, has client received the services he or she needs during and after the intervention period?

In addition to the social worker and client, the beliefs and values of the members of the interdisciplinary team must also be considered. Social workers need to be aware of value conflicts that might arise among the other team members. These team members need to be aware of how their personal feelings and resultant opinions might inhibit them from addressing all of the possible options with a client. For example, in the case of the unmarried pregnant woman, a physician, nurse, or any other member of the health care delivery team who did not believe in abortion would also be obligated to refer the client. This is not to assume that social workers are more qualified to address this issue or that they always have an answer. Social workers should always be available to assist these professionals and always advocate for how to best serve the needs of the client. Values and beliefs can be influential in identifying factors in the individual decision-making strategy and remain an important factor to consider and identify in the assessment process.

4. *Issues surrounding culture and race should be addressed openly in the assessment phase.* The social worker needs to be aware of his or her cultural heritage as well as of the clients' to ensure that the most open and receptive environment is created. Dziegielewski (2003) suggests that the social worker (a) needs to be aware of his or her own cultural limitations; (b) needs to be open to cultural differences; (c) needs to recognize the integrity and the uniqueness of the client; (d) needs to use the client's learning style, including his or her own resources and supports; and (e) needs to implement the biopsychosocial approach to practice from as integrated and as nonjudgmental a format as possible. For example, when completing a mental health assessment, cultural factors are identified and addressed prior to any type of assessment or intervention.

5. *The assessment must focus on client strengths and highlight the client's own resources for providing continued support.* One of the most difficult tasks for most individuals to complete is to find, identify, and plan to use their own strengths. People, in general, have a tendency to focus on the negatives and rarely praise themselves for the good they do. With the advent of behavioral managed care, health care social workers must quickly identify the individual and collectively based strengths that each client possesses. Once this has been achieved, these strengths must be stressed and implemented as part of the intervention plan. Identifying an individual's strengths can be directly linked

to self-determination and the individual's support networks. In this time-limited intervention environment, individual resources are essential for continued growth and maintenance and can continue as a sign of wellness long after the formal intervention period has ended.

It is assumed that the assessment begins with the first client–social worker interaction. The information that the health care social worker gathers will provide the database that will assist in determining the requirements and direction of the helping process. In assessment, it is expected that the social worker will gather information about the client's present situation and history regarding the past, and anticipate service expectations for the future. This assessment should be multidimensional and always include creative interpretation of perspectives and alternatives for service delivery.

Generally, the client is seen as the primary source of data. This information can come from either a verbal or written report. Information about the client is often derived through direct observation of verbal or physical behaviors or interaction patterns between other interdisciplinary team members, family, significant others, or friends. Viewing and recording these patterns of communication can be extremely helpful in later establishing and developing strength and resource considerations. In addition to verbal reports, written reports are also employed. Often background sheets, psychological tests, or tests to measure health status or level of daily function may be used. Although the client is perceived as the first and primary source of data, social work traditionally emphasizes including information from other areas. This means talking with the family and significant others to estimate planning support and assistance. It might also be important to gather information from other secondary sources, such as the client's medical record and other health care providers. Furthermore, to facilitate assessment, the social worker must be able to understand the client's medical situation. The social worker, although not expected to act as a physician or nurse, needs to be aware of what medical conditions a client has and how these conditions can influence behavior.

In completing a multidimensional assessment, there are four primary steps that can be well adapted to the health care setting. First, the problem must be recognized. Here the health care social worker must be active in uncovering problems that affect daily living and in engaging the client in self-help or skill-changing behaviors. It is important for the client to acknowledge that the problem exists, because once this is done "the boundaries of the problem become clear, and exploration then proceeds in a normal fashion" (Hepworth, Rooney, & Larsen, 2001, p. 205).

Second, the problem must be clearly identified. The problem of concern is identified as what the client sees as important; after all, the client is the one who is expected to create change behavior. In the health care field, it is common to receive referrals from other health care professionals. These same referrals often provide the basis for reimbursement as well. Caution needs to be exercised to prevent the referral source from determining how the problem is viewed and what should constitute the basis of intervention. It is a good idea clinically and from a cost-effectiveness stance for the health care social worker to look at each individual case and process this referral information. In addition, when striving to help the client, referral information and suggestions should always be part of your discussion with the client.

Third, the problem strategy and a plan for intervention must be developed. According to Sheafor, Horejsi, and Horejsi (1997), the plan of action is the "bridge between the assessment and the intervention" (p. 135). Here the health care social worker must help to clearly focus on the goals and objectives that will be followed in the intervention process. In the initial planning stage, emphasis on the outcome to be accomplished is essential.

Lastly, once completed an assessment plan must be implemented. The outcome of the assessment process is the completion of a plan that will guide, enhance, and in many cases determine the course of the intervention to be implemented. With the complexity of human beings and the problems that they encounter, a properly prepared multidimensional assessment is the essential first step for ensuring quality service delivery.

CHAPTER SUMMARY AND FUTURE DIRECTIONS

The helping relationship is a complex one that cannot be measured completely through the information gathered, through either the systematic approach as used in the PIE or the more diagnostic approach presented with the DSM-IV-TR multiaxial system. The information gathered from these diagnostic schemes is designed to support and assist the assessment process. This information is meant to serve as the basis for the development of intervention strategy. Therefore, a diagnostic impression or assessment needs to be intervention-friendly, thereby outlining and providing the ingredients for the treatment planning and strategy to follow. The practitioner should always consider incorporating a number of evidenced-based tools such as direct behavioral observation techniques and self-anchored rating scales. Whether social workers truly subscribe to or support the distinction between assessment and diagnosis, they still must be able to relate to other professionals and/or service providers who do. In the current health care profession, social workers must be able to show clearly that they are able to complete the task at hand—no matter what it is called. Regardless, all diagnostic or assessment activity in the health care field should be related to the needs of the client.

The social work profession has embraced the necessity for diagnosis in practice—however, this need has been recognized with caution. In accepting the requirement for completion of a diagnosis, much discontent and dissatisfaction still exist. Some social workers feel that diagnosis, when linked to the traditional definition of a medical perspective, is inconsistent with social work's history, ethics, and values. Today, however, this view is changing. Many health care social workers, struggling for practice survival in this competitive cost-driven health care system, disagree. They think that practice reality requires that a traditional method of diagnosis be completed to receive reimbursement. Their argument rests within the practice reality that it is this capacity for reimbursement that influences and determines who will be offered the opportunity to provide service (Dziegielewski, 2002a).

To compete in today's current social work environment, the role of the social worker is twofold: (a) to ensure that quality service is provided to the client; and (b) to ensure that the client has access to services and is given an opportunity to see that his or her health needs are addressed. Neither of these tasks is easy or popular in today's environment. The push for health care practice to be conducted with limited resources and services and the resultant competition to be the provider have really changed and stressed the role of the health care social work professional. However, amid this turbulence, the role and the necessity of the services the social worker provides in the area of assessment and intervention remain clear. Social workers must know the tools for assessment and diagnosis that are being used in the field, and must be familiar and able to use them. Assessment and diagnosis are often viewed as the first step in the intervention hierarchy, a step in which that social work professionals should become well versed.

There are numerous tools and methods of diagnosis currently being used. The PIE, the ICD-10, and the DSM-IV-TR represent only a small portion of what is available. These forms of systematic assessment can help to provide social workers with a framework for practice. Particularly, the ICD-9 and the DSM-IV are most reflective of the dominant view in the United States, which is rooted in the medical model. Many social workers fear that these methods may result in a label being placed on clients that is difficult to remove. Regardless, social workers have a unique role in assessment and diagnosis. As part of the interdisciplinary team, the social worker brings a wealth of information regarding the environment and family considerations essential to practice strategy. Social workers, with a focus on "skill building" and "strength enhancing," are well equipped not only to play a key role in the psychosocial assessment of the client but also to establish the intervention plan that will guide and determine the course and quality of service delivery that will be received by the public.

REFERENCES

Adkins, E. A. (1996). Use of the PIE in a medical social work setting. In J. M. Karls & K. M. Wandrei (Eds.), *Person-in-environment system: The PIE classification system for social functioning problems* (pp. 67–78). Washington, DC: NASW Press.

American Psychiatric Association. (2000). *Diagnostic and statistical manual of mental disorders* (4th ed.) Text revision. Washington, DC: American Psychiatric Press.

Carlton, T. O. (1984). *Clinical social work in health care settings: A guide to professional practice with exemplars.* New York: Springer Publishing Co.

Corey, G. (2001). *Theory and practice of psychotherapy* (6th ed.). Belmont, CA: Brooks/Cole.

Davis, S. R., & Meier, S. T. (2001). *The elements of managed care: A guide for helping professionals.* Belmont, CA: Brooks/Cole.

Dziegielewski, S. F. (1997). Time-limited brief therapy: The state of practice. *Crisis Intervention and Time-Limited Treatment, 3,* 217–228.

Dziegielewski, S. F. (2002a). *DSM-IV-TR™ in action.* New York: Wiley.

Dziegielewski, S. F. (2002b). Herbal preparations and social work practice. In A. Roberts and G. Green (Eds.), *Social workers' desk reference.* (pp. 651–657). New York: Oxford University Press.

Dziegielewski, S. F. (2003). *Clinical, advanced, intermediate: Preparation for the social work licensure exam.* Orlando, FL: Siri Productions.

Dziegielewski, S. F., & Holliman, D. (2001). Managed care and social work: Practice implications in an era of change. *Journal of Sociology and Social Welfare, 28*(2), 125–138.

Dziegielewski, S. F., & Leon, A. (2001). *Social work practice and psychopharmacology.* New York: Springer Publishing Co.

Ethics meet managed care. (1997, January). *NASW NEWS, 42,* 7.

Hepworth, D. H., Rooney, R. H., & Larsen, J. (2001). *Direct social work practice: Theory and skills* (6th ed.). Pacific Grove, CA: Brooks/Cole.

Karls, J. M., & Wandrei, K. M. (Eds.). (1996a). *Person-in-environment system: The PIE classification system for social functioning problems.* Washington, DC: NASW Press.

Karls, J. M., & Wandrei, K. M. (1996b). *PIE manual: Person-in-environment system: The PIE classification system for social functioning problems.* Washington, DC: NASW Press.

Kutchins, H., & Kirk, S. A. (1986). The reliability of DSM-III: A critical review. *Social Work Research & Abstracts, 22,* 3–12.

Kutchins, H., & Kirk, S. A. (1988). The business of diagnosis. *Social Work, 33,* 215–220.

Kutchins, H., & Kirk, S. A. (1993). DSM-IV and the hunt for gold: A review of the treasure map. *Research on Social Work Practice, 3,* 219–235.

Meyer, C. H. (1995). Assessment. In R. Edwards (Ed.), *Encyclopedia of social work* (19th ed., pp. 260–270). Washington, DC: NASW Press.

PDR: Medical dictionary (1st ed.), (1995). Montvale, NJ: Medical Economics.

Pollak, J., Levy, S., & Breitholtz, T. (1999). Screening for medical and neurodevelopmental disorders for the professional counselor. *Journal of Counseling Development, 77,* 350–357.

Sheafor, B. W., Horejsi, C. R., & Horejsi, G. A. (1997). *Techniques and guidelines for social work practice* (4th ed.). Needham Heights, MA: Allyn & Bacon.

Steps taken to watchdog managed care. (1997, January). *NASW NEWS, 42,* 12.

Wandrei, K. M., & Karls, J. M. (1996). Structure of the PIE system. In J. M. Karls & K. M. Wandrei (Eds.), *Person-in-environment system: The PIE classification system for social functioning problems* (pp. 23–40). Washington, DC: NASW Press.

Whiting, L. (1996). Forward. In J. M. Karls & K. M. Wandrei (Eds.), *Person-in-environment system: The PIE classification system for social functioning problems* (pp. xiii–xv). Washington, DC: NASW Press.

GLOSSARY

Assessment: The process of determining the nature, cause, progression, and prognosis of a problem and the personalities and situations involved therein; it is the thinking process by which one reasons from the facts to tentative conclusions regarding their meaning.

Axis I: This is the first level of coding with the DSM multiaxis diagnostic system. According to the DSM-IV classification system, the following diagnostic categories are included: pervasive developmental disorders, learning disorders, motor skills disorders, communication disorders, and other disorders that may be focus of clinical treatment.

Axis II: This is the second level of coding with the DSM multiaxis diagnostic system. According to the DSM-IV classification system, the following diagnostic categories are included: personality disorders and mental retardation.

Axis III: This is the third level of coding with the DSM multiaxis diagnostic system. According to the DSM-IV classification system, general medical conditions that can affect the mental health condition of the client are recorded.

Axis IV: This is the fourth level of coding with the DSM multiaxis diagnostic system. According to the DSM-IV classification system, the psychosocial and environmental problems/stressors, such as problems with primary support, problems related to social environment, educational problems, occupational problems, housing problems, economic problems, problems with access to health care services, problems related to interaction with the legal system, and other psychosocial problems, are recorded here.

Axis V: This is the fifth level of coding with the DSM multiaxis diagnostic system. According to the DSM-IV classification system, the level of functioning a client has is recorded on this axis.

Coping index: A coding classification within the PIE considering the degree to which a client can handle a problem with his or her internal resources.

Diagnosis: The process of identifying a problem (social and mental as well as medical) and its underlying causes and formulating a solution.

Diagnostic product: This is generally identified as what is obtained after the health care social worker uses the information gained in the diagnostic process.

Diagnostic process: Examination of the parts of a problem to determine the relationships between them and the means to their solution.

DSM-IV-TR: The *DSM-IV-TR* is a manual that presents a classification system designed to assist professionals in assigning a formal diagnostic pattern.

Duration index: A coding classification within the PIE in which the occurrence and duration of the problem is documented.

Factor I: This is the first of the four levels for problem classification used in the PIE. This constitutes a measurement of social functioning.

Factor II: This is the second area for classification used in the PIE. Emphasis here is placed on the identification of environmental problems.

Factor III: This is the third area for classification using the PIE. This category deals with mental health problems and uses the codification of the DSM-IV to describe it.

Factor IV: This is the fourth category of the PIE classification system. This area explores the physical problems and diagnoses that can affect the client.

Generalized Assessment of Functioning: A scale used on Axis V of the DSM-IV to incorporate a recording measure for a client's highest level of functioning over a certain period.

Global Assessment of Relational Functioning: This assessment is used to address family or other ongoing relationship status on a hypothetical continuum from competent to dysfunctional.

Labeling: The process of assigning a clinical diagnosis to a client that will stay with that client indefinitely.

Person-in-Environment: This is a formal method of codification that was designed by and for social workers to assist in the assessment process.

Social and Occupational Functioning Assessment Scale: A scale that can be used to address an individual's level of social and occupational functioning that is not directly influenced by overall severity of the individual's psychological symptoms.

QUESTIONS FOR FURTHER STUDY .

1. Based on the current trends and reimbursement patterns for assessment and diagnosis, what do you see as the future role for health care social workers regarding this process?
2. Do you believe that the PIE will continue to gain in popularity in the health care professions other than social work?
3. Do you believe health care social workers will abandon the use of the *DSM-IV* diagnostic categories in the future because of the potential problem that labeling can cause for clients?
4. Do you believe that a diagnostic, assessment, and intervention planning framework to guide social work practice is required for reimbursement of social work services to increase?
5. Identify what you believe are the major strengths and weaknesses in the diagnostic and assessment process used today in health care service delivery.

WEBSITES

Mental Health Net
Guide to mental health online, featuring over 6,000 individual resources; winner of several awards.
http://www.cmhc.com/

Mental Health Resources for Social Workers
Medical information on mental health for the health care social worker.
http://www.neuroscience.miningco.com

NetPsych.com
Explores new uses of the internet to deliver psychological and health care services.
Try pressing the HUH? button on this site.
http://www.netpsych.com

Psychiatric Times
Full text of news and clinical articles for mental health professionals.
http://www.mhsource.com/psychiatrictimes.html

PART III

Fields of Clinical Social Work Practice in Health Care Settings

This page intentionally left blank

CHAPTER 9

Practice of Social Work in Acute Health Care Settings

Sophia F. Dziegielewski and Diane Holliman

ACUTE HEALTH CARE SETTINGS

The history of health care social work, traced earlier in this book, lends credence to the role of the health care social worker as an integral part of health care service delivery. Throughout history, social work has been at the forefront in providing health care services to clients in the acute care setting. Today, acute care settings remain the single largest employer of clinical social workers involved in health care delivery (Poole, 1995).

The importance of acute care social work intervention was first highlighted in 1903 at Massachusetts General Hospital when Dr. Richard C. Cabot appointed Garnet Isabel Pelton, a trained nurse, to act as a clinic social worker. Dr. Cabot, as did many other physicians of his time, realized the importance of psychosocial factors in medical illness and understood that as the role and responsibilities of the physician grew, psychosocial responsibilities would have to be delegated to other helping professionals. The medical social worker was assigned duties focusing on the economic, emotional, social, and ecological needs of patients and families and was expected to relay all information gathered back to the physician (Cabot, 1919).

To accomplish the assigned tasks in the late 1800s and early 1900s, the health care social worker was required to have adequate medical knowledge, an understanding of disease and factors that affected mental health, and a firm comprehension of public health. For social workers in the acute health setting, responsibilities initially included reporting problematic domestic and social conditions to the physician, assisting and ensuring treatment compliance with the established medical regime, and providing linkages between the acute care setting and the appropriate community agencies.

With the medical advances of the late 1950s came the promotion of cardiac surgery, transplant surgery, dialysis, and neonatal intensive care. Medical social workers not only were identified as instructors for sick clients and their families, but they developed challenging roles as educators of interdisciplinary health care professionals.

In the 1960s, the nation's interest in health care increased dramatically when Medicaid and the Community Mental Health Projects were developed. With the public's resurgent regard for health matters in the United States, social work in health care began its own rebirth. "The medical social worker is in the best position of anyone on the hospital staff to bridge the gap between the hospital bed, the patient's home and the world of medical science" (Risley, 1961, p. 83).

Today, in the area of acute health care social work, there are numerous roles and services that social workers provide. There are also numerous areas or fields of practice where they are employed. Three major areas of practice for the health care social worker that will be discussed in this section are acute care medical hospitals, acute care mental health hospitals, and social work in the nephrology setting. Areas of service provision in these acute health care settings include case consultation, case finding, case planning, psychosocial assessment and intervention, case consultation, collaboration, treatment team planning, group therapy, supportive counseling, organ donation coordination, health education, advocacy, case management, discharge planning, information and referral, quality assurance, and research (Holliman, 1998). Examples of acute care settings in the field of social work can vary; yet, generally, social workers work in hospitals and other short-term care facilities, such as substance abuse treatment facilities, community mental health centers, and health and wellness outpatient services (NASW, 1995a). Table 9.1 provides a definition and brief description of the role of social work professionals in the major acute clinical practice settings.

To integrate further the actual tasks completed by the acute care social worker and the expectations within the field of practice, three

TABLE 9.1   Acute Care As a Field of Practice

Acute care medical hospitals	The provision of services that includes problems related to completion of daily activities, environmental problems, patient and family adverse reactions, or dysfunctional adjustment to illness and changes in functional status, problems related to physical, sexual, and emotional maltreatment, vocational and educational problems, legal problems, and so on. Major functions include psychosocial assessment, high-risk case finding and screening, preadmission planning, discharge planning, psychosocial counseling, financial counseling, health education post-discharge follow-up, consultation, outpatient continuity of care, patient and family conferences patient and family advocacy, and so forth.
Acute care psychiatric hospitals	Methods and services provided to patients and their families to ensure that a patient's illness, recovery, and safe transitions from one care setting to another are considered. Psychosocial factors are highlighted that include living arrangements, developmental history, economic, cultural, religious, educational, and vocational background that may impinge on the understanding, treatment, and relapse prevention of the psychiatric disorder. Functions and services provided include intake or admission evaluation, psychosocial assessment and treatment planning, high social risk case finding, education and advocacy, individual, group, family counseling, crisis intervention, consultation, expert testimony, discharge and after-care planning, and so on.
Nephrology settings	Methods and services provided to improve the quality and appropriateness of psychosocial services for patients with end-stage renal disease. Major services provided include psychosocial evaluations, casework, group work, information

(continued)

TABLE 9.1 *(continued)*

Nephrology settings *(continued)*	and referral, facilitation of community resources, team care planning and collaboration, advocacy for clients, and patient and family education.

ªAll definitions taken from NASW standards for the practice of NASW Indicators for Social Work and Psychosocial Services in Nephrology Settings, 1994. NASW Clinical Indicators for Social Work and Psychosocial Services in the Acute Psychiatric Hospital, 1994. NASW Brochures, 1994, Washington, DC: NASW.

popular and prominent areas where acute health care social workers are employed will be explicated. A case exemplar is provided that is designed to highlight acute care social work and the processes that are involved in treatment, as well as areas of strength and concern in the present state of practice delivery.

CASE STUDY

Ted (age 74) was waiting at home for his wife Martha (age 64) to return from her shopping trip. As he looked through the window, Ted was surprised to see his wife Martha walking toward their home. She had left earlier that day to go shopping and had taken the family car. Ted looked concerned as he asked her, "Where is the car?" Martha did not answer right away and continued staring off in a daze. He quickly realized that something was wrong. Martha began to cry as she replied that she could not find it. "Someone must have moved it," she said. Ted began to get excited as he asked if it had been stolen. Martha was not sure. Ted asked her if she had notified the police. Martha stated that she did not and expressed no reason for not doing so. Ted picked up the telephone to call the police. Immediately after he picked up the telephone, a thought struck him that terrified him so much he immediately put the telephone down. Ted realized this situation was much more serious than a missing car.

He asked Martha to tell him what happened. Martha said she could not and became restless as she struggled to remember the events leading to her arrival home. Ted knew she could not have gone too far from home because of her fast return. He suspected that the car had to be nearby. As they tried to retrace her steps, they found the car approximately a block away from the house. The keys were in it, and the windows were down. This event served as the catalyst for the long difficult journey Martha and Ted were about to face.

Ted immediately took Martha to the local hospital emergency room. While waiting, his thoughts were racing, making it seem like an eternity. After being evaluated, Martha was immediately admitted to the hospital. In the rush of being taken to her room, Ted could not help but feel lost within the process. No one stopped to talk with him or explain anything that was happening. The only thing he was told by the nurses was that the physician would speak with him later. At one point during the admission process, the physician told him that she had had a stroke. Later her condition was formally diagnosed as a neurological condition called vascular dementia. During the first day in the hospital, Martha's condition seemed to worsen. She was having increased difficulty speaking and was occasionally incontinent of bowel and bladder. The admitting physician was no longer attending her, and another physician had been assigned. Ted met him in the hallway after leaving his wife's hospital room.

Ted did not see a social worker until after the third day in the hospital. On arrival, Ted stated that he was dissatisfied with the care his wife was receiving. He felt as though everyone was so busy that no one seemed interested in explaining things to him. His wife was fine when he brought her in, and now she was doing poorly. "She is wetting herself and everyone acts like that is okay, and she is ready to go home." The social worker asked Ted if he had time to come and talk with her in the office. Ted joined her eagerly. The social worker listened calmly, allowing him to ventilate his frustrations. The social worker could see how Ted was struggling. While in the office, Ted put his head in his hands and began to cry. He said, "I believe this is my worst nightmare coming true." The social worker realized that he needed to talk about what he was experiencing in this process and tried not to be distracted by the fact that she had three other clients who needed placement.

Once Ted was able to process what had happened over the last few days, he was able to discuss and formulate a discharge plan. The social worker stated that, based on the recent managed care guidelines implemented by the hospital, Martha no longer had a reason that constituted her medical necessity to stay in the hospital. The physician, however, was still somewhat concerned about her and recommended a less restrictive placement until she could be further stabilized. The physician hoped Ted's wife could be placed in a supervised environment for the next few months. Ted stated that his wife had no insurance at this time because she was due to go on Medicare next year. When he retired from his job, he did not have family coverage. They did have a small savings account. The social worker explained to Ted that nursing home beds in the area were difficult to find, especially for those that were private pay. Ted seemed shocked, since he knew that not having insurance could be a problem, but he did have enough money to pay for the needed care. The social worker stated that many nursing homes allow only a few beds to be filled with private-pay individuals and that would make finding a bed more difficult. Ted was angry as he said, "That is crazy—if I can pay for it, why would they not take her?" The social worker explained that she was not really sure of all the reasons why such policies had been adapted. Her personal opinion was that insurance often remains the preferred method of reimbursement because it is more predictable than private dollars. Unfortunately, private dollars often run out much sooner. The social worker asked if Ted believed he could handle his wife at home with support. She explained the services that would be available from a home health care agency. Ted was not sure, but the physician had told him she was going to have to be discharged tomorrow, so he felt he had no choice.

Later in the day, the social worker told the physician that Martha's husband had agreed to take her home but was concerned about his ability to care for her properly. She also explained to the physician that he was concerned with the decline in his wife's condition that occurred since her admission and that no one had directly addressed this with him. The physician stated that he would be available to talk with Ted by telephone if necessary. In closing, the physician inquired about the discharge status of the two other patients who would be discharged tomorrow. The social worker stated that she had spent so much time with Ted that she had not gotten a chance to work on the other patients' placement yet. The physician was visibly agitated when he said, "That's just great" (Dziegielewski, 1996).

Unfortunately, situations similar to this one continue to occur for the acute care hospital social worker. Acute care social workers often report that they feel torn between what is best for their client, the needs of the agency, and the restrictions placed on them as part of service delivery. It is clear that in situations such as this, the price of this seemingly "cost-effective" managed care strategy far exceeded the dollar emphasis placed on it (Dziegielewski, 1996; Dziegielewski & Holliman, 2001). Martha and Ted and so many other clients can become silent victims, making the role of the acute care social worker as broker and advocate an essential one. For hospital social workers and many other professionals working in these types of short-term health care facilities, reports of such cases are becoming increasingly more common. Today, attending physicians are pressured to seek quick or early discharges for clients. In the press for time, the "humanistic" aspects of patient care which may include listening and supportive counseling can be sacrificed for maintaining the more "technical" ones such as stabilizing the patient's medical condition and prescribing medications.

ACUTE CARE MEDICAL HOSPITALS AND SOCIAL WORK PRACTICE

The current state of practice in the health care setting mirrors the turbulence found in the general health care environment (Dziegielewski, 1996; Dziegielewski & Holliman, 2001; Lens, 2002). For those who work in hospitals, this setting has always been considered a place where the pace is fast and where there is repeated and continuous access to emotionally charged areas of practice (Holliman, 1998; Mankita & Alalu, 1996).

Today, hospital social workers are, like other health care professionals, being forced to deal with numerous issues that include declining hospital admissions, reduced lengths of stay, and numerous other restrictions and methods of cost-containment (Braus, 1996). Struggling to resolve these issues has become necessary because of the inception of prospective payment systems, managed care plans, and other changes in the provision and funding of health care (Lens, 2002; Ross, 1993; Simon, Showers, Blumenfield, Holden, & Wu, 1995). Previous research has linked not receiving services to higher rates of high-risk patient relapse (Christ, Clarkin, & Hull, 1994; Hudson, 2001; Lockery, Dunkle, Kart, & Coulton, 1994).

In most hospitals, the goal of discharge planning is the arrangement of an appropriate follow-up service plan for return to a lesser level of care. Many times the role of the social worker is assumed to end once the client is discharged from the facility (Simon et al., 1995). Hospital social workers often complain that they are being forced to discharge clients from services more quickly, and clients are being returned to the community in a weaker state of rehabilitation than ever before (Bywaters, 1991; Holliman, 1998). Also, these discharge plans often have little systematic feedback about the postdischarge implementation (Resnick & Dziegielewski, 1996; Simon et al., 1995).

Acute care hospital social workers also may have different expectations of what they perceive as their role in the practice environment (Blumenfield & Epstein, 2001; Davidson, 1990). These different expectations may lead to blurring and overlap of the services that these health care professionals provide. Therefore, when health care administrators are forced to justify each dollar billed for services, there is little emphasis placed on the provision of what some term as "expendable services," such as mental health and well-being services and thorough discharge planning, in the hospital setting (Dziegielewski, 1996). Unfortunately, the services that the hospital social worker provides are often placed in this category, and, as a result, they have been forced to adjust to the brunt of initial dollar-line savings attempts.

As discussed earlier, just the sheer numbers of allied health care professionals who are moderately paid provide an excellent hunting ground for administrators pressured to cut costs. These administrators may see the role of the hospital social worker as adjunct to the delivery of care and may decide to cut back or replace professional social workers with nonprofessionals with less training in human behavior and critical thinking. These substitute professionals do not have either the depth or breadth of training when compared with the hospital social worker, and the services provided may be reflective of a different and possibly substandard level of care. For example, a trained paraprofessional in hospital discharge planning may simply facilitate a placement order. Issues such as the individual's sense of personal well-being, ability to self-care, or level of family and environmental support may not be considered. Therefore, the employment of this type of paraprofessional can be cost-effective but not quality care driven. If these personal/social and environmental issues are not addressed, clients may be put at risk for harm. The client who is discharged home to a family that does not want them is more at risk of abuse and neglect. A client who has a negative view of self and a hopeless and hapless view of his or her condition is at greater risk for depression or even suicide. Many paraprofessionals or members of other professional disciplines can differ from social work professionals because they may not recognize the importance of culture and environmental factors. Examples of situations when cultural and environmental factors play a part in patient care is when a client's family objects to a blood transfusion for religious reasons or when an elderly wife who has never driven a car is devastated that her husband is being placed in a nursing home over 50 miles away from their home. The deemphasis or denial of this consideration can result in the delivery of not only "cheap" but also substandard care.

FUTURE OF ACUTE CARE HOSPITAL-BASED SOCIAL WORK

In today's environment of behaviorally based managed care, capitation, fee for service, and decreased number of hospital inpatient beds, health care social work continues to hold a place in the acute care hospital setting. The traditional roles and tasks that are ascribed for social workers in this area, however, have and will continue to change. According to Kadushin and Kulys (1994), the future challenge for acute medical hospitals is to combine the humanitarian objective of practice with the hospitals' agenda for cost control and rationing of resources.

Hospital social work departments are moving away from traditional linear management, and the result is fewer, less structured administrative positions (Berkman, 1996). Social work services are often put under nursing or as part of nursing. This has happened in VA hospitals where social work services have been decentralized and social workers now work in service lines such as mental health or long term care.

To increase marketability, several social work programs have now begun to enter areas and provide services that are not considered traditional. For example, a program in Oregon had hospital social workers assist as financial assistance workers by helping to facilitate the efficiency and accurate identification of Medicaid and other eligibility assistance programs. By providing this service, hospital revenues were directly affected (Spitzer & Kuykendall, 1994). In addition to developing new avenues for emphasis, the relationship between cost and benefit for a program or service is also being stressed (Christ, Siegel, & Weinstein, 1995). As new programs and services are being considered, cost-benefit ratios are also being calculated as part of development and service evaluation. Cost-benefit information is of interest to administrators and hospitals because these programs must be viewed as viable and cost enhancing to get the initial support needed to be considered for implementation.

SOCIAL WORK IN THE ACUTE MENTAL HEALTH SETTING

"In many ways, acute psychiatric services represent the mental health service sector that has experienced the greatest 'boom and bust' from the 1960s to the present" (Lyons et al., 1997, p. 147). It is believed that primarily as a result of the deinstitutionalization that occurred during the community mental health movement, many individuals who were seriously mentally ill and unable to be handled in the community, had been released. This was also during the advent of psychiatric medications that allowed individuals with mental illness to live more safely and enjoy a better quality of life (Holliman, 1998). However, the mental health problems experienced by these individuals were often too serious to be handled in the community and with the pressure to return for inpatient stabilization a "revolving door" phenomenon occurred. Acute inpatient stabilization became repeatedly necessary as outside of the facility the community system remained underdeveloped and ill prepared. Many of these individuals with mental illness also became homeless or part of the prison population or criminal justice system (Draine & Solomon, 2001).

When examining health care social work service provision in the inpatient acute psychiatric center, the short duration of stay cannot be overlooked. These acute services are clearly time limited and are generally reserved for those in crisis who are in need of immediate stabilization related to either suicidal or homicidal behavior. After stabilization, these clients are generally transferred as quickly as possible to less intensive and expensive outpatient settings (Lyons et al., 1997).

FUTURE OF ACUTE INPATIENT MENTAL HEALTH SERVICES

Managed care strategies and managed health benefit programs are now considered a part of most U.S. corporations (NASW, 1995a). The current focus on health and wellness and the decreased stigma associated with the treatment of mental health problems have clearly created an increased in service requisition (Epstein & Aldredge, 2000; NASW, 1996; Lyons et al., 1997). Before the onset of managed care service delivery, most mental health services were operated on a fee-for-service basis. This meant that fee negotiations occurred between the consumer and the provider. In today's health care environment, this has changed. Today, one basic concept of managed care intervention is that the managed care provider now serves as the gatekeeper, overseer, and advocate for the services the client will be eligible to receive (Lyons et al., 1997). Because inpatient mental health treatment is considered the highest level of care and the most costly for the mental health disorders, case managers for managed care organizations are reluctant to approve it.

Considering the primary purpose of managed care, which is cost containment, one learns that "shorter" acute inpatient mental health treatment has become practice reality. The actual cost of inpatient mental health treatment, historically, is known to be variable. Thus, emphasis on cost containment is expected to continue to grow, along with the increased acceptability and desire for mental health services. Health care social workers in practice over the last 20 years have witnessed unprecedented service curtails and cutbacks—which will continue to occur. Inpatient facilities are being forced to become creative in the way they deliver services. Many of these facilities are now offering intermediate-level care programs, where less expense is associated with the treatment. Oftentimes, mental health and substance abuse programs are developing service associations, and in many cases they are offering interventions to address both problems under the same agency. In addition, most programs are continuing to develop more community-based systems where medication management and compliance are the primary service issues. In this managed system of health care, service delivery care within the formal acute inpatient setting will continue to decrease. This decrease will result in the increase of more home-based service systems, hospital day care programs, or other inpatient diversion programs. Outpatient detoxification programs and intensive outpatient substance abuse treatment programs will become more common. Considering the severe degree and unpredictability of certain mental health problems, it is not believed that acute psychiatric services will ever stop completely; however, services of this nature are sure to be more tightly controlled and severely curtailed in the future.

TODAY'S HEALTH CARE SOCIAL WORKER

Name: Michele Saunders, LCSW
List State of Practice: Florida
Title of Current Position: Vice President, Community Relations,
                             Acute Care Services
                             Licensed Clinical Social Worker

Duties in a typical day:

I represent an acute care facility where I am involved with community organizing and planning for the improvement of the service system for people with mental illnesses and/or substance use disorders. This involves strategic planning meetings with other providers, key stakeholders, and funders of services. I am also involved with program development for our organization, exploring new service opportunities to help our clientele and writing business plans or grants for funding.

I provide education through workshops, resource fairs, and community forums to the community about mental illnesses, the efficacy of treatment, and the need for the community to support these programs. I do a variety of training around mental illness issues. I also participate in legislative advocacy to improve policies and financial appropriations to people with mental illnesses and/or substance use disorders.

What do you like most about your current position?

I enjoy being involved with so many of the other community providers and stakeholders for system change and improvements. I enjoy working on the macro level of social work to impact policy decisions. I find it very rewarding to help bring around changes and improvements that will help many people. I also enjoy the advocacy and education components.

What do you like least?

Sometimes the politics involved with policy changes and system improvement can create barriers that slow down progress. Also, I have learned that not everyone involved plays fairly and there are many different (and sometimes opposing) agendas to deal with.

What "words of wisdom" do you have for the new health care social worker who is considering working in a similar position?

I would suggest they have good communication skills, learn good negotiation skills, get to know their community and its needs, and be able to build good relationships and sustain good relationships across the board. Have lots of energy and passion; and be optimistic, yet realistic. Know how to separate out the issues from what is agency-based and don't allow the issues to become personal.

What is your favorite health care social worker story?
My favorite health care social worker story related to my current position is when I was able to convene a group of providers, family members, and law enforcement officers to develop a crisis response model (based on one in Memphis, TN) called Crisis Intervention Team (CIT). Through my facilitation and direction, the group developed an effective police-based crisis response system in which specially trained officers are diverting people with mental illnesses and/ or substance use disorders into treatment and away from jail when they are in crisis. It is very rewarding to see all groups working together for the betterment of the consumer, their family, and the community as a whole.

SOCIAL WORK IN THE NEPHROLOGY SETTING

Kidney dialysis (artificial kidney treatment) and organ transplant are two medical treatments designed to help individuals who suffer from permanent kidney failure. In some cases, dialysis may also be used for acute kidney failure. Basically, the kidneys are bean-shaped organs that provide three primary functions necessary for life: (a) to help remove waste; (b) to filter the blood; and (c) to help regulate blood pressure (National Kidney Foundation, 1996). When neither of these organs is capable of working adequately, severe and often fatal illness may result.

Individuals require kidney dialysis when they develop end-stage renal disease (ESRD), where about 85% to 90% of the normal kidney function is lost. Others, who are considered good candidates may elect to have a kidney transplant, where the goal is to replace current kidney function with another human kidney that can improve the overall quality of life for the client (National Kidney Foundation, 1996). However, finding a family member who is a match or enduring the transplant waiting list is sometimes tedious and difficult. Generally, kidney dialysis services are offered in a hospital, in a dialysis unit or clinic that is not part of the hospital, or at home.

There are two types of dialysis: hemodialysis and peritoneal dialysis. Hemodialysis, where the client's blood is pumped through an artificial kidney machine, can be completed either in the acute care setting or at home. Oftentimes, treatments are done three times a week and last three to four hours. This procedure can be given at home; however, it is essential that a family member or friend is standing by to assist. In peritoneal dialysis, a solution called dialysate flows from a bag into the peritoneum, and waste products and excess fluids pass from the blood into this solution. The used solution is later removed from the body by gravity or machine. Oftentimes, when using the machine, this procedure can be done at night by connecting the tube to the machine before going to bed and disconnecting it in the morning. If it is done by gravity, the client usually changes the bag solution several times throughout the day (National Kidney. Foundation, 1996).

The process of dialysis is an intensive, time-consuming one. The resulting health care intervention for the nephrology client is generally considered a team effort. Interdisciplinary team members often include the nephrologist (physician), the transplant surgeon, the nephrology nurse, the renal nutritionist, patient care technicians, financial counselors or billing personnel, donor coordinators (when waiting for a transplant), the clinical transport coordinator (link for transportation to treatments), and the nephrology social worker. The nephrology social worker is considered an essential, necessary, and a service-reimbursable part of this health care delivery team. Because these treatments are expensive and can be draining on the social and emotional well-being of the client and his or her family, social workers are expected to help provide direct counseling and referral to help clients and their family members cope. They are also designated to help the client develop treatment plans and sources of emotional support to improve quality of life. Client compliance issues are paramount, particularly in the areas of diet and following the outlined treatment protocol. In addition, the nephrology social worker must be aware of what services are available to the client within the federal, state, and community agencies and help link the client to them whenever necessary (Dobrof et al., 2001).

Dialysis treatment was approved for Medicare reimbursement with the passage of Public Law 92603 (Sec. 2991) in 1972. In these earlier years, there was little coordination of service, and most dialysis programs were run autonomously with no coordination from the Medicare system. In 1978, however, this changed, and the ESRD network was formed (Forum of ESRD Networks, 1995). This body was to provide an oversight system to unite and regulate the care given by dialysis providers. The goal of the ESRD networks is to (a) provide immediate access to treatment; (b) treat clients with quality medical care; and (c) help individuals to maintain a quality of life that enables them to remain functioning members of the community (Forum of ESRD, 1995). In today's managed care environment, because these expensive treatment services, including those provided directly by the social worker, remain Medicare reimbursable, coordination and control to minimize excess waste and expenditures are considered essential.

To help maintain quality of life, the role of the social worker is considered integral. The functions of the nephrology social worker can include psychosocial evaluations (assessment for the treatment plan), casework (counseling and supportive intervention), group work (education and self-help), information and referral, facilitation of community referrals, team planning and coordination, patient and family education, and advocacy for clients on their behalf within the setting or beyond that with local, state, and federal agencies (NASW, 1995b). In addition, with the numerous service cutbacks and cost-effectiveness strategies, many nephrology social workers are now being required to expand their duties. Many are being asked to serve as financial counselors to ensure that the client and the service agency will receive adequate reimbursement for services needed. These services can involve assisting clients to apply for Medicare disability—to seeking outside insurance carriers to cover additional services not directly covered under Medicare guidelines (medicines, eye glasses, transportation etc.).

COMPLETION OF THE PSYCHOSOCIAL ASSESSMENT

For the nephrology social worker in today's managed care environment, of the outcomes-based psychosocial assessment can be the most difficult and time-consuming task that must be faced. However, its completion is essential to the present and future care that the nephrology client will receive. When tasked with the completion of an outcomes-based psychosocial assessment, social workers should first ask themselves the following questions: Why am I gathering this information (be clear about the purpose)? What will this psychosocial assessment tell me about the client? How will I best use this information in the establishment of specific outcomes-based objectives that will help my client once collected? In gathering information, key areas to be noted include pertinent family history, family history of illness, important people and significant others in the client's life, impact of the illness, physical functioning, occupational functioning, and emotional factors that are related to functioning level. See Table 9.2 for an outline that lists factors to be considered in the development of an outcomes-based assessment.

CHAPTER SUMMARY AND FUTURE DIRECTIONS

Berkman (1996), Dziegielewski (2002), and Holliman (1998) believe that social workers have essential skills and practice techniques that are needed in today's acute care settings. The role of the health care social worker in the acute care setting remains clear. Regardless of the acute care setting, health care social workers are integral in providing assistance with treatment plans and compliance issues; assisting clients and families with discharge planning and referral; providing counseling and support for clients and significant others in the areas of health, wellness, mental health, bereavement, and so on; assisting clients and their families to make ethical and morally difficult decisions that can affect health and mental health; educating clients, their families, and significant others to psychosocial issues and adjusting to illness; assisting in resolving behavioral problems; assisting in identifying and obtaining entitlement benefits; securing nonmedical benefits; assisting with risk management and quality assurance activities; and lastly, advocating for enhanced and continued services to ensure continued client well-being. In working with clinical social workers in the acute care setting, the practice issue that seems to cause the most concern can most simply be stated as: There is great pressure to prove (with outcomes-based interventions) that more can be done with less; all this can be accomplished in the least restrictive environment using the most time-limited strategy possible.

TABLE 9.2   Nephrology Outcomes-Based Psychosocial Assessment

Assessment category and information to be gathered:

Family of origin, nuclear family, and other information

Family Information	List and briefly describe the following: • Incidence of family illness • Myths, attitudes, beliefs about condition • Myths, values, and beliefs about health care system • Previous education about the illness • Religious, ethnic, cultural beliefs about condition • Coping strategy for dealing with illness • History of alcohol or other substance abuse • History of previous psychiatric problems Outcome indicators developed should include: • Recommendations for specific education and prevention services needed • Recommendations for "ethnic sensitive" practice
Family presence and level of involvement	List and briefly describe the following: • All family members active within the family system • Dependence and interdependence patterns of involvement • Family members viewed as helpful to the client • Family members viewed as essential to client functioning • Family members the client cares the most about Outcome indicators developed should include • Identify available family supports • If limited support, make concrete recommendations on how to increase family support network

Level of physical functioning

List and briefly describe the following:
• Predialysis level of functioning
• What is different now in level of functioning
• Present level of functioning
• Client's perception of long-term effects and illness complications
• What does client want to achieve

(continued)

TABLE 9.2   *(continued)*

Assessment category and information to be gathered:

Outcome indicators developed should include
- Establish a baseline level of functioning
- Identify return to a desirable level of functioning
- Educate about advanced directives
- Educate regarding realistic outcomes of disease

Level of social functioning

List and briefly describe the following:
- Predialysis level of social functioning (church, school, clubs, friends, hobbies, etc.)
- Present level of social functioning (what can and cannot be done)
- Long-term effects of the illness on social functioning

Outcome indicators developed should include
- Establish a baseline of social functioning
- Determine a desirable level of functioning
- Determine ways to increase client involvement

Level of emotional functioning

List and briefly describe the following:
- Predialysis level of functioning
- Previous coping skills (acceptance, understanding)
- Level of self-esteem and contentment
- Unresolved grief and loss issues
- Ability to appropriately express feelings
- Suicidal ideation and intent
- Spirituality beliefs
- Identify problems with intimacy, sexuality, sensuality, body image, etc.
- Long-term effects of the illness on emotional functioning

Outcome indicators developed should include
- Establish a baseline for emotional functioning
- Identify emotional issues that need to be addressed
- Educate and assist in development of appropriate coping skills as needed

TABLE 9.2 *(continued)*

Occupational level of functioning

List and briefly describe the following:
- Predialysis level of functioning
- Employment history
- Current employment status
- Present level of occupational functioning
  - As perceived by client
  - As perceived by family members
  - As perceived by health care team
- Understanding of long-term effects of illness
- Future employment expectation

Outcome indicators developed should include
- Establish a baseline level of functioning
- Factors that will help client return to a satisfactory level of functioning
- Outline future career considerations for enhanced functioning (education, change of job area, etc.)

Other considerations

Financial
- Identify present financial situation
- List insurance and income availability

Transportation issues
- Identify transportation barriers or service limitations

REFERENCES

Berkman, B. (1996). The emerging health care world: Implications for social work practice and education. *Social Work, 41,* 541–549.

Blumenfield, S., & Epstein, I. (2001). Introduction: Promoting and maintaining a reflective professional staff in a hospital-based social work department. *Social Work in Health Care, 33*(3/4), 1–13.

Braus, P. (1996, February). Who will survive managed care? *American Demographics, 18,* 16.

Bywaters, P. (1991). Case finding and screening for social work in acute general hospitals. *British Journal of Social Work, 21,* 19–39.

Cabot, R. C. (1919). *Social work: Essays on the meeting ground of doctor and social worker.* New York: Houghton Mifflin.

Christ, G. H., Siegel, K., & Weinstein, L. (1995). Developing a research unit within a hospital social work department. *Health and Social Work, 20,* 60–69.

Christ, W. R., Clarkin, J. F., & Hull, J. (1994). A high risk screen for psychiatric discharge planning. *Health and Social Work, 19,* 261–270.

Davidson, K. W. (1990). Role blurring and the hospital social worker's search for a clear domain. *Health and Social Work, 15,* 228–234.

Dobrof, J., Dolinko, A., Lichtiger, E., Uribarri, J., & Epstein, I. (2001). Dialysis patient characteristics and outcomes: The complexity of social work practice with the end stage renal disease population. *Social Work in Health Care, 33,* 105–128.

Draine, J., & Solomon, P. (2001). Threats of incarceration in a psychiatric probation and parole service. *American Journal of Orthopscyhiatry, 71,* 262–267.

Dziegielewski, S. F. (1996). Managed care principles: The need for social work in the health care environment. *Crisis Intervention and Time-Limited Treatment, 3,* 97–110.

Dziegielewski, S. F. (2002). *DSM-IV-TR™ in action.* New York: Wiley.

Dziegielewski, S. F. & Holliman (2001). Managed care and social work: Practice Implications in an Era of Change. *Journal of Sociology and Social Welfare, 28,* 125–139.

Epstein, M. W., & Aldredge, P. (2000). *Good but not perfect.* Boston: Allyn and Bacon.

Forum of ESRD Networks. (1995, March). *The end stage renal disease network system* [Brochure]. Los Angeles, CA: ESRD Clearing House.

Holliman, D. (1998). *Discharge planning in Alabama hospitals.* DAI-59-09A 3647 Ann Arbor: UMI: Unpublished Dissertation.

Hudson, C. G. (2001). Changing patterns of acute psychiatric hospitalization under a public managed care program. *Journal of Sociology and Social Welfare, 28,* 141–176.

Kadushin, G., & Kulys, R. (1994). Patient and family involvement in discharge planning. *Journal of Gerontological Social Work, 22,* 171–199.

Lens, V. (2002). Managed care and the judicial system: Another avenue for reform? *Health and Social Work, 27*(1), 27–35.

Lockery, S., Dunkle, R., Kart, C., & Coulton, D. (1994). Factors contributing to the early re-hospitalization of elderly people. *Health and Social Work, 19,* 182–191.

Lyons, J. S., Howard, K. I., O'Mahoney, M. T., & Lish, J. D. (1997). *The measurement and management of clinical outcomes in mental health.* New York: Wiley.

Mankita, S., & Alalu, R. (1996, spring). Hospital social work—challenges, rewards. *New Social Worker,* 4–6.

National Association of Social Workers (NASW). (1995a). *A brief look at managed mental health care* [Brochure]. Washington, DC: NASW Press.

National Association of Social Workers (NASW). (1995b). *NASW/NKF clinical indicators for social work and psychosocial services in nephrology settings* [Brochure]. Washington, DC: NASW Press.

National Association of Social Workers. (1996). *Code of ethics/NASW.* Washington, DC: Author.

National Kidney Foundation. (1996). *What everyone should know about kidneys and kidney disease* [Brochure]. New York: National Kidney Foundation.

Poole, D. (1995). Health care: Direct practice. *In Encyclopedia of social work* (Vol. 2, pp. 1156–1167). Washington, DC: NASW Press.

Resnick, C., & Dziegielewski, S. F. (1996). The relationship between therapeutic termination and job satisfaction among medical social workers. *Social Work in Health Care, 23,* 17–35.

Risley, M. (1961). *The house of healing.* London: Hale.

Ross, J. (1993). Redefining hospital social work: An embattled professional domain [Editorial]. *Health and Social Work, 18,* 243–247.

Simon, E. P., Showers, N., Blumenfield, S., Holden, G., & Wu, X. (1995). Delivery of home care services after discharge: What really happens. *Health and Social Work, 20,* 5–14.

Spitzer, W. J., & Kuykendall, R. (1994). Social work delivery of hospital-based financial assistance services. *Health and Social Work, 19,* 295–297.

GLOSSARY

Acute care medical hospitals: Hospitals that provide services to treat problems related to completion of daily activities; environmental problems; patient and family adverse reactions or dysfunctional adjustment to illness and changes in functional status; problems related to physical, sexual, and emotional maltreatment; vocational and educational problems; legal problems; and so on. Major functions include psychosocial assessment, high-risk case finding and screening, preadmission planning, discharge planning, psychosocial counseling, financial counseling, health education, postdischarge follow-up, consultation, outpatient continuity of care, patient and family conferences, patient and family advocacy, and so on.

Acute care nephrology settings: Methods and services provided to improve the quality and appropriateness of psychosocial services for clients with end-stage renal disease. Major services provided include psychosocial evaluations, casework, group work, information and referral, facilitation of community resources, team care planning and collaboration, advocacy for clients, and family education.

Acute care psychiatric facilities: Methods and services provided to clients and their families to ensure that a client's illness, recovery, and safe transition from one care setting to another is considered. Psychosocial factors are highlighted that include living arrangements, developmental history, and economic, cultural, religious, educational, and vocational background that may impinge on the understanding, treatment, and relapse prevention of the psychiatric disorder. Functions and services provided include intake or admission evaluation; psychosocial assessment and treatment planning; high social risk case finding; education and advocacy; individual, group, and family treatment and counseling; crisis intervention; consultation; expert testimony; discharge and after-care planning; and so on.

Acute care setting: A restrictive inpatient setting that is generally of a time-limited nature.

Artificial kidney: A device that removes waste products and excess fluids from the human body when the kidneys are unable to do so.

Caregivers: Individuals who assist their family members to stay in the least restrictive environment possible.

Dialysate: A solution used in dialysis to remove excess fluids and waste products from the blood.

Dialysis: Process of maintaining the chemical balance of the blood when an individual's kidneys are not able to do so.

End-stage renal disease (ESRD): The stage at which permanent kidney failure has occurred and dialysis or kidney transplant is needed to maintain life.

Hemodialysis: A form of dialysis using an artificial kidney machine to remove fluids and waste products from the bloodstream.

Medicaid: A federal-state supported program that pays for medical services for those who meet certain means-tested criteria.

Medicare: Medical insurance provided by the federal government under the Social Security Act.

Nephrologist: A physician who specializes in dealing with clients who suffer from kidney diseases.

Peritoneal dialysis: A form of dialysis that uses the client's abdominal cavity or peritoneum for dialysis treatment.

QUESTIONS FOR FURTHER STUDY

1. Do you believe that the role of the hospital social worker will continue to change? If so, what future changes do you anticipate happening?
2. Do you agree with the author's statement about linking all services provided in the health care area to include a cost-benefit ratio? How can a cost-benefit ratio be computed for social workers in the acute care setting?
3. Do you believe that services presently offered to nephrology dialysis clients will increase or decrease in the future? Why?

WEBSITES

The American Medical Association
The AMA promotes the art and science of medicine and the betterment of public health.
http://www.ama-assn.org

Health Resources and Services Administration
HRSA directs national health programs vulnerable and in-need populations.
http://www.hrsa.dhhs.gov

Med Help International
Helping those in need find qualified medical information and support for patients.
http://www.medhlp.netusa.net/

National Cancer Institute
The NCI is the federal government's principal agency for cancer
   research and training.
http://www.nci.nih.gov/

Social Work, Health & the Caring Profession
Articles, links, and information for professionals in social work and/
   or health care.
http://www.careandhealth.co.uk

CHAPTER 10

Long-Term Health Care and Restorative Health Settings

Sophia F. Dziegielewski

LONG-TERM AND RESTORATIVE CARE

It is clear in today's environment that there are numerous fields of practice for health care social workers. Clinical health care practice in long-term and restorative care settings cannot be simply defined; it refers to clinical settings that range from rehabilitative care to continued care. Recent attention has been brought to this area of health care for several reasons. One is that medical respite and long-term care services continue to increase (Dyck, 2001). Although there are numerous reasons postulated for this increase probably the most significant one is to defray or decrease hospital acute or short-term costs (Salit, Kuhn, Hartz, Vu, & Mosso, 1998). For the most part, long-term care or respite programs can help to reduce or save money for hospitals by reducing acute care services such as those provided in the emergency department. Therefore, respite programs and facilities can provide a diversion from emergency room use. This is especially important as a means toward cost reduction because emergency rooms appear to be seeing increasing numbers of individuals who are homeless, poor, and uninsured (Genignani, 1999). What complicates this further is that many of the individuals receiving emergency department care lack the means or ability to adhere to medical advice, making their health conditions worse (Ross & Mirowsky, 2000). Respite or long-term care programs can also assist with diversion from hospital admissions or decrease hospital stay by offering individuals with medical problems alternative options to inpatient acute care (Clark & Kuzmickas, 1997; Respite Conference Notes, 2000). Yet, this type of patchwork continuum requires a level of comprehensive and interrelated care that requires collaboration from an interdisciplinary perspective (Rivers, McCleary, & Glover, 2000). This intensive coordination can leave clients with unmet needs as well as increased controversy between local, state, and federal governments regarding who bears the responsibility for funding these services (Feder, Komisar, & Niefeld, 2000). Furthermore, lack of adequate and timely health care, lack of available drugs, lack of health professionals, and unaffordable user fees can have a negative impact on disease outcomes. These circumstances can escalate the problems for those who require these types of services (Amoah et al., 2000; Bassili, Omar, & Tognoni, 2001; Bjork, 2001). Without resources for medical or social services, a remediable health problem can become a permanent condition.

Poole (1995) stated that the guiding principles for restorative and long-term care were that (a) services should be provided in the least restrictive environment possible; (b) services should help and support clients in autonomous decision making; and (c) services should maximize a client's optimal level of physical, social, and psychological function and subsequent well-being. Poole (1995) suggested that there are numerous settings that could be addressed under this heading, including rehabilitative hospitals and clinics, nursing homes, intermediate care facilities, and supervised boarding homes, as well as home health care agencies, hospices, hospital home care units, and so on. Just as the settings in this area are variable, so are the services that these health care social workers provide. To integrate the actual tasks completed by the clinical social worker and the expectations within the field of practice further, two popular and prominent restorative and long-term practice areas within the health care area will be explicated.

HISTORY OF HEALTH CARE USE AND COST-CONTAINMENT MEASURES

In 1965, Title XVII (Medicare) was implemented to provide health insurance for the elderly, a high-risk group in terms of vulnerability to illness and poverty (Axinn & Levin, 1982). Medicare was one of the amendments to the Social Security Act of 1935. It was found that an increase in service use, primarily health care admissions of the elderly, did occur once the Medicare program was implemented. Rhodes (1988) linked the increase in hospital usage by the elderly to the implementation of the Medicare program.

With the implementation of the Medicare program, many elderly and disabled individuals could afford health care that they could not afford previously; physicians and hospitals also benefited, as greater flexibility in providing needed health care services was secured. In 1983, Congress mandated a radical change in the payment structure for hospital care to rescue the Hospital Insurance Trust Fund from imminent bankruptcy (Lee, Forthofor, & Taube, 1985). In the original system that was "fee for service," Medicare paid what hospitals charged for a particular service. Astoundingly, it was found that many of the same services were costing different amounts, depending on who provided it. The government wanted to achieve some regulation, and in an attempt to do so, the payment system based on diagnostic-related groups (DRGs) was developed (Begly, 1985).

DIAGNOSTIC-RELATED GROUPS

The DRG system was originally created to produce an equitable and standard payment scale across all hospitals. In this system, service recipients were grouped together who had similar conditions and resources. These groups made up the hospital product called the *case mix*. Case information was gathered, and time-limited outcomes were developed. Once completed, these cases were classified into units called DRGs. Originally, three classes of DRGs were designated: surgical, medical, and psychiatric. Each diagnostic category was designated with a particular length of stay (e.g., gallbladder removal, 7 days).

This new system presented several problems for health care providers. First, because the DRG payment schedule was fixed, acute hospitals and inpatient settings knew how much money they would receive for each individual case. This provided little incentive for hospitals to treat individuals who might extend beyond the current average number of allowable days for a particular diagnosis. In this system, hospitals were given incentives to avoid or refuse to accept patients who might require an extended stay. Unfortunately, elderly and disabled individuals, who generally had chronic or complicating conditions, were highly affected by this practice. When dealing with this type of client, where it was expected that the hospital stay might be longer than the allowable DRG days, hospitals received no motivation *not* to discharge the client as quickly as possible.

This "quick" discharge process created two problems for the health care social worker employed in the restorative or long-term setting. First, many of these frail individuals were low-income elderly who had minimal supports in the community for restorative extended home care assistance (Blazyk & Canavan, 1985). Second, many individuals were being discharged to long-term care facilities in sicker condition than they were previously. Nursing home social workers, in particular, complained about the increase in serious illnesses from which their new clients were suffering. Nursing staff was also stressed because these new patients required much more care and observation. Considering the for-profit motive behind most restorative home care or long-term care facilities, increases in staff rarely occurred to accommodate the additional needs of these new more labor-intensive clients. At times, readmission to the acute care setting, which is more costly for the individual and the hospital, was required (Berkman & Abrams, 1986).

The advent of the DRG and the relationship it has to managed care can still cause problems for health care social workers because they generally handle the discharge and placement options for elderly individuals in both restorative and long-term care settings. Because of managed care pressures, health care social workers must be aware of and have immediate access to community support services to facilitate "quick" discharge back into the community. Family members and other essential caregivers need to be aware of the client's medical condition, including signs, symptoms, and how to deal with emergency situations. Education about the needed medical treatment can generally be handled by the physician or the home health care nurse. However, responsible social work practice requires initiating this process and ensuring that it has been completed.

Discharging frail individuals who are sicker because of limited DRG days may place additional stress on the family or extended care staff. In discharges back into the community, family stress is often viewed as a major contributing factor to long-term care admission (Pratt, Wright, & Schmall, 1987). Measures should be taken to allow families to communicate needs, problem-solve, and have available support groups. Health care social workers provide excellent ports of entry for supportive and educational services for both clients and their families.

A frail client who needs a 'great deal of individual attention through restorative home care or in the long-term inpatient treatment facility can create increased stress for staff members. Support groups and regular inservice training on how to treat these individuals become mandatory. If additional staff is needed to facilitate service needs, recommendations for such support should be made.

TODAY'S HEALTH CARE SOCIAL WORKER

Name: Holly Bailey, LBSW
List State of Practice: Alabama
Professional Job Title: Director of Social Services
                              Long Term Care Facility

Duties in a typical day:
To ensure that the residents' needs are met my weekly duties include facilitation of care planning meetings, which consist of input regarding a client's progress toward individual care objectives. I work as part of an interdisciplinary team that consists of nurses, nurse's aides, a dietitian, and an activity director. I am also responsible for quarterly assessments, which are submitted to the state on the care provided. I am also responsible for making phone calls and coordinating the needs of our clients with families and their support systems. I work closely with the nurses on developing and implementing any behavioral management objectives that are needed.

What do you like most about your position?
I work in a close-knit agency where staff and clients and family all work together to support the clients we serve. We are a Christian-affiliated facility and many of the clients and their families share a common bond with other residents and their families. I also love helping clients to become more independent or secure the services they need to meet their own needs.

What do you like least about your position?
One negative aspect of my position is what I refer to as "jackpot justice." Since many attorneys advertise to the community to encourage lawsuits against nursing homes, this advertisement encourages certain individuals to look for problems or magnify problems that might otherwise be easily addressed.

What "words of wisdom" do you have for the new health care social worker who is considering working in a similar position?
I find this work very rewarding. I feel like my job has purpose when I can help a client who has to live in chronic pain every day to gain more independence and self-respect. No matter how busy you get always remember to take time to allow for one-to-one interaction with the clients you serve. Just listening and making efforts to help can make a client feel so much better.

What is your favorite health care social work story?
My favorite case example happened when I helped a client who suffered from muscular dystrophy. This resident reached the point where he could no longer sit in his own wheelchair. He was forced to spend most of the day in a reclining geriatric chair, and he constantly told everyone how unhappy he was. After consultation with others I found that a special wheelchair could be purchased but it was not covered by insurance and was so expensive that his family could not afford it. After making some phone calls, I was able to find a sponsor. The local Easter Seals Association purchased the chair and helped us to adjust it to the resident's needs. Now the resident can be seen self-propelling by in his new wheelchair. To add to the final touch, our activities director made a license plate for the back of his wheel chair that says "Roll Tide." This is the motto for the Alabama State University football team.

THOSE IN NEED OF RESTORATIVE AND LONG-TERM CARE

Any discussion of long-term care facilities and restorative home care services would be incomplete without a discussion of the elderly, since they are the primary recipients of such services in the United States. For many frail elderly individuals, long-term care has become or will become a way of life (Garner, 1995). As the sheer numbers of elderly individuals increase, so does the possibility of dealing with impaired health status (Childs, 2000). This trend is expected to continue, especially as infants born after World War II (often referred to as the "baby boomers," or the "baby-boom cohort" born from 1945 to 1965) continue to age (Butler, 1994; Garner, 1995; Rhodes, 1988). With the increased emphasis on health and well-being, outlined clearly in Healthy People

2000, the healthy life span is expected to grow (U.S. Department of Health and Human Services, 1995). It is further predicted that death rates will continue to decline, leaving more aged individuals in society, especially among the "old" old, or those over age 75. Growth within the elderly population combined with strides within the scientific community have led to increased interest in promoting and understanding the factors that lead to longer and healthier life spans (Belsky, 1988; Mosher-Ashley, 1994; Rhodes, 1988). This is an area for clinical social work advocacy and intervention in the long-term and restorative settings that cannot be ignored.

In general, elderly individuals are now seeking, and in many cases expecting, relief from their health care concerns. They use acute hospital services, physician services, and long-term care services more than any other age group (Rhodes, 1988). This is an interesting development, when the elderly only make up 12% of the total population of the United States yet account for 30% of the nation's annual health care costs (McCullough & Cody, 1993). This trend has made elderly individuals the focus of much discussion in the managed health care environment.

HEALTH ISSUES IN LONG-TERM AND RESTORATIVE HOME CARE

When working with clients in restorative home care or long-term care settings, health issues considered important can generally be divided into two types: chronic physical impairment and mental health concerns. With the elderly, there is probably no factor of more immediate concern than the potential loss of physical health (Brody & Brody, 1987). Many of these individuals fear the chronic loss of unaided activity or perceived independence. A chronic condition is generally defined as a disease that is of long duration, constituting a long, drawn-out progression (Taber's Cyclopedic Medical Dictionary, 1977). An acute condition, conversely, generally has a rapid and severe onset that lasts for a short duration (Taber's Cyclopedic Medical Dictionary, 1977).

There are many studies relating the financial costs of chronic diseases to the quality of life of ill people and their families. The costs related to the chronic conditions generally include direct costs, indirect costs, and hidden costs (Bjork, 2001; Shobhana et al., 2000; Chew, Goh, & Lee, 1999). The costs directly related to chronic illnesses include charges for medical care or self-treatment that are borne by the patient, government, organized health care providers, or insurance companies. Examples are inpatient care, emergency visits, physician services, ambulance use, drugs, devices, and outpatient and diagnostic tests. The burden of any chronic disease weighs not only on those who are ill. It also has a significant indirect cost because it has a pronounced effect on their families, on state or local authorities who provide social assistance (if such exists), and on any others who assist and support the chronically ill (Guico-Pabia, Murray, Teutsch, Wertheimer, & Berger, 2001).

Unfortunately, the elderly or disabled individual is often affected by chronic physical or mental conditions, as opposed to acute ones. From a psychosocial perspective, suffering from a chronic condition is generally the elderly person's worst fear because this type of condition often results in a loss of activity or of unaided mobility (Rhodes, 1988). Further, physical and mental health conditions are often related and interdependent. For example, a physical (physiological) condition, such as a stroke, may develop into a mental health (psychological) condition known as dementia.

PHYSICAL AND MENTAL HEALTH ISSUES IN THE LONG-TERM CARE SETTING

In the long-term health care setting, the fear of activity loss, and the actual occurrence of such loss are areas that should be addressed by the health care social worker. Because many of these individuals suffer from chronic conditions, the probability of the condition getting better is unlikely. In this society, there is a tendency to deny that problems may be terminal. Family members and other interdisciplinary team members may tell aged people that the condition will get better rather than helping the individual develop ways to cope with the existing condition.

It is important for clinical health care social workers working in the long-term care setting to be knowledgeable of these chronic conditions, their signs and symptoms, and the expected progression of various diseases. Further, there is considerable evidence to support the importance of involvement and support by family members in creating a general sense of well-being in the elderly individual (Dziegielewski, 1990, 1991; Rubinstein, Lubben, & Mintzer, 1994). A definition of the methods and roles of the health care social worker in the long-term setting is provided in Table 10.1. The health care social worker can help in educating clients and family members to cope with and understand changes that will occur. A comprehensive assessment of the individual, considering health conditions and environmental factors, remains critical.

ISSUES FOR SOCIAL WORKERS IN THE LONG-TERM CARE SETTING

Health care clients suffer many life stresses, including widowhood, social and occupational losses, and physical health problems that are often of a progressive nature. In addition, many health care social workers are expected to provide service to mentally impaired clients who are admitted to restorative home care or long-term care facilities (Marks, Flannery, & Spillane, 2001). With the availability of nursing home beds, this trend could continue to increase. One reason for this increase is deinstitutionalization; over the past 33 years, state mental hospitals have shrunk to one third their former size (Talbott, 1988). In the last 30 years, many privately run long-term care facilities, including adult congregate living facilities (boarding homes) and intermediate-and skilled-level care nursing homes, have been opened. For example, of the 1.6 million nursing home residents in 1996, 17% of them required assistance with two or more activities related to self-care (Grando et al., 2002). These homes can also provide a discharge option for mentally impaired elderly clients that other population groups do not have. Most of the patients admitted to extended care facilities are over age 65. Several authors (Diamond, 1986; Dobelstein & Johnson, 1985; Lusky, 1986; Swan, 1987; Talbott, 1988) have suggested that old-age homes are convenient but inappropriate placement options for the mentally impaired elderly, since they do not provide mental health services. Marks, Flannery, and Spillane (2001) argued that there is little empirical support to guide families and others in placement decisions, and the national trend to place mentally impaired elderly in these facilities without adequate support continues. Although some authors argue that Americans' use of nursing home care is decreasing. These arguments are based on the fact that many individuals are seeking alternatives to institutionalized care (Bishop, 2000). This means that individuals admitted to these facilities often have more serious conditions and are unable to access other types of supportive care.

TABLE 10.1   Definition of Services in the Long-Term Care Setting

Long-term care health care social worker services	A method of providing services of assessment, treatment, rehabilitation, supportive care, and prevention of increased disability of people with chronic physical, emotional or developmental impairments. These areas of practice generally are multidisciplinary and can include general hospitals, chronic disease hospitals, nursing homes (skilled nursing facilities and intermediate care facilities), rehabilitation centers, hospices, residential centers for the developmentally disabled, day care programs, home health care programs, and so on.

Note. Definition taken from NASW standards for the practice of NASW Standards for Social Work Services in Long-term Care Facilities, 1991, Washington, DC: NASW Press.

Regardless, few long-term care facilities provide psychosocial interventions, and medication is heavily emphasized as the sole method of treatment. Therefore, health care social workers need to question the practice of using the long-term care setting as a placement for the mentally impaired elderly. It is important to note that although each facility is different, it cannot be assumed that mental health services will be provided. Social workers need to be aware of what long-term facilities exist in an area and the services that these facilities can offer to the mentally impaired elderly client.

RESTORATIVE HOME CARE SOCIAL WORK[*]

CASE STUDY

Mary is 73 years old. Her husband Jack is 78 and has recently suffered from a stroke. Jack and his wife retired to Florida and have been living there for the past 5 years. They have no family in the state; however,

---

[*] The author would like to thank Dr. Cheryl Resnick for her contributions in writing this section on restorative home care social work.

they do have several friends and acquaintances that live nearby. Mary has also had several health problems and is recovering from an episode of shingles that surfaced after a recent episode of the flu.

On discharge from the hospital, Jack was released home with the assistance of home health care services. Services that he has been receiving include speech therapy, physical therapy, and nursing assistance. Today, the social worker has been asked to visit the home because physical therapy is about to be discontinued. There will also be a withdrawal of the home health aides that have been going to the home and assisting with bathing and so on. Mary has requested the appointment. She called the home health care agency in tears, stating that she does not know what she will do because she cannot possibly handle Jack without this support. Mary remembered how helpful the social worker was in implementing the treatment services after discharge to the hospital and felt comfortable asking her once again for advice and support.

Home-based services have become more popular because of the personal care involved and the emphasis on cost savings over institutionalized care. Based on these factors, it is easy to see why home health care has experienced an enormous burgeoning in the past decade; home health care is viewed as a humane and compassionate way to deliver health and supportive services (Walker, 1996). In fact, it has been recognized as the fastest-growing component of Medicare spending, with 2.2 million Medicare recipients receiving $7 billion worth of services in 1991. A tripling of expenditures from the $2.1 billion spent in 1987 has been illustrated (Ingoldsby et al., 1994).

The transformation of hospital reimbursement in "managed care" often necessitates the swift discharge of patients from the hospital setting to home. In addition, they are likely to be more acutely ill on discharge from the acute care facility. This had led many to think that elderly patients are being discharged from hospitals "quicker and sicker" (Proctor et al., 1996; Schwartz et al., 1990; Stewart et al., 1995; Simon et al., 1995; Wimberley & Blazyk, 1989). Those opposed to institutional care are vulnerable in that home health services rarely, if ever, provide the around-the-clock nursing and monitoring that rehabilitative settings and nursing homes do (Proctor et al., 1996). In addition, this population is known to suffer with an increasing number of chronic illnesses (Schwartz et al., 1990).

The prevailing economic climate has greatly altered the face and nature of home health care (Stewart et al., 1995). The resultant movement toward the incorporation of home health services has created and recreated meaningful roles for health care social workers.

HISTORY AND DEVELOPMENT OF RESTORATIVE HOME CARE

As noted previously, the profession of social work has a strong history grounded in home visitation. In the days of the Charity Organization Societies, friendly home visitors frequently interacted with individuals in need in the home environment (Norris-Shortle & Cohen, 1987). Traditionally, home visitation provided one way to offer services to nonvoluntary clients and those less likely to frequent agency offices because they were socially isolated, ostracized, ill, incapacitated, or homebound (Norris-Shortle & Cohen, 1987; Wasson, Ropeckyj, & Lazarus, 1984). Home visitation enabled social workers to intercede with populations who otherwise would be less likely to receive interventions and services.

Perhaps, partly for the previously stated reasons, Hancock and Pelton claim that "the conference and the friendly visiting were considered the most valuable components of the helping process" (1989, p. 21). In fact, home health services in the United States date back to the late eighteenth century (Levande et al., 1988). When the Community Mental Health Act of 1963 shifted care toward the community, the government mandated that local communities provide services to meet the basic mental health needs of residents. Title XVIII amendments to the Social Security Act inspired Medicare services in 1965. Medicare mandated service delivery within the home and reimbursed social work services offered through certified home health agencies (Axelrod, 1978).

Silverstone (1981) defines long-term care as "one or more services provided on a sustained basis to enable individuals whose functional capacities are chronically impaired to be maintained at their maximum levels of health and well-being" (p. 85). Levande et al. (1988) describe an increasing need for home health social workers to work with dependent elders. They indicate that such intervention is both cost-effective and provides timely long-range planning for the elderly population by linking older persons with resources, informal networks, and potential family care options (Levande et al., 1988). In today's managed care milieu, with increasing focus on cost containment and expense reduction, home social work visitation provides an economical, viable option in service delivery. In fact, home health care often serves as a mechanism to offset institutionalization, deferring rehospitalizations, rehabilitative hospital stays, and nursing home placements.

POPULATION RECEIVING SERVICES

In this environment of deliberation about the financial solvency of Medicare, the well-being of our aged population may stand in the balance. Health care organizations are intensifying efforts to coordinate appropriate discharge plans for the aged in an effort to link this population with necessary community services (Wimberley & Blazyk, 1989). It is anticipated that relevant linkage with community resources will result in decreased hospital readmission rates.

Prescott et al. (1995) indicate that 22% of Medicare hospitalizations experienced readmission within 60 days of discharge between 1974 and 1977. They cite references that demonstrate that the readmission rate may be as high as 27%. Their research additionally establishes that 48% of the readmissions were potentially preventable.

Those 60 years and older exhibited a greater need for home health care, displayed longer hospital lengths of stay, and suffered a greater number of diagnoses. Several social variables appeared to play an important role in hospital readmission. These social factors encompassed issues regarding nursing home placement, inadequacy of community social support systems, mental impairment among many of the elderly, poor functional status, poverty, and survival of those of advanced age (85 years and older) (Prescott et al., 1995). Ironically, these groups were not only the most likely to experience hospital recidivism but were also those most in need of appropriate home health services. Those needing services are often unaware of exactly what community resources exist and may not understand how to access such services. Proctor et al. (1996) noted that up to 50% of hospital readmissions are due to inadequate supportive services in the home. Home health social workers serve a critical need both before hospital discharge and most certainly afterward. Wimberley and Blazyk (1989) found that 34.7% of their sample had three or more hospital admissions in the past year, and 10% of all patients were readmitted to the hospital within 7 days of discharge. Their results indicate that those needing community services were likely to be admitted to the hospital more frequently and those who overstayed the DRG required more referrals to community agencies.

Under the current reimbursement systems, skilled home care needs are more likely to be reimbursable through insurance than are custodial care needs. Those needing home health aides to assist with activities of daily living may find themselves ineligible in the absence of skilled service needs, and with recent cutbacks in funding of social services, community resources are not always readily available. To alleviate this situation, the Social Work Department at Mount Sinai Medical Center established an interim home care program (Schwartz et al., 1990). Through grant funding, hospital funds, and partial patient payment, home health aide services were provided for 4 to 12 hours for 6 to 8 weeks. Continuity of care was achieved in 95.2% of cases, 96.2% of the patients achieved independence after the interim care services, and only 6.6% experienced hospital readmissions within a 30–day period (Schwartz et al., 1990). Therefore, the time-limited home health assistance of intensive posthospital care administered to elderly clients resulted in decreased hospital lengths of stay and decreased hospital readmissions, and assisted the elderly population in maximizing their levels of independence. Integration of adequate home care services has a great potential to reduce hospital readmission rates, simultaneously maximizing the potential recovery and independence of the elderly patient population.

Ingoldsby et al. (1994) employed a three-division classification system to depict home health care participants. Their study delineated individuals who are post acute, medically unstable, and primarily chronic. Post acute was defined as individuals receiving recuperative care (e.g., recovering from a stroke, fracture, recent surgery, etc.). Medically unstable was defined as individuals with a medical condition, making them vulnerable to additional medical complications (e.g., diabetes, respiratory problems, and congestive heart failure). The third group was defined as those with chronic long-term illnesses that resulted in a steady decline in function (e.g., dementia, Parkinson's disease, and general frailty) (Ingoldsby et al., 1994, pp. 27–28). These three groups of identified home health clients are the population most likely to obtain home health care services.

FAMILY AS CAREGIVER

Hospital discharges do not always work out as planned. In one study, more than 23% of the chronically ill and elderly hospitalized patients were discharged with discharge plans rated as barely adequate or worse (Simon et al., 1995). When these frail elderly cannot access formal community support systems, not only are they put at enormous risk (for readmission to the hospital, long-term institutionalization, and extreme emotional consequences), but family/friend caregivers then bear the consequences of inadequate discharge planning.

Caregivers are usually family members and friends, most often women, usually a spouse, daughter, or daughter-in-law, who are likely to accept responsibilities to the detriment of their own work and families. These caregivers must juggle their own commitments when adding caregiver responsibilities to other roles and functions (Stone et al., 1987). Spousal caregivers are more likely to be older and unemployed and to view provision as a normative expectation of marriage. They provide a greater number of care hours and a higher number of services. Child providers evidence a greater degree of role strain and show interesting gender patterns of care provision (Young & Kahana, 1989). Men are more likely to assist with home repairs, household chores, and driving functions, whereas women cook, clean, shop, and become involved in the more intimate operations (e.g., bathing, personal care, etc.). In Young and Kahana's study (1989), 61% of caregivers experienced low energy, 21% endured a decline in general health, and 37% sustained mental health aftereffects.

Several important factors impact caregiving. Among them are: the number and level of patient demands, additional caregiver responsibilities, the physical condition of the caregiver (when the caregiver is an elderly spouse, she or he may be frail and sick), whether or not the caregiving function is temporary or permanent, the amount of social support available (e.g., respite), and the number of family conflicts surrounding the caregiving situation (e.g., one sibling assuming major caregiving responsibilities) (Morrow-Howell et al., 1993). Clearly, professional help can only benefit overburdened informal systems.

Research also demonstrates that caregiver burden, caregiver strain, caregiver inner emotional conflict, as well as a lack of community support greatly impact family/friend and elderly well-being (Hasselkus, 1988; Young & Kahana, 1989; Zarit et al., 1986). Because people are being discharged from hospitals "quicker and sicker," as has been stated previously, caregivers are being asked to know and do more in a greatly technologically advanced, medical environment. As Morrow-Howell et al. (1993) point out, "families may be coerced into caregiving because of economic and moral pressures without concern for their caregiving abilities"; they go on to remind us that "willingness does not ensure adequate care" (p. 189).

Family burden may be great when insufficient discharge planning results in delayed implementation of home health services; "delays in delivery were correlated with reported deterioration in patient functional abilities and poorer ratings of the emotional health of household members" (Simon et al., 1995, p. 10). When caregivers feel excessive burden, they are more likely to promote institutionalization as a caretaking option (Penning, 1995; Zarit et al., 1986).

Well-coordinated, excellent home health service capable of providing caregiver respite and training is critical to the containment of emotional as well as financial burdens. This must be a collaborative effort between staff and family/friends—one in which a realistic evaluation of caregiver capabilities can be made. Sensitivity is shown by the professional so as to enable and encourage the caregiver's perception of "ownership" of the caretaking tasks (Hasselkus, 1988). These balancing tasks are not easy and can be both realized and sustained through professional social worker intervention.

RESTORATIVE HOME HEALTH CARE AS A FIELD OF PRACTICE

Social work roles in home health care can be varied as well as demanding. They include dealing with parent/child relations; recognizing, reporting, and intervening with elder abuse; counseling regarding family/marital issues; assisting with personality adjustment and adjustment to diagnoses and consequences of medical illness; advocating in legal and housing predicaments; and obtaining community resources and material assistance. The role of the social worker involves frequent, complex telephone interaction, consultation with interdisciplinary staff, facilitation of interagency interactions, and service provision as well as referral communications (Vincent & Davis, 1987).

Assessment, a primary social work function, requires a thorough comprehension of the medical, emotional, mental, social, and environmental factors impacting a client. Recognition of these elements is essential in formulating decisions as to whether or not the client will adjust and adequately function at home. Axelrod (1978) outlines four major functions of home health social workers: casework, counseling, and advocacy, as well as program coordination. She defines the parameters as the assessment of function, development, and implementation of a treatment plan. Through this process, both family/caregiver and client can receive therapeutic interventions that will enable them to develop skills of coping and independence.

Home care visits are short term and time limited in nature, necessitating proper referrals and interdisciplinary cooperation. Axelrod (1978) describes another potential social work function—that of program coordinator. Many social workers in home care have assumed such supervisory responsibilities. They are "accountable to the agency for assurance that service is being delivered in keeping with administrative directives" (Burack-Weiss & Rosengarten, 1995, p. 191). The supervisor must ensure that social work services are provided for clients and their caregivers in ways that will maximize the ability of clients to perform activities of daily living and experience a higher quality of life. The social work supervisor in home care has additional responsibilities of training and consultation and the ongoing provision of support to staff. Interdisciplinary team members must coordinate efforts to optimize client recovery and movement toward independent function. Development and organization of new programs, such as volunteer training and activation of volunteer units, can be a primary role of the home health social worker. Axelrod (1978) also alludes to social work roles in writing grants, locating funding sources, and advocating through legislative testimony. This makes the role of the home care supervisors critical, since they have the supplementary obligation to ensure that efficient discharge planning from home care services occurs.

Discharge planning from home care services is as critical as discharge planning from the hospital. It entails teaching caregivers and patients to manage independently. The home health social worker is crucial to this process. Stewart et al. (1995) found that although patients are sicker on admission to home care services, most improve and do not remain homebound. When patient and caregiver abilities to cope are maximized, independent functioning after discharge from home care services is often the result (Cox, 1992).

Persons with unmet home health needs are known to have more poor outcomes than those receiving adequate services (Proctor et al., 1996). As demonstrated earlier, family and friends may not be properly trained and can provide only so much in the way of caregiving assistance. In fact, "for too many patients, formal providers did not provide the care or services expected by the hospital-based social worker" (Proctor et al., 1996, p. 37). These gaps in service often reflect a failure of family and friends to provide all that the discharge planner hoped might be available through these sources. Home health services alleviate caregivers' stress, a necessary element in maximizing recovery for older home health clients.

Restorative Home Care and Case Management

The role of the managed care case manager regarding home care services must be understood. Case management in social work has typically been defined as a method of providing services whereby a professional social worker assesses the needs of the client and the client's family. When appropriate, the social worker also arranges, coordinates, monitors, evaluates, and advocates for a package of multiple services to meet the specific client's complex needs (NASW, 1995). In managed care, however, this traditional definition has been modified. Today case managers (many of whom are not social workers) generally serve as gatekeepers who are capable of referring, initiating, or disallowing service provision. Therefore, the primary role of the managed care case manager is to link the client to the most cost-effective and efficacious service possible.

A home health referral is generally triggered when there is a need for a diagnostic profile, and when the client's case meets the use review referral criteria; or there are unmet discharge planning needs. Home health care social workers need to be aware of the role of the case manager and keep open the lines of communication. Being accessible by telephone, fax, mail and e-mail are just some of the ways that communication between the two can be highlighted. Each case manager will expect that the referral source is accredited by JCAHO (Joint Commission on Accreditation of Hospitals) and that there is a understanding of these principles. For example, the social worker must be aware of the importance of coordination of care while implementing the basic standards for a continuum of quality care. She or he must also be able to outline the service that will be provided so that insurance benefits are understood. Outcome data must highlight treatment effectiveness whether the health care social worker deals directly with the managed care case manager or not; many times the case manager will be the entry point for service delivery. When working in the restorative health care setting, the social worker needs to familiarize herself or himself with the individuals serving in this role and the influence that these communications can have on service referral and delivery.

PLANNING FOR DEATH IN LONG-TERM AND RESTORATIVE HOME CARE

Much of the confusion in our society regarding death can be linked to the denial, secrecy, and fear of death that we have created (LaRue, 1985). Death is an inevitable part of life, yet many individuals in our society spend most of their time ignoring and avoiding this fact, at least until it affects them directly. It is usually at this time that an individual struggles with feelings of loss, separation, guilt, fear, and anger. Many individuals fear the unknown that death will bring and the loss of independence that often comes with a chronic illness. Family members fear making decisions about a loved one, especially regarding continuing or discontinuing one's life (Dziegielewski & Harrison, 1996). The elderly individual and the family member often turn to science and medicine for the answers. Physicians, as representatives of the scientific and healing community and leaders of the interdisciplinary team, are often sought out and expected to have the answers and make sense of decisions. However, physicians are taught from the day they enter medical school to preserve life, and many physicians are not prepared to deal with the psychosocial aspects of dying (Nolan, 1987). The training of physicians has prepared them to be "rescuers from pain, and many times these physicians see themselves as arch rivals from death" (LaRue, 1985, p. 11). Since physicians cannot always handle the full responsibility of dealing with the possibility of death, and since they are part of an interdisciplinary team, the social worker is often sought after to help the individual or the family cope with death.

Before the health care social worker can successfully help the family or the individual to deal with factors related to death and dying, several areas must be examined. First, the health care social worker must become aware of her or his own feelings regarding death. Many social work practitioners, not unlike their medical counterparts, are uncomfortable with the subject of dying (Dziegielewski & Harrison, 1996). To assist in understanding the concept of death, it may help for the social worker to become acquainted with how death is viewed in other countries and by certain religions. For example, the Roman Catholic Church has been responsive in its quest for more literature regarding an individual's right to die (LaRue, 1985). By becoming aware of the alternative conceptions of death and the legitimating of the role of death, social workers may become somewhat desensitized to the perception or mysticism surrounding death in this country. Once desensitized, the health care social worker is able to relate these alternative concepts to individual clients or their family and friends.

The second concern in helping individuals deal with death is to know the resources or services available in the community that might assist the individual to prepare for death. One such service is the hospice program. Hospice services, which are funded by Medicare, offer services to individuals who are suffering from terminal illness and are expected to have 6 months or fewer to live (Crichton, 1987). These programs do not focus on prolonging life beyond its natural end. Often the social worker serves as part of an interdisciplinary team designed to assist the individual and family members in preparation for natural death.

LIVING WILL

The health care social worker must also be familiar with the implementation of a *living will*. Most individuals are aware of the need for, and do complete, a will that declares who will receive their money, property, and other worldly goods. However, a living will is less often contemplated and implemented (Paterson, Baker, & Maeck, 1993). The living will is a document that allows an individual to state, in advance, preferences relating to the use of life-sustaining procedures in the event of a terminal illness. In completing a living will, many individuals are given the chance to state when they want to avoid unwanted life-sustaining measures. This type of will can be especially helpful to family members, who are frequently left with the burden of making this decision when their medically ill relative is mentally incapacitated (Dziegielewski & Harrison, 1996). Without such a will, family members may avoid making this type of decision because they may believe that initiating such a procedure gives them too much control and responsibility over the medically ill person. A living will is generally created by simply expressing one's wishes while in a state of sound mind and body, and having the document legally witnessed.

REFERENCES

Amoah A. G., Owusu, S. K., Acheampong, J. W., Agyenim-Boateng, K., Asare, H. R., Owusu, A. A., Mensah-Poku, M. F., Adamu, F. C., Amegashie, R. A., Saunders, J. T., Fang, W. L., Pastors, J. G., Sanborn, C., Barrett, E. J., & Woode, M .K. (2000). A national diabetes care and education programme: The Ghana model. *Research and Clinical Practice. 49*, 149–157.

Axelrod, T. B. (1978). Innovative roles for social workers in home care programs. *Health and Social Work, 3*, 48–66.

Axinn, J., & Levin, H. (1982). *A history of American response to need.* New York: Harper & Row.

Bassili, A., Omar, M., & Tognoni G. (2001). The adequacy of diabetic care for children in a developing country. *Diabetes Research and Clinical Practice, 53*, 187–199.

Begly, C. (1985). Are DRGs fair? *Journal of Health and Human Resources Administration, 8*, 80–89.

Belsky, J. (1988). *Here tomorrow: Making the most of life after fifty.* Baltimore, MD: Johns Hopkins Press.

Berkman, B., & Abrams, R. (1986). Factors related to hospital readmission of elderly cardiac patients. *Social Work, 31*, 99–103.

Bishop, C. E. (2000). Where are the missing elders? The decline in nursing home use. *Health Affairs, 19*, 249–250.

Bjork S. (2001). The cost of diabetes and diabetes care. *Research and Clinical Practice, 54*(1), S13–S18

Blazyk, S., & Canavan, M. (1985). Therapeutic aspects of discharge planning. *Social Work, 30*, 489–495.

Brody, E., & Brody, S. (1987). Aged. In A. Minaham (Ed.), *Encyclopedia of social work* (18th ed., pp. 106–126). Silver Spring, MD: NASW.

Burack-Weiss, A., & Rosengarten, L. (1995). Challenges for the home care supervisor. *Journal of Gerontological Social Work, 2*, 191–211.

Butler, R. N. (1994). Baby boomers: Aging population at risk. *Geriatrics, 49*, 13–14.

Chew, F. T., Goh, D. Y., & Lee, B. W. (1999). The economic cost of asthma in Singapore. *Austria New Zealand Medicine, 29*, 228–33.

Childs, N. (2000). Covering the costs of graying America. *Provider, 26*(2), 51–52.

Clark, B., and Kuzmickas, D. (1997). Respite care programs offer a safe place to heal. *Health Care for the Homeless Information Resource Center.* Available online: *www.prainc.com/hch/newsletter/mar 97 c.htm.*

Cox, C. (1992, March). Expanding social work's role in home care. *Social Work, 37*, 179–183.

Crichton, J. (1987). *The age care source book: A resource guide for the aging and their families.* New York: Simon & Schuster.

Diamond, T. (1986). Social policy and everyday life in the nursing home: A critical ethnography. *Social Science Medicine, 23,* 1287–1295.

Dobelstein, A., & Johnson, B. (1985). *Serving older adults: Policy, programs and professional activities.* Upper Saddle River, NJ: Prentice Hall.

Dyck, M. J. (2001). A public policy concern: Access to long-term care. *Journal of Gerontological Nursing, 27*(7), 13–22.

Dziegielewski, S. F. (1990). *The institutionalized dementia relative and the family member relationship.* Unpublished doctoral dissertation, Florida State University, Tallahassee.

Dziegielewski, S. F. (1991). Social group work with family members of elderly nursing home residents with dementia: A controlled evaluation. *Research on Social Work Practice, 1,* 358–370.

Dziegielewski, S. F., & Harrison, D. F. (1996). Social work practice with the aged. In D. F. Harrison, B. A. Thyer, & J. Wodarski (Eds.), *Cultural diversity and social work practice* (2nd ed., pp. 138–175). Springfield, IL: Charles C Thomas.

Feder, J., Komisar, H. L., & Neifeld, M. (2000). Long-term care in the United States: An overview. *Health Affiliates, 19*(3), 40–56.

Garner, J. D. (1995). Long-term care. In R. Edwards (Editor-in-Chief), *Encyclopedia of social work* (Vol. 2, pp. 1625–1634). Washington, DC: NASW Press.

Genignani, J. (1999). Workers' triple whammy: Low paid, unhealthy and uninsured. *Business and Health, 17*(10), 53–54.

Grando, V. T., Mehr, D., Popejoy, L., Maas, M., Rantz, M., Wipke-Tevis, D. D., & Westhoff, R. (2002). Why older adults with light care needs enter and remain in nursing homes. *Journal of Gerontological Nursing, 28*(7), 47–53.

Guico-Pabia, C. J., Murray, J. F., Teutsch, S. M., Wertheimer, A. I., & Berger, M. L. (2001). Indirect cost of ischemic heart disease to employers. *American Journal of Managed Care, 7*(1), 27–34.

Hancock, B. L., & Pelton, L. H. (1989). Home visits: History and functions. *Social Casework, 70,* 21–27.

Hasselkus, B. R. (1988). Meaning in family caregiving: Perspectives on caregiver/professional relationships. *Gerontologist, 28,* 686–691.

Ingoldsby, A., Kumar, N., Cohen, M. A., & Wallack, S. S. (1994). Medicare home health care: The struggle for definition. *Journal of Long-Term Home Health Care, 13,* 16–31.

LaRue, G. A. (1985). *Euthanasia and religion.* Los Angeles, CA: The Hemlock Society.

Lee, E., Forthofor, R., & Taube, C. (1985). Does DRG mean disastrous results for psychiatric hospitals? *Journal of Health and Human Services Administration, 8,* 53–78.

Levande, D., Bowden, S. W., & Mollema, J. (1988). Home health services for dependent elders: The social work dimension. *Journal of Gerontological Social Work, 11,* 5–17.

Lusky, R. (1986). Anticipating the needs of the U.S. elderly in the 21st century: Dilemmas in epidemiology, gerontology and public policy. *Social Science Medicine, 23,* 1217–1227.

Marks, L., Flannery, R. B., Spillane, M. (2001). Placement challenges: Implications for long-term care for dementia sufferers. *American Journal of Alzheimer's Disease and Other Dementias, 16*(5), 285–288.

McCullough, P. K., & Cody, S. (1993). Geriatric development. In F. S. Sierles (Ed.), *Behavioral science for medical students* (pp. 163–167). Baltimore, MD: Williams & Wilkins.

Morrow-Howell, N., Proctor, E. K., & Berg-Weger, M. (1993). Adequacy of informal care for elderly patients going home from the hospital: Discharge planner perspectives. *Journal of Applied Gerontology, 12,* 188–205.

Mosher-Ashley, P. M. (1994). Diagnoses assigned and issues brought up in therapy by older adults receiving outpatient treatment. *Clinical Gerontologist, 15,* 37–64.

National Association of Social Workers (NASW). (1995). *A brief look at managed mental health care.* Washington, DC: Pamphlet, NASW Press.

Nolan, K. (1987). In death's shadow: The meanings of withholding resuscitation. *Hasting Center Report, 17,* 9–14.

Norris-Shortle, C., & Cohen, R. R. (1987). Home visits revisited. *Social Casework, 68,* 54–58.

Paterson, S. L., Baker, M., & Maeck, J. P. (1993). Durable powers of attorney: Issues of gender and health care decision making. *Journal of Gerontological Social Work, 21,* 161–177.

Penning, M. J. (1995). Cognitive impairment, caregiver burden, and the utilization of home health services. *Journal of Aging and Health, 7,* 233–253.

Poole, D. (1995). Health care: Direct practice. In *Encyclopedia of social work* (Vol. 2, pp. 1156–1167). Washington, DC: NASW Press.

Pratt, C., Wright, S., & Schmall, V. (1987). Burden, coping and health status: A comparison of family caregivers to community dwelling institutionalized Alzheimer's patients. *Social Work, 10,* 99–112.

Prescott, P. A., Soeken, K. L., & Griggs, M. (1995). Identification and referral of hospitalized patients in need of home care. *Research in Nursing and Health, 18,* 85–95.

Proctor, E. K., Morrow-Howell, N., & Kaplan, S. J. (1996). Implementation of discharge plans for chronically ill elders discharged home. *Health and Social Work, 21,* 30–40.

Respite Conference Notes. (2000, September). *Chicago gathering for respite care with the homeless.* Conference conducted at the Egan Conference Center, DePaul University, Chicago, IL.

Rhodes, C. (1988). *An introduction to gerontology: Aging in American society.* Springfield, IL: Charles C Thomas.

Rivers, P. A., McCleary, K. J., & Glover, S. H. (2000). Long-term care financing: Are current methods enough? *Journal of Health and Human Services Administration, 22*(4), 472–494.

Ross, C. E., and Mirowsky, J. (2000). Does medical insurance contribute to socioeconomic differentials in health? *Milbank Quarterly, 78,* 291–321.

Rubinstein, R. L., Lubben, J. E., & Mintzer, J. E. (1994, March). Social isolation and social support: An applied perspective. *Journal of Applied Gerontology, 13,* 58–72.

Salit, S. A., Kuhn, E. M., Hartz, A. J., Vu, J. M., & Mosso, A. L. (1998). Hospitalization costs associated with homelessness in New York City. *New England Journal of Medicine, 338,* 1734–1740.

Schwartz, P. J., Blumfield, S., & Simon, E. P. (1990). The interim home care program: An innovative discharge planning alternative. *Health and Social Work, 15,* 152–160.

Shobhana, R., Rama, R. P., Lavanya, A., Williams, R., Vijay, V., Ramachandran, A. (2000). Expenditure on health care incurred by diabetic subjects in a developing country—a study from southern India. *Diabetes Research and Clinical Practice, 48*(1), 37–42.

Silverstone, B. (1981). Long-term care. *Health and Social Work, 6,* 285–345.

Simon, E. P., Showers, N., Blumfield, S., Holden, G., & Wu, X. (1995). Delivery of home care services after discharge: What really happens. *Health and Social Work, 20,* 5–14.

Stewart, C. J., Blaha, A. J., Weissfeld, L., & Yuan, W. (1995). Discharge planning from home health care and patient status post-discharge. *Public Health Nursing, 12,* 90–98.

Stone, R., Cafferata, G. L., & Sangl, J. (1987). Caregivers of the frail elderly: A national profile. *Gerontologist, 27,* 616–626.

Swan, F. (1987). The substitution for nursing home care for in-patient psychiatric care. *Community Mental Health Journal, 23,* 1.

Taber's cyclopedic medical dictionary. (1977). Philadelphia: F. A. Davis.

Talbott, J. (1988). Taking issue. *Hospital and Community Psychiatry, 39,* 115.

U.S. Department of Health and Human Services. (1995). *Healthy people 2000: Midcourse Review* (1995 revisions). Washington, DC: U.S. Public Health Service.

Vincent, P. A., & Davis, J. M. (1987). Functions of social workers in a home health agency. *Health and Social Work, 12,* 213–219.

Walker, A. (1996). The cost-effectiveness of home health: A case presentation. *Geriatric Nursing, 17,* 37–40.

Wasson, W., Ropeckyj, A., & Lazarus, L. (1984). Home evaluation of the psychiatrically impaired elderly: Process and outcome. *Gerontologist, 24,* 238–242.

Wimberley, E. T., & Blazyk, S. (1989, November). Monitoring patient outcome following discharge: A computerized geriatric case-management system. *Health and Social Work, 14,* 269–276.

Young, R. F., & Kahana, E. (1989). Specifying caregiver outcomes: Gender and relationship aspects of caregiver strain. *Gerontologist, 29*, 660–666.

Zarit, S., Todd, P. A., & Zarit, J. A. (1986). Subjective burden of husbands and wives as caregivers: A longitudinal study. *Gerontologist, 26*, 260–266.

GLOSSARY

Caregivers: Individuals who assist their family members to stay in the least restrictive environment possible.

Case management: A method of providing services whereby a professional assesses the needs of the client and the client's family, when appropriate, and arranges, coordinates, monitors, evaluates, and advocates for a package of multiple services to meet the specific client's complex needs.

Home health care social work: Providing services to the client in the home or the least restrictive living environment possible.

Restorative home care services: This term is used interchangeably with home health care services.

Social work in long-term care settings: Provision of services in the area of assessment, treatment, rehabilitation, supportive care, and prevention of increased disability of people with chronic physical, emotional, or developmental impairments. These practice settings are generally multidisciplinary and can include general hospitals, chronic disease hospitals, nursing homes (skilled nursing facilities and intermediate care facilities), rehabilitation centers, hospices, residential centers for the developmentally disabled, day care programs, home health care programs, and so on.

QUESTIONS FOR FURTHER STUDY

1. Do you believe that the role of the restorative home care social worker will continue to change? If so, what future changes do you anticipate happening?
2. Do you believe that the health care social work in the long-term setting will continue to change? If so, what future changes do you anticipate happening?

WEBSITES

The ALZHEIMER Page
Links to everything you need to know on the above topic; also good
for patient's families (large type).
http://www.biostat.wustl.edu/alzeheimer

Alzheimer's Association
Information about chapters, caregiver resources, medical and public
policy
information, and links.
http://www.alz.org

American Public Health Association
APHA is an association with members from over 50 occupations in
the public health field. A unique, multidisciplinary environment
of professional exchange and study.
http://www.alpha.org/

The Center for Independent Living
CIL is a national leader in helping people with disabilities live
independently and productively.
http://www.cilberkley.org/

Chronic Illness Network
The first Internet multimedia source dedicated to chronic illnesses,
including AIDS, Persian Gulf War Syndrome, autoimmune disorders, and a host of others.
http://www.chronicillnet.org/

DeathNET
Specializes in information concerning euthanasia, suicide, living
wills, and terminal illnesses. Dying with dignity theme, houses
archives of Dr. Jack Kevorkian.
http://www.IslandNet.com:80/ ~deathnet

Disability Information and Resources
One of the largest collections of resources on all types of disabilities.
http://www.eskimo.com/ ~jlubin/disabled.html

Electronic Rehabilitation Resource Web Site
A lot of information about handicaps and rehabilitation. Papers,
    databases, listings of support organizations, and funding sources.
http://www.sjuvm.stjohns.edu/rehab/

Family Caregiver Alliance
Information about statistics and research, public policy, publications,
    and more.
http://www.caregiver.org/

Grief Network
Bereavement, grief, death, and dying resources.
http://www.rivendell.org/

HIV/AIDS
The Detroit Community AIDS Library (DCAL) offers some of the
    most information on this topic.
http://www.libraries.wayne.edu/dcal/aids.html

Institute for Health, Health Care & Aging Resources
Local, state, and national health care and policy issues.
http://www.ihhcpar.rutgers.edu

CHAPTER 11

New Horizons: Health and Wellness Counseling

Sophia F. Dziegielewski and George Jacinto

HEALTH PROMOTION AND SOCIAL WORK PRACTICE

> A paradigm shift in medicine away from disease and illness and toward an emphasis on wellness and health is occurring.
> —J.L. Randall

The current shift in the medical paradigm toward an emphasis on wellness and health fits well with the holistic approach of social work. In health settings throughout history, health and wellness interventions have been a form of counseling in which social workers have engaged. In the past, this type of service was viewed as an adjunct to other methods of intervention. With the influence of behaviorally based managed care services and the paradigm shifts that have occurred, providing this type of counseling has become an expected part of practice. Whether this service is provided directly to clients or to fellow members of the interdisciplinary team, social workers are making vital contributions.

Generally, when most professionals think of health and wellness counseling, they think of providing it to individual clients; however, this type of counseling can be more inclusive and involve an individual, family, group, or community. In today's environment, the need for health and wellness counseling is expanding, and what was usually thought of as the domain of the public health social worker has increased to include other social work settings such as community-based agencies. While a number of approaches have been suggested, most incorporate the "whole" person in the context of the individual's environment as the focus of intervention. The goal of the wellness approach is to assist individuals in planning to live more fully in every aspect of functioning by integrating body, mind, and spirit in a meaningful manner (Smith, Myers, & Hensley, 2002). Many health care professionals are now being called on to provide one-to-one counseling in this area and to provide workshops and other forms of health maintenance and awareness services. Community-focused health promotion programming involves group as well as individual strategies. Many times social workers are challenged to provide educational information as part of the counseling dimensions of wellness programming. For instance, one may provide a seminar on wellness and then meet with small groups or individuals to assist individuals in applying the newly learned information to their life routines.

This holistic type of specialized education and counseling varies from assisting with weight reduction programs and smoking cessation programs to providing information and techniques to address stress management. Health and wellness counseling offers social workers another area for expansion that will help many social workers do what they really like—provide counseling. A holistic approach to counseling requires that one perceives the client in the environment and pays attention to interpersonal exchanges. The environment comprises one's family, neighborhood, employment setting, and the larger community. The interactions of many people in the community affect the health and well-being of entire populations. While wellness promotion has been primarily used with middle-class White clients, a shift toward use in poor ethnic neighborhoods has shown success as well. For instance, The Well, a neighborhood-based health promotion for Black women located in a housing project in central Los Angeles, provided an office for a nurse practitioner with a database for scheduling clinic visits with hospitals and health practitioners, an exercise and fitness room, and a lounge/library (Brown, Jemmott, Mitchell, & Walton, 1998). The services of The Well included self-help groups, health education, a walking-for-wellness program, facts and feelings workshops, exercise classes, family planning, a birthing project, prevention, economic development activities, "sister circles" and health advocacy services. The Well employed social work counseling and empowerment techniques. The program was owned by neighborhood residents, and it had a convenient neighborhood-based location, a working relationship with a university, and a number of community partnerships.

Social workers can also enter into partnerships with formal health counseling programs and can assist in providing professional services. For example, *employee assistance programs* (EAPs) have gained tremendously in popularity. The premise that employee assistance programs are built on is simple: "When employees are struggling with problems in their personal lives, these problems can have a negative impact in the workplace" (Levitt, 1994, p. 428). There are numerous advantages for health care agencies and providers to support these types of intervention with their workers. It is beyond the scope of this chapter to explain the historical and current role of social work in EAP; however, its relevance and applicability are important for establishing further marketability of health care social work.

SOCIAL WORKERS CONTRIBUTE TO WELLNESS PROMOTION EFFORTS

Whether this service is provided directly to clients or fellow employees, there are three specific benefits that social workers who engage in the provision of health counseling can provide. First, social workers have expertise in working with and integrating the behavioral bio-psycho-social-spiritual factors related to an individual, and they can use their expertise to demonstrate how these factors can positively affect health and wellness. Maintenance of health and wellness includes a number of multifaceted tasks such as individual and group counseling, family planning, prevention efforts, economic development activities, community organization, advocacy, empowerment, psychoeducational workshops, marketing, and exercise classes, to name a few (Altpeter, Earp, & Schopler, 1998; Brenner, 2002; Brown et al., 1998; Myers, Sweeney, & Witmer, 2000). These tasks are interrelated approaches that are well suited for the trained social work professional who can understand and incorporate these factors into the overall intervention process.

Second, social workers are skilled in counseling and understanding individual and family dynamics. Many times in instruction of health education, the simple presentation of information is not enough. Clients may need the additional assistance that only a trained professional can provide. For example, a client was recently diagnosed with adult-onset diabetes. He was immediately referred for health and dietary advice because the physician wanted to initiate a trial of dietary control before placing him on medications. After the client's numerous failures to self-regulate dietary needs, a referral to the health care social worker was made. On interviewing the client, it became obvious to the social worker that the client knew exactly what he was supposed to eat and why. The dietary education that was provided appeared adequate. In exploring this further, it appeared that the client was angry over his diagnosis and in a misguided way was rebelling against it. In addition, he stated that he did not prepare the meals his wife did. When asked how he felt about his diet, the client stated, "I tell my wife what to cook and she doesn't listen." In this situation, the social worker was able to help the client recognize the need to resolve issues regarding acceptance of his own medical limitations and vulnerability. She also invited the client's wife to attend an intervention session, and together they discussed the implications of his diabetes, and how it was affecting their relationship. At the conclusion of the session, the social worker helped to arrange for the wife and the client to both meet with the dietitian one more time. After two meetings with the social worker, diet compliance improved significantly, and the client was able to maintain his condition without medication supplementation. This example helps show how the social worker can be a valuable asset in recognizing individual problems and family considerations that could otherwise impede progress.

A third area, which is probably the most important, is that social workers are trained in formal diagnosis, assessment, and intervention. If an individual is experiencing a mental health problem that is beyond his or her control, the social worker has the capability to address it or make an appropriate reference. Schools of social work generally train social workers in the basics of diagnosis, assessment, and intervention planning. In practice, these skills are adapted to assist the client who is intervention noncompliant or in need of attaining more involved health and wellness services. Social workers who are part of the interdisciplinary health team are also trained in this area and can easily provide this service. Because rapport with clients is seen as essential in social work practice, this process can be further used to allow clients to feel more comfortable and be able to address intervention issues in a quicker or possibly more efficient manner.

The last area of benefit for inclusion of social work in health care counseling is a logistic one. Social workers are already part of the health care delivery team. Although agencies may recognize the need for employee assistance, agencies may not have the economic resources to hire someone to provide counseling services. Using clinical social workers who are already familiar with a program and the health care setting can allow health care agencies and service providers to dispense services to their own employees at a limited cost.

This need for counseling is highlighted with the recognition of *vicarious traumatization*. In this phenomenon, health care professionals are exposed to individuals who have been *traumatized* and repeatedly are exposed to the details that surround the trauma. Therefore, the health care provider also experiences repeated episodes of trauma (Figley, 1995). In some cases, the helper himself or herself may also need assistance with letting the trauma go. Several examples of this include the emergency room team that tries to save the life of a child but cannot; the paramedic who must assist in several tragic events in the course of his or her day, including multiple traffic accidents, drownings, suicide, or homicide attempts; the hospice worker who continually cares for the terminally ill client, and so forth. Programs for debriefing health care professionals are being formulated (Mitchell & Everly, 1996); the use of social workers in facilitating this type of "stress-debriefing" or identification of critical incidents in the group setting is increasing (Donigian & Hulse-Killacky, 1999).

AWARENESS IN HEALTH COUNSELING

The key task that will increase awareness in health counseling is assisting individuals to become cognizant of what factors are important to maintaining their own health and wellness. The purpose of health promotion counseling programs is to help communicate needed information that will assist the individual in making needed changes; assist individuals in using this information to develop self-help skills that can empower them to address health needs; and assist individuals to gain access to the techniques or technology that can help them in meeting their needs. Social workers can provide assistance to the individual in helping to accomplish the tasks of health promotion programs. This makes health care social work a service that cannot be overestimated. In addition, the social worker can enhance wellness education and skill building by adding therapeutic counseling designed to address barriers that might impede progress.

THEORETICAL FOUNDATIONS

Of the many different theoretical frameworks used in establishing and conducting health and wellness counseling, two appear to have had the most significant influence. The first framework is based in social learning theory, and the second is within a health belief model or health counseling approach.

SOCIAL LEARNING THEORY

The roots of *social learning theory* can be traced back to the work of Lewin (1951). It was further postulated by Albert Bandura in the 1960s (Bandura, 1971, 1977). In health counseling, reinforcement patterns of behavior are socially learned, determined, or maintained. Individuals are recognized as social beings; therefore, it is the "social" and "cultural" environment that actively influences and mediates individual behavior. Bandura (1977) postulated that individuals change their behavior in response to situational circumstances. He believed that individuals learn best by observation, specifically by watching others perform and after watching this performance, *modeling* the behavior. He believed that individuals watch which behaviors are rewarded and punished and "vicariously" embrace the implications of what they witness.

According to this theoretical framework, individuals learn not only from *direct reinforcement* but from *self-reinforcement* as well. In self-reinforcement, the individual reinforces himself or herself without an external stimulator. In health counseling, generating this awareness is necessary for behavior change to occur. Once the motivation for a behavior is learned, social learning principles are outlined and employed to achieve skill building and to change dysfunctional behaviors.

HEALTH BELIEF MODEL

A second model that is often related to health and wellness counseling is the *health belief model*. In this model, "fear" or recognition of one's "susceptibility" to an adverse health outcome or illness motivates the individual to partake in health change behavior (Becker, 1974;

Rosenstock, 1974). In general, the health belief model postulates that individuals must (a) see themselves as vulnerable to certain health problems; (b) see this vulnerability as leading to a potentially serious problem; (c) believe that intervention or prevention activities are effective, yet not overly burdening regarding time, effort, or expense; and (d) receive a stimulus of some type that initiates them to seek action (Elder, Geller, Hovell, & Mayer, 1994).

To develop health change behaviors, specific skill development as well as the transfer of information is considered essential. Many times at the center of the change strategy is the client's desire to obtain his or her own sense of *self-control* regarding the health issues he or she is experiencing. This makes interventions designed to address self-efficacy, self-awareness, and self-control essential. In general, this model is similar to social learning because it applies to the concept of awareness. In both models, awareness leads to a sense of susceptibility that, in turn, helps to motivate the development of change behavior (Chapman, 1994).

PREVENTION IN WELLNESS

Health awareness programs seek to promote continued health as well as prevent health problems from becoming worse. Therefore, prevention is an essential part of wellness counseling. *Epidemiology*, which is the basic study of the frequency and distribution of a specified phenomenon such as disease (Barker, 1999), has evolved immensely over the years. For example, we can now predict the approximate number of deaths that will occur each year that are preventable or avoidable. Actually, according to Colvez and Blanchet (1981), 80% of the diseases in the United States are preventable. The major factors related to mortality, morbidity, and disability are circulatory disease, neoplasms, trauma, respiratory disease, muscoskeletal disabilities, and mental illness (Bracht, 1995). These conditions can lead to increased health care expense, and disease prevention is clearly indicated as an overall health care cost reduction strategy.

Health counseling with a focus on prevention has been divided into three areas. The first area is *primary prevention*. This direct form of intervention reduces the susceptibility of individuals to disease (Burger & Youkeles, 2000). It is in this area that most directed health education strategies fall. The emphasis is on educating individuals so that they will be less likely to engage in health-defeating behaviors. Examples of primary prevention programs are those designed to achieve better community sanitation or warn the population of the danger of cigarette smoking. Other examples can include sex education in the schools or any other programs designed to prevent conditions from occurring.

In *secondary prevention*, approaches are designed and employed for early detection before irreversible damage has occurred (Burger & Youkeles, 2000). In secondary prevention, a problem is identified, and then a strategy is employed to keep it from spreading. Secondary prevention requires active case finding on the part of the health care social worker. This ensures that the effects of the condition are minimized and the spread to other individuals, families, or communities is minimal. The duty of the social worker to initiate early intervention practices is considered essential. For example, when working with HIV-infected clients, secondary prevention strategies are crucial in helping the client learn how to address and identify, the factors that will reduce the spread.

The third type of prevention is referred to as *tertiary prevention*. In tertiary prevention, the goal is to manage disease to minimize disability (Burger & Youkeles, 2000). This type of prevention is often addressed in rehabilitative/restorative inpatient and outpatient settings. In this form of prevention, the health care social worker helps a client who has already experienced the problem to recuperate or recover from it. In addition to directly intervening in the problem, the social worker must also focus on building strengths in the client to assist him or her if the problem is exacerbated.

HUMOR AND PROMOTING WELLNESS

Humorous laughter is an ageless phenomenon that scientists have always had difficulty understanding (Ziv, 1984). They do not comprehend the cognitive, physiological, philosophical, and psychological aspects of humor. Humor is one of the most effective yet overlooked forms of communication that humans employ. Unfortunately, however, humor is generally not fully recognized as a critical tool for use in the professional setting. In fact, there is little research on the use of humor as an essential component of interpersonal relationships. This paucity of supportive evidence can be related to subjective and varied perceptions of humor as an intervention.

Most people agree that humor plays a role in nearly every situation in which people interact. In many formal medical settings, humor, especially when it is in the form of laughter, is viewed as unprofessional. This stigma has squelched some attempts to include it in formal research. To date, the effects of humor have been cited in areas such as education (Hill, 1988), psychotherapy (Salameh, 1993), and training in leadership (Ziv, 1984). In the medical setting, humor has been used for combating stressful illnesses such as hypertension and stroke (McGhee, 1979). Furthermore, the Bible refers to humor as a medicine to guide an individual to health (Proverbs 17:22). In our society, attempts have been made to utilize and understand laughter as a tension reducer that promotes group cohesion and goal attainment (Ziv, 1988). For example, during formal training on HIV/AIDS, instructors are encouraged to use humor as part of health education training whenever possible (Dremburg & Walker, 2001). According to these trainers, the use of humor in working with client education in the medical setting can be an effective icebreaker; it can be utilized as a bonding tool, and it can serve to relieve the immense tension from the serious situations that clients face. Therefore, humor can be utilized to allow people to let down their guard and relax.

HUMOR IN MEDICAL SETTINGS

Humor is a multifaceted concept that is receiving increasing attention in the health care setting. The use of humor can serve as a method toward maintaining, enhancing, or improving the physical and/or emotional well-being of an individual. Granick (1995) explained that many therapists regard humor to be a valuable productive vehicle that has enabled clients to progress effectively with personal, social, and emotional problems. According to Salameh (1993), "Therapeutic humor has an educative, corrective message.... [It] promotes cognitive-emotional equilibrium . . . and the therapist can draw attention to behaviors while affirming the essential worth of the client." Humor "acts as an interpersonal lubricant" (p.113).

Kush (1997) believed that is one attribute of a fully functioning person. The sign of a healthy psyche is when a person is able to utilize humor when acknowledging problems that can impede wellness. Falk and Hill (1992) believed that many theorists, regardless of theoretical orientation, find humor useful. Falk and Hill (1992) stated that counselor "humor can be constructive in forming and furthering the therapeutic alliance . . . [and] breaking through resistive defenses . . . [and] aiding in catharsis, but also can enable clients to avoid conflicted areas" (p. 40). Lastly, humor can also be used as a coping mechanism to avoid conflict allowing the person to remain safe until he or she is ready to deal with the painful events in life.

Humor when utilized within the health setting as part of the therapeutic relationship can promote self-esteem, stimulate creative thinking, and broaden perspectives. Health care social workers can assist clients to convert experiences that are upsetting and help them learn to laugh about them in order to regulate unsatisfactory responses. Granick (1995) described a session during which a client was tense and irritated with himself because he lost his temper with his children. At that moment Granick utilized a prop to illicit humor, thus reducing the client's tension. This anecdote illustrates one feature of humor in the therapeutic process that allows the client to experience an upsetting situation as comical and benign. Humor can help reorient perceptions, attitudes, and behaviors and can lead to more balanced interactions.

Furthermore, humor can be integrated in the medical setting as a method of enhancing catharsis. Humorous comments can stimulate a client to share his or her most inner thoughts, feelings, and conflicts. It also provides an opportunity to stimulate new ways of perceiving and understanding attitudes, behaviors, and situations (Gladding, 1995). This broadening of perceptions allows for the opportunity to change. Since the stimulation of laughter has been associated with relief of tension and depressed feelings, clients have the capacity to revise their problem-solving approach under less pressure. Humor can be used as a vehicle to stimulate meaningful insights, such as words of wisdom, through recollections of past events or similar situations. In terms of health and wellness, writers have reported that humor has helped individuals survive emotional and physical suffering, imprisonment, illnesses, loss, and suffering (Granick, 1995).

Solomon (1996) believed that humor allows people to gain control by redefining the situation as less threatening and less embarrassing and thus under control. Although people may not be able to change or control some events, they can redefine the meaning of those events and thus influence the perceived consequences. Humor in a therapeutic context allows clients to feel a sense of control over their mood when circumstances may be out of their hands and in the hands of the providers (McGhee, 1998). This suggests that individuals who use humor to cope with life stressors do so to positively evaluate self-efficacy and self-control. There has been an extensive amount of research done on the concept of perceived control and its relationship to physical and psychological conditions. The results of these studies indicate that people more often than not experience positive outcomes from perceiving that they have control of what impacts them and experience negative outcomes, such as depression, when they perceive a lack of control. In turn, this perceived control was associated with better emotional well-being, better methods of coping with stress, better health and physiological outcomes, and improved performance (Martin & Lefcourt, 1983).

The research has indicated that humor has also been utilized as a diagnostic aid in a variety of mental health conditions. Goldin and Borden (1999) compiled literature reporting that the humor has been used to predict patient adjustment after hospitalization; to measure the extent of a client's depression; and even for assessing schizophrenic patient difficulties in socialization. Several instruments have been developed for the specific purpose of measuring humor (Fry & Salameh, 1987). For example, Martin and Lefcourt 1983, 1984) developed the Coping Humor Scale as well as a Situational Humor Response Questionnaire, thus providing a tool that allowed for an in-depth assessment of client humor.

Additionally, humor has been found to be diagnostically significant with children in understanding the natural development of adaptive mechanisms (Buckman, 1994). Ziv (1984) and Buckman (1994) explored the developmental progression of humor and how children could share humor with adults as a way of receiving comfort for fears. Therefore, in clinical settings, humor can be used to assess a child's capacity to identify reality and to set the stage for further psychological or social adjustment.

Overall, humor can have a liberating effect on people, providing comfort while helping to soothe the pains of misfortunes, and thereby enabling the client to deal with situations in a mature, intelligent, and constructive fashion. Humor also strengthens the rapport between the client and the therapist. Health care social workers can encourage the use of humor to make painful experiences seem less painful. As noted by Abel (1998), "Humor affords an opportunity for exploring cognitive alternatives in response to stressful encounters and perhaps for reducing the negative affective consequences of a real or perceived threat" (p. 267). Finally, the therapist may be able to add to a client's social repertoire and thus provide a stress control method (Goldin & Bordan, 1999). One must note, however, that the crucial element is timing and humor must fit the situation for it to be effective.

INCORPORATING HUMOR IN THE THERAPEUTIC ENVIRONMENT

When individuals take emotional disturbances too seriously humor does not evoke pleasant feelings and can result in obsessions and anxiety (Gladding, 1995). Additionally, Freiheit, Overholser, and Lehnert (1998) noted that "adolescents who are depressed may have an impaired ability to appreciate the humor in situations" (p.33). These clients may perceive the therapist's jokes or humorous comments as unsympathetic; this can endanger the therapeutic relationship and this makes evaluating when it is best to incorporate humor critical. The health care social worker must judge when the appropriate time arises for utilizing humor. According to Gladding (1995), humor in counseling is improper when: "the counselor uses it to avoid dealing with client anxieties, a client views it as irrelevant to his or her reasons for being in counseling, it is experienced as a put-down, or it is inappropriately timed" (p. 411; as cited in Goldin & Bordan, 1999).

Humor creatively involves "the ability to perceive relationships between people, objects, or ideas in an incongruous way, as well as the ability to communicate this perception to others" (Ziv, 1984, p.111). Timing, client perception, and therapeutic relationships are all essential elements to determining when to use humor within the counseling arena.

It has been theorized that humor is important in releasing or lessening tensions and conflicts within the group setting. For a group to be strong and productive, it must have cohesion (Ziv, 1984). Shared laughter and pleasure can increase the group's well-being, thus enhancing the productivity of the group. Therefore, using humor can build and maintain teamwork in "stress-laden milieus" (Kuhlman, 1993, p. 19).

Basically, the use of humor as evidenced by laughter in the group setting can have both short-term and long-term benefits in the area of stress management (Kuhlman, 1993). Laughter can serve to release tension, allowing members to behave impulsively without breaking societal taboos (McGhee, 1979). This openness may allow for creative problem solving while encouraging team building. Humor helps to release tension and gives the participant a feeling of belonging. Furthermore, the use of humor in the form of private jokes or "inside jokes" can serve as a defense against strangers infiltrating a group (Morgan et al., 1986). These jokes create a shared experience allowing the group to remain superior over the newcomer.

In summary, interest in the use of humor it has led to the creation of a growing number of workshops and courses on how to develop or improve a sense of humor. As mentioned earlier, humor is a key component in training programs; such a program has been used for counseling HIV/AIDS clients (Dremburg & Walker, 2001). Dremburg and Walker's participants' guide (*Client-Centered Counseling, Testing, Partner Counseling and Referral Services*) includes a list of ten basic counseling skills that are used within the counseling session; humor is one of these. While using humor with such a fatal disease may seem questionable, Dremburg and Walker (2001) believe that "humor is a significant tool to lighten the conversation, as a tool to stress a point or build rapport"(p.13). They go on to state within the training manual:

> It is okay to interject humor during a counseling session, but it must be done appropriately and with sensitivity to the client. Every client is different, and not every client will appreciate a humorous moment during the counseling session . . . Try to be spontaneous and not appear to be repeating a memorized script . . . don't repeat the use of humor just because one client accepted it. . . . The next person may not receive it the same way. (p. 13)

Humor as part of health and wellness counseling should be utilized to create a nonthreatening environment, facilitate communication, and ensure the development of a trusting relationship between client and therapist or any persons involved (Granick, 1995). In the classroom setting, affording students the opportunity to release tension with nonthreatening humor may open their minds to more complicated subjects. Within the therapy session, humor can be utilized to decrease tension and build rapport. Within teams humor is utilized to increase team building and bonding among members. After all, as Kush (1997) noted, humor adds a "colorful dimension to our personality . . . and . . . is a desirable characteristic of a healthy personality" (p. 22). Overall, humor seems to be one of the most overlooked tools that would benefit interpersonal communication.

In terms of the future, more research is needed to define how and when to best encourage the use of humor in not only the therapy setting, but within any realm of life where stress may become overwhelming or where tensions are high. Humor is clearly a factor to be considered in diminishing the effects of stress with performance, and more research is needed to determine the level at which stress actually degrades or improves performance. Laughter has been cited as a form of communication, but little is known on exactly how much humorous communication is necessary for a group to be productive.

IMPLEMENTATION OF HEALTH COUNSELING

Once health care social workers are made aware of the process of health counseling, the theoretical underpinnings, and the strategies needed, they felt more prepared to provide formal training, assistance, support, and direct counseling services in numerous health settings. A few of the many areas for health education and maintenance activities include health counseling regarding weight control, cigarette smoking, health and nutrition, sex education, parenthood, preparation for childbirth, family member or significant other illness, terminal illness, and eventually preparation and acceptance of one's own death or the death of others.

The factors that can motivate clients to seek and initiate health counseling can vary. Many times the actual symptoms may bring clients in. Kurtz and Chalfant (1991) warn, however, that symptom identification alone may not be enough to initiate help-seeking behavior. In support of this contention, they remind us that only a small proportion of individuals who suffer from health problems actually seek intervention.

Zola (1966) listed five factors that influence an individual's desire to seek health and wellness counseling. The first is experiencing an interpersonal crisis. The crisis experience itself calls attention to the symptoms that motivate the individual to seek intervention. The second is impairment in social relations. In these cases, social activities once found to be rewarding lose their appeal, and the individual is motivated to seek help. The third factor important for motivating individuals to seek help is when it is requested by loved ones. In these cases, someone close to the individual asks them, or insists, that they seek intervention to facilitate or maintain the current level of social connection. A fourth factor is that individuals may become frightened by the illness, and this fear of what might happen forces them to seek help. Lastly, help-seeking behavior is affected by the nature or quality of the symptoms experienced. Present symptoms that are generally not similar in severity, duration, or onset to what has been experienced in the past may also initiate help-seeking behavior.

In understanding client help-seeking behavior, it is not only the psychological, anatomical, or biological factors that influence action toward seeking help. It is primarily the psychosocial influences that reflect the client's daily life as a social human being (Kurtz & Chalfant, 1991). Therefore, social workers need to be mindful that in implementing a health counseling approach to practice, providing educational information alone is not enough. Interaction between the social worker and the client that focuses on the development of specific skills is necessary. In health counseling, the focus is on increasing psychoeducation while taking this knowledge and developing concrete skills to address the problem (Lewis, Sperry, & Carlson, 1993). There are three basic areas that generally constitute the process of health counseling: (a) a focus on educational skill building; (b) a focus on personal control; and (c) a focus on the social environment (Lewis, Sperry, & Carlson, 1993)

UNDERSTANDING THE DYNAMICS IN HEALTH COUNSELING

There are several educational strategies that can assist the health care social worker in providing education as part of wellness counseling. The provision of health education is essential in helping to shape the beliefs of adults their ability to build motivation for self-change.

To facilitate implementation of the educational process, Chapman (1994) suggests the following strategies. First, when trying to educate someone, use the following three-step strategy: show, discuss, and apply. The goal here is to create an environment where experiential learning can occur. When an individual understands the basics and can see how they are applied, he or she is able to adjust to the new behavior and incorporate it more quickly (Plescia, Koontz, & Laurent,

2001). For example, in teaching clients to use relaxation training or the technique of deep breathing to relieve stress, one can use the many stress reduction tapes that depict these techniques. Yet, none of these marketed tapes is considered the first choice for educating the client. In practice, the social worker has the flexibility to customize the experience for the client, which, in turn, facilitates learning. In educating an individual to the process of deep breathing, whether in an individual or group session, first the process is discussed; second, the benefits of the technique and the uniqueness of these benefits to the client are emphasized; third, the social worker has the ability to customize the education program to meet the needs of those involved. Simply stated, explaining stress reduction techniques and the process of deep breathing, demonstrating how they can be completed, and assisting the individual to apply the techniques in a protective and supportive environment can help an individual to understand the process quickly.

A second educational strategy to assist with health and wellness counseling is "repetitive exposure to the information" (Chapman, 1994). This is based on the simple premise that the more times individuals hear something, the more likely they are to remember and apply it. This makes repeating and reemphasizing key points a necessity. The technique of summarization should always be applied. Basically, in this technique, the client is asked to summarize at the beginning and end of the session what occurred. The use of this technique incorporates the principle of repetition in the educational learning format. Further, it also stresses that the client summarize the session in his or her own words. The actual self-stating of the goals and objectives covered in a session can help the client assimilate more quickly. Whether it is a formal therapeutic session or a brief encounter, repeating what was covered or what is expected to be completed can help to clear up misunderstandings or misinterpretations that might otherwise impede change behavior.

The third technique to facilitate education is to always remember to teach an individual through small increments of change (Chapman, 1994). When physicians are trained to use medications with the elderly, the rule of thumb is usually "dose low and go slow." The same principle applies here. Dose low, by keeping the steps small, and go slow, by watching the client, ensuring that he or she is following the information that is being presented.

The fourth strategy is to emphasize the benefit to be gained by participating in the program. Clear goals, objectives, and outcome-based criteria will help. In addition, these goals and objectives must be reviewed periodically to ensure that adequate progress is being made. Individuals are more likely to stick to a program when they believe it can benefit their lives by reducing their susceptibility to disease or illness.

The fifth strategy involves maximizing and directing session time to facilitate education. Oftentimes, reading material or note taking can reinforce what is learned. In the health counseling encounter, this is often not possible; therefore, it is not uncommon for the social worker to prepare handouts or notes for the client. Handouts are used that stress the basic points of what was covered. They can also serve to reinforce the factors presented in the time-limited encounter. Chapman (1994) gave several suggestions for using printed materials. Those that are most relevant to the provision of health education counseling have been modified and listed in Table 11.1.

A HOLISTIC MODEL FOR WELLNESS COUNSELING

The use of educational strategies can be found in the work of Myers, Sweeney, and Witmer (2000), who developed what they call *The Wheel of Wellness*, which incorporates 16 characteristics of a healthy individual. The 16 characteristics are illustrated graphically on four concentric circles and spokes. The four circles have within them the following five life tasks: (a) spirituality, (b) self-direction, (c) work and leisure, (d) friendship, and (e) love. They suggest that a practitioner can use the wheel in counseling through four phases as follows: (a) by using a life span focus to introduce the concepts of the Wheel of Wellness model; (b) by conducting an assessment of the individual using the five life tasks; (c) by implementing interventions designed to enhance wellness in selected areas of the Wheel; and (d) by providing ongoing evaluation of progress, follow-up, and as-needed continuation of phases (b) through (d) above.

COMMUNITY INTERVENTION PROGRAM FOR HEALTH PROMOTION IN POOR AND ETHNIC COMMUNITIES

Brenner (2002), Altpeter, Earp, and Schopler (1998), and Auslander, Haire-Joshu, Houston, Williams, and Krebill (2000) describe several

TABLE 11.1   Guidelines for Providing Written Materials

1. Use a handout that the individual can take home that includes the important points regarding what was covered.
2. Use written material that can be taken home and reviewed. In the beginning, give all material to the client; do not expect him or her to go get it from the library bookstore, and so on.
3. Try to keep handouts to approximately one page each. Be sure to bullet the major points. Keep the handout in outline form, not full sentences of written text.
4. Be sure that once identified, the goals and objectives are clearly stated on the handout material.
5. If the individual is going to create lists as homework, it is a good idea to place these on index cards. These cards are more duable than paper and can be easily folded in half and placed in a wallet or pocket.
6. On the handout, list references for continued growth—particularly, books and other materials that address self-help strategy that can be employed after ending the formal encounter.
7. Get the individual to assist with what should be placed on the handout(s). In this way, the individual will feel part of the process.
8. Advise the individual of the importance of keeping the written material and how it can be used at a later date to reinforce intervention strategy.

successful wellness promotion programs within three ethnic communities. Brenner directed the East Harlem Healthy Heart program using a community intervention model that focused on multiple risk factors. The various aspects of the approach included (a) targeting members of the community who reported multiple risk factors such as a high fat and cholesterol diet, hypertension, and smoking; (b) targeting every segment of the community with information about the project, including churches, schools, associations, retail outlets, supermarkets, tenant associations, day care centers, mass media, and elected officials; (c) developing community ownership and involvement in the health promotion programs; (d) developing volunteer recruitment and training; and (e) developing social marketing strategies. Altpeter, Earp, and Scholper (1998) assert that implementing programming for health promotion can be an overwhelming task. They highlight the complexity of using several theoretical approaches. In addition, the study provides insights into ways in which both lay and professional communities can effectively work together. Auslander et al. (2000) report that use of a health promotion that individually targeted the intervention material in combination with community organization techniques demonstrated potential in reducing the risk of diet-related diseases among African American women.

TIME-LIMITED HEALTH COUNSELING

Health counseling as a form of time-limited brief intervention is different from traditional psychotherapy. Acknowledgment of these differences is the first step in getting health care social workers to feel more comfortable in implementing this as a practice strategy. First, health counseling, like other time-limited brief interventions, is more action oriented than traditional psychotherapy. Clients are expected to participate actively and engage in motivated self-change behavior to achieve interventive success. If reduction in health risk requires lifestyle changes, participation is essential. To make these lifestyle changes, the social worker must be skilled in how to initiate the client change process and maintain it.

Second, health counseling, like the other forms of time-limited intervention, is always brief in duration. Third, and somewhat unlike most other forms of social work intervention, the primary focus of intervention should always be prevention. Lastly, in traditional psychotherapy, rapport is an ongoing and building process; in health counseling, however, it must be established in the first session. In this method, rapport in itself is only important because it can be used to help facilitate change behavior.

METHOD FOR TIME-LIMITED HEALTH COUNSELING

Lewis, Sperry, and Carlson (1993) establish three criteria for initiating the practice of health counseling: (a) complete a functional assessment; (b) identify personal or change interest; and (c) establish what is the expected outcome. In establishing a functional assessment, the social worker tries to understand the client's present health behaviors in terms of personal and contextual factors. Many times a formal assessment procedure, such as a complete social and developmental history, is not practical and a more basic assessment can suffice. From a limited perspective, information about personality style, health beliefs, current level of functioning, and past or current coping behaviors can assist in formulating a plan. It is also important to assess someone's level of knowledge regarding the problem and whether the client is open to change.

As recommended by Lewis, Sperry, and Carlton (1993), one question to be asked to establish the present level of disability is

- How does your _____interfere with your daily life? (Name the problem.)

The second area to be addressed is to identify the individual's interest to initiate change. Here the individual is interviewed to establish why he or she believes the problem is happening. Focus is placed on ascertaining what he or she believes can be done to address the problem, and what he or she is willing to do to change it. A question that can facilitate gathering this information is

- What do you believe are the reasons for your problem (e.g., stress, obesity, smoking, etc.)?

The last area to be addressed in problem assessment is identification of the expected outcome. Here the individual is assessed to see how willing, realistic, and open he or she is to the change process suggested. Questions to establish this inquiry include

- What specific changes do you expect to make?
- When do you expect to accomplish this?
- What kind of involvement do you want from me as the social worker?

CHAPTER SUMMARY AND FUTURE DIRECTIONS

Health counseling is not a new method of health care practice. Actually, it has been used in numerous health care settings, in many different forms, and can be traced back to the early beginnings of health care practice. For health care social workers, however, this method of practice is increasingly viewed as a necessary and viable approach. New approaches to address wellness such as the *Wheel of Wellness* provide frameworks with which to conduct practice that holistically conceptualizes the person (bio-psycho-social-spiritual)-in-environment. The use of efficient assessment frameworks will be cost effective and provide services that are needed by clients. Social workers need to assist clients in as timely, cost-containing, and efficient ways as possible. This holistic approach allows just that. When using a holistic approach, counseling, education, and aspects of community organization and needs assessment may be required to deliver effective programming. Over the years, there has been increased emphasis on the provision and inclusion of education as part of the intervention regime. Education is viewed as an integral service within the holistic approach to wellness promotion. Health and wellness counseling can initiate client skill building, while emphasizing the importance of prevention and wellness services. Health care social workers are encouraged to approach this type of service delivery seriously. It can provide a viable, necessary, and marketable way for health care social workers to provide clinical service.

REFERENCES

Abel, M. (1998). Interaction of humor and gender in moderating relationships between stress and outcomes. *Journal of Psychology, 132,* 267–276.

Altpeter, M., Earp, J. A. L., & Schopler, J. H. (1998). Promoting breast cancer screening in rural, African American communities: The "science and art" of community health promotion. *Health and Social Work, 23,* 104–115.

Auslander, W., Haire-Joshu, D., Houston, C., Williams, J. H., & Krebill, H. (2000, January). The short-term impact of a health promotion program for low-income African American women. *Research on Social Work Practice, 20*(1), 78–97.

Bandura, A. (1971). *Social learning theory.* Morristown, NJ: General Learning Press.

Bandura, A. (1977). *Social learning theory.* Upper Saddle River, NJ: Prentice Hall.

Barker, R. L. (1999). *The social work dictionary* (4th ed.). Washington, DC: NASW Press.

Becker, M. H. (1974). The health belief model and personal health behavior. *Health Education Monographs, 2,* 324–473.

Bracht, N. (1995). Prevention and wellness. In R. Edwards (Ed.), *Encyclopedia of social work* (19th ed., pp. 1879–1886). Washington, DC: NASW Press.

Brenner, B. (2002). Implementing a community intervention program for health promotion. *Social Work in Health Care, 35*(1/2), 359–375.

Brown, K. A. E., Jemmott, F. E., Mitchell, H. J., & Walton, M. L. (1998). The Well: A neighborhood-based health promotion model for black women. *Health and Social Work, 23,* 146–152.

Buckman, E. (1994). *The handbook of humor: Clinical applications in psychotherapy*. Malabar, FL: Krieger.

Burger, W. R., & Youkeles, M. (2000). *Human services in contemporary America* (5th ed.). Pacific Grove, CA: Brooks/Cole Thomson Learning.

Chapman, L. S. (1994). Awareness strategies. In M. P. O'Donnell & J. S. Harris (Eds.), *Health promotion in the work place* (pp. 163–184). Albany, NY: Delmar.

Colvez, A., & Blanchet, M. (1981). Disability trends in the United States population. *American Journal of Public Health, 71*, 464–471.

Donigian, J., & Hulse-Killacky, D. (1999). *Critical incidents in group therapy* (2nd ed.). New York: Wadsworth.

Dremburg, M., & Walker, K. (March 2001). Personal interview & HIV/AIDS pre/post test counseling course. *Participants' guide: Client-centered counseling, testing, partner counseling and referral services.* Sponsored by the Orange County Health Department.

Elder, J. P., Geller, E. S., Hovell, M. F., & Mayer, J. A. (1994). *Motivating health behavior.* Albany, NY: Delmar.

Falk, D., & Hill, C. (1992). Counselor interventions preceding client laughter in brief therapy. *Journal of Counseling Psychology, 39*(1), 39–45.

Figley, C. R. (Ed.). (1995). *Compassion fatigue: Coping with secondary traumatic stress in those who treat the traumatized.* Bristol, PA: Brunner/Mazel

Freiheit, S., Overholser, J., & Lehnert, K. (1998). The association between humor and depression in adolescent psychiatric inpatients and high school students. *Journal of Adolescent Research, 13* (1), 32–48.

Fry, W., & Salameh, W. (1987). *Handbook of humor and psychotherapy. Advances in the clinical use of humor.* Sarasota, FL: Professional Resource Exchange.

Gladding, S. (1995). Counseling: Wit and humor. *Journal of Humanistic Counseling, Education & Development, 34*(1), 3–10.

Goldin, E., & Bordan, T. (1999). The use of humor in counseling: The laughing cure. *Journal of Counseling and Development, 77*, 405–415.

Granick, S. (1995). The therapeutic value of humor. *USA Today Magazine, 124*(2604), 72–75.

Hill, D. (1988). *Humor in the classroom: A handbook for teachers (and other entertainers).* Springfield, IL: Charles C Thomas.

Kuhlman, T. (1993). Humor in stressful milieus. In W. Fry & W. Salameh (Eds.), *Advances in humor and psychotherapy* (pp. 19–45). Sarasota, FL: Professional Resource Press.

Kurtz, R. A., & Chalfant, H. P. (1991). *The sociology of medicine and illness* (2nd ed.). Boston: Allyn & Bacon.

Kush, J. (1997). Relationship between humor appreciation and counselor self-perceptions. *Counseling and Values, 42*, 22–29.

Levitt, D. B. (1994). Employee assistance programs. In M. P. O'Donnell & J. S. Harris (Eds.), *Health promotion in the work place* (pp. 429–458). Albany, NY: Delmar.

Lewin, K. (1951). Frontiers in group dynamics. In D. Cartwright (Ed.), *Field theory in the social sciences*. New York: Harper & Row.

Lewis, J., Sperry, L., & Carlson, J. (1993). *Health counseling*. Pacific Groves, CA: Brooks/Cole.

Martin, R. A., & Lefcourt, H. M. (1983). Sense of humor as a moderator of the relation between stressors and moods. *Journal of Personality and Social Psychology, 45*, 1313–1324.

Martin, R., & Lefcourt, H. M. (1984). The situational humor response questionnaire: A quantitative measure of the sense of humor. *Journal of Personality and Social Psychology, 47*, 145–155.

McGhee, P. (1979). *Humor: Its origin and development*. San Francisco: W. H. Freeman.

McGhee, P. (1998). Rx: Laughter. *RN, 61*(7), 50–53.

McWhinney, I. R. (1989). *A textbook of family medicine*. New York: Oxford University Press.

Mitchell, J. T., & Everly, G. S. (1996). *Critical incident stress management: The basic course workbook*. Ellicott City, MA: International Critical Incident Stress Foundation.

Morgan, B., Jr., Glickman, A., Woodard, E., Blaiewes, A., & Salas, E. (1986). *Measurement of team behaviors in a Navy environment* (NTSC Tech. Rep. No. TR-86–014). Orlando, FL: Naval Training Systems Center.

Myers, J. E., Sweeney, T. J., & Witmer, J. M. (2000, Summer). The wheel of wellness counseling for wellness: A holistic model for treatment planning. *Journal of Counseling and Development, 78*, 251–266.

Plescia, M., Koontz, S., & Laurent, S. (2001, May). Community assessment in a vertically integrated health care system. *American Journal of Public Health, 91*(5), 811–814.

Randall, J. L. (1996). Evolution of the new paradigm. *Primary Care, 23*, 183–198.

Rosenstock, I. M. (1974). Historical origins of the health belief model. *Health Education Monographs, 2*, 328–335.

Salameh, W. (1993). Introduction. In W. Fry & W. Salameh (Eds.), *Advances in humor and psychotherapy*. Sarasota, FL: Professional Resource Press.

Smith, S. L., Myers, J. E., & Hensley, L. G. (2002, Spring). Putting more life into life career courses: The benefits of a holistic wellness model. *Journal of College Counseling, 5*(1), 90–95.

Solomon, J. (1996). Humor and aging well. *American Behavioral Scientist, 39*, 249–272.

Ziv, A. (1984). *Personality and sense of humor*. New York: Springer Publishing Co.

Ziv, A. (1988). Teaching and learning with humor: Experiment and replication. *Journal of Experimental Education, 57*, 5–15.

Zola, I. K. (1996, October). Culture and symptoms: An analysis of patients' presenting complaints. *American Sociological Review, 31*, 615–630.

GLOSSARY

Confidentiality: The information that is obtained about the client in the conduct of direct practice; this includes client identity, content of verbalizations, professional opinions about the client, and material from records.

Employee Assistance Program: Services offered by employers to employees to help them address personal, social, or occupational problems that may impede work performance.

Epidemiology: The basic study of the frequency and distribution of a specified phenomenon, such as disease.

Health belief model: In this model for addressing health and wellness, "fear" or recognition of one's "susceptibility" to an adverse health outcome or illness motivates the individual to partake in health change behavior. Often the individual views himself or herself as in a vulnerable but solvable situation that can be addressed.

Informed consent: This is where client permission is obtained to participate in the health and wellness counseling being provided.

Modeling: In social learning theory, modeling relates to how individuals learn; they watch which behaviors are rewarded and punished, and "vicariously" embrace implications of what they witness.

Primary prevention: This is the first area of direct prevention services; the objective is to reduce the susceptibility of individuals to disease or to prevent social problems from occurring.

Relative or limited confidentiality: This is the form of confidentiality that most social workers ensure. In this form, information is kept confidential that the social worker is not ethically or morally bound to reveal.

Secondary prevention: These prevention strategies evolve around early detection so that methods of behavior change can be employed before irreversible damage has occurred.

Self-control: In the health belief model, this refers to an individual's desire to secure and maintain command of his or her state of health or wellness.

Self-reinforcement: Where the individual reinforces himself or herself without an external stimulator, such as in direct reinforcement.

Social learning theory: A intervention model that highlights the importance of social learning through modeling and direct or self-reinforcing behaviors.

Stress: Any influence that interferes with normal functioning by producing internal stress or strain.

Stressor: A stimulus that causes, evokes, or is otherwise related to the stress response.

Tertiary prevention: In tertiary prevention, the goal is to manage disease so as to minimize disability.

Trauma: Any event, particularly those outside the realm of usual experience, that causes the development of marked distress.

Traumatic stress: Intense arousal of feelings related to a particular event or situation.

Vicarious: The feelings or emotions that develop from sharing the experience of another person.

Vicarious traumatization: In this phenomena, helping professionals who work with individuals in crisis are repeatedly exposed to trauma through vicarious (i.e., imagining what it is like) means and may also begin to feel the effects of the trauma.

QUESTIONS FOR FURTHER STUDY

1. In what other areas of health care social work practice can health counseling be used?
2. Make a list of several different types of client problems that can be addressed through health education counseling.
3. What roles for the expansion of health care counseling do you see in the future?
4. What components would you include in developing a health promotion for people with juvenile diabetes?
5. What aspects of health promotion are most appealing to you?
6. What additional skills do you need to provide this kind of holistic counseling?

WEBSITES

Agency for Health Care Policy and Research
http://www.ahcpr.gov

All Health
http://www.allhealth.com

American Health Information Management Association
http://www.ahima.org

American Journal of Health Promotion
http://www.healthpromotionjournal.com

American Public Health Association and American Journal of Public
   Health
http://www.apha.org

Association of State and Territorial Directors of Health Promotion
   and Public Health Education
http://www.astdhpphe.org

This page intentionally left blank

PART IV

Special Topics and Exemplars in Clinical Health Care Practice

This page intentionally left blank

CHAPTER 12

Emergency Room Social Work Services

Sophia F. Dziegielewski and Delbert Ernest Duncklee, Jr.

EMERGENCY ROOM SOCIAL WORK

Social work services are offered in many hospital emergency rooms across the country; yet, in this fast-paced environment the actual services provided can differ greatly. According to Bristow and Herrick (2002), the services that social workers provide in this setting include psychosocial assessments, bereavement counseling and support, substance abuse assessment and referral, discharge planning, referrals for community resources, emotional support, and educating and advocating for patients.

Five social workers working in a large regional hospital's department of emergency services were questioned. They all worked together as part of an emergency team. Although their tasks varied, all of the social workers stressed the importance of being able to provide crisis intervention techniques and supportive counseling services to clients and their families.

The emergency room, is generally perceived as a fast-paced setting. In this setting, crises, deaths, and severe client problems need to be assessed and addressed as quickly and efficiently as possible. The pressure for immediate action in this setting is intense, and the social worker must remain in a constant state of readiness, prepared for what might come through the door next. According to Van Wormer and Boes (1997), the emergency room setting is different from other settings in the hospital because of the speed and intensity of which services must be assessed and provided. According to Ponto and Berger (1992), referrals to the emergency room social worker often involved complex problems. Specific cases included (1) an acute psychiatric episode involving suspected or threatened self-inflicted injuries, anxiety attacks, or emergent psychotic episodes; (2) an acute medical crisis involving long-term mental illness, chemically dependent individuals, or homeless or transient patients; (3) cases of domestic violence or rape; (4) suspected cases of child abuse or neglect, including sexual abuse; and, (5) any traumatic injury or illness that involved the police or other agencies, including assault, sexual assault, domestic violence, intoxication, or temporary disabling conditions (Ponto & Berger, 1992).

A TYPICAL DAY IN THE EMERGENCY ROOM: CASE APPLICATION

The following scenario is not that unusual in the emergency room setting. A trauma alert pager goes off to inform the social worker that a trauma victim will be arriving in less than 10 minutes. The social worker calmly finishes with the client she or he has been talking to in regard to a vehicular accident. Once separated from this client, the social worker rushes into the trauma room. The trauma team is busy preparing for the arrival of the next client. As the medical evacuation nurse brings the client in, the social worker listens to pick up vital information to locate the client's family. The security guard goes through the client's clothes and/or purse to find any identification or phone numbers for the social worker. This time the social worker is lucky and is able to get some identification for the client, who is unable to speak. The social worker rushes to the phone to see if she or he can get a phone number for the client's family. The social worker then calls the family and calmly informs them that they need to come to the hospital as soon as possible. The social worker also gets all of the information possible about the client for the treatment staff in case the client has any significant health problems or allergies that the team needs to be aware of.

Once the family arrives, the social worker is called to the main entrance to speak with the family members, who are often distraught. They then wait together for the physician to bring them information about their loved one's condition. The social worker talks to the family about the general condition of the client and assesses how the family will handle any bad news. The social worker then returns to the trauma room to notify the doctor that the client's family has arrived and to request that he speak with them whenever possible.

The social worker then accompanies the doctor to the quiet room where the family is waiting. The doctor informs the family of their relative's condition. Once the doctor has given them the news, the social worker helps the family by giving them emotional support. In the event that the client dies, the social worker helps the family reminisce and process the loss, while arranging for the family to see the body. The social worker provides support as needed while the family comes to terms with the death. This continues until the family is ready to leave the hospital. The social worker then provides the family with resources for dealing with their grief and the funeral.

This is only a brief excerpt of what an emergency social worker may deal with in just the first few hours of her shift. While situations like this are happening, other less pressing issues that demand the social worker's attention continue. The role of the emergency room social worker is complex, and it is not uncommon for multiple crisis situations to occur needing immediate attention and assistance.

INTERDISCIPLINARY AND MULTIDISCIPLINARY TEAMWORK

For many social workers in the emergency room setting, it is not uncommon to work as part of an interdisciplinary or multidisciplinary team. Teams in this setting often involve a variety of professionals—comprised of physicians, nurses, respiratory technicians, health unit coordinators, x-ray technicians, nurse case managers, social workers, and other health care professionals. Some emergency departments divide this team further into what is often termed a *case management subteam or dyad* that utilizes the combined services of a nurse and a social worker (Bristow & Herrick, 2002). In this setting, the case management subteam members work together to provide social services and discharge planning and to ensure that continuum of care needs are met for each client served.

Historically, the presence of a social worker in the emergency room setting has been important from both a supportive and clinical perspective. It also provides direct case management and discharge planning services. The supportive services social workers provide are critical for helping clients that have more than medical issues that need to be addressed. This can include discharge planning or counseling services to assist with the loss of a loved one. Many of these clients can be in a crisis state, or the situation of the client can precipitate a crisis reaction by the family or support system. In the emergency room, the problems clients seek treatment for are multifaceted and complex, and the types of problems addressed are diverse, ranging from auto accidents to other types of accidental and nonaccidental injuries. Many individuals may have acute or chronic episodes of an illness or first or repeated episodes of a physical or mental illness or there may be suicide attempts related to health and/or emotional issues.

In the supportive role, the social worker in this setting is often confronted with life and death decisions where high-risk screening is warranted (Bergman et al., 1993). These decisions are difficult under the best of circumstances, but in this type of trauma setting, the process is magnified immensely. Wells (1993) provided the following guidelines for social work intervention when dealing with sudden death situations. She defined the first step in the helping process as finding and providing the family with a private room to wait in, while also making sure that the family has been given as much preliminary information pertaining to their loved one's condition as possible. Wells (1993) believed that keeping the family informed was the first step to helping the families feel supported. This supportive function lays the groundwork and can benefit the entire team because when the client and his or her family feel supported they are more likely to feel that the whole team is concerned.

In addition, social workers also need to make sure that information provided to the family is given in such a way that the family understands what is being told to them. Helping to clarify difficult terms will help to avoid confusion and lessen the stressful time spent by all professionals with the family. An emergency room social worker often repeats what the physician has said to the family and allow the family to discuss it further if need be. Creating a caring and nonpressured haven for the family in the mist of a chaotic environmental situation can help the family to better adjust to the current situation.

Once the family has been notified of the death, the social worker will need to guide the family through the initial grief reaction. This includes comforting the family, helping them complete paperwork, supporting and encouraging concrete planning and decision making, providing referrals, and offering to contact clergy—that is, providing as supportive a discharge environment as possible (Wells, 1993). If family members are in denial, the social worker can assist by reviewing the events that have transpired and help the family begin the adjustment process that will follow. Finally, the social worker will offer to accompany the family members to view the body and provide support. Because sudden death related to trauma is common in the emergency room setting, the social worker must be prepared to address events of this nature. The social worker must also be well versed in these tasks in order to minimize stress on the family members of a deceased patient.

The emergency room social worker can assist with case management by gathering contact information for family and friends, as well as by finding additional means for meeting the client's health needs. Unfortunately, some believe the emergency room has become a dumping ground for those that lack insurance or are homeless. This group of individuals needs short-term intensive support designed to facilitate the discharge process and decrease the chance of recidivism. Since many individuals who seek care in the emergency room often lack or have inadequate health care coverage, this factor may force clients to seek emergency rooms as a means for obtaining nonemergency or episodic care (Spitzer & Kuykendall, 1994). Ponto and Berger (1992) make the argument that providing social worker services in the emergency room setting could actually have cost benefits in terms of helping identify such cases and facilitating the redirection to other services. Unfortunately, since social workers have not been quick to apply cost benefits to service provision, the cost-saving features of this activity have not been clearly identified.

Another group that often uses emergency room services is the homelessness, including homeless men, homeless women, and homeless women with children (Zugazaga, 2002). Boes and Van Wormer (1997) as well as Zugazaga (2002) report that the incidents of homelessness among women are continuing to increase. The factors often leading to homelessness in women include difficulties with domestic violence, mental illness, addictions, and finances.

In cases of domestic violence, screening procedures such as risk assessments (Friend & Mills, 2002) and protocol such as documentation and pictures of the injured areas are sometimes expected. For a more detailed assessment and examples of how to address the needs of the battered woman in the emergency room, the reader is referred to the work of Boes (1998) and Boes & McDermott, (2002). Regardless of the differences that may occur in protocol among the different hospitals for working with this population, one goal always remains paramount, and that is discharging the client to a safe place. To address problems of this nature, Boes and Van Wormer (1997) recommend that emergency room social workers consider using a strengths-based feminist perspective in helping these individuals. In this type of effort, the support networks a client has are identified along with the client's individual strengths.

Ponto & Berger (1992) point out three advantages to having social work services available in the emergency department. First, social workers generally have an extensive knowledge of the resources available and so are able to assess, process, and link clients to the needed services in a much more timely manner. Second, because the social worker is close and on call, the client's problem can be immediately addressed, reducing the burden on other team members and in many ways freeing the other team members to deliver the needed medical services to others. Lastly, Ponto & Berger (1992) believe that the social work they observed enabled clients to move back into the community with more than concrete resources. Clients were actually supported in the referral process, thereby decreasing the need for readmission.

Finally, the authors looked at revenues from billing for social work services versus expenses from providing services. Of the 198 cases reviewed, 74% paid for their bill, leaving a significant deficit for the hospital to cover (Ponto & Berger, 1992). Unfortunately, these researchers did not look at and compare this loss of revenue to the cost that might be saved for providing social work services. They also did not look at the savings that these services produced by linking patients with follow-up care, thus decreasing return visits. This remains a critical area for future research.

According to Keehn, Roglitz, and Bowden (1994), emergency department social workers need to take a proactive stance with patients complaining of nonmedical issues. Their study, which looked at 1,758 patients seen by social workers over a 12-month period, revealed that most of the interventions provided were support oriented (i.e., tangible services, patient support, family support) or proactive (e.g., crisis intervention, discharge planning, psychosocial assessment, consultation). In addition, they reported that "the greatest decline in recidivism occurred in those categories where social work used a proactive intervention strategy as opposed to a more support-oriented intervention" (1994, p. 73). Team members need to be educated about the role of the social worker as a contributing member to the team as well as about the essential services they can provide.

The emergency department social worker role includes psychosocial assessments, bereavement counseling, substance abuse counseling, and crisis intervention. Social workers are trained to be a resource for information regarding medical legal issues, guardianship, discharge planning, and community resources. Social workers provide emotional support during placement of family members in nursing homes, rehabilitation facilities, and psychiatric or emergency shelters during a crisis. In addition, as part of the team, social workers/nurse case managers can help locate community resources for patients and families (Bristow & Herrick, 2002). With the extensive trauma that occurs in this setting, it is not uncommon for the social worker to also take a supportive role, assisting other team members for what has been termed secondary or vicarious trauma (Dane & Chanchkes, 2002).

As part of a subteam, the social worker and nurse case manager can work together to help the hospital administration realize that the application of a social worker and nurse case manager can prevent unnecessary hospital and emergency room admissions. This service can also decrease unnecessary costs and decrease fragmentation in patient care (Bristow & Herrick, 2002). Using a team approach to emergency room services that includes a social worker allows for a more holistic approach to patient care.

OPINIONS OF SOCIAL WORKERS IN THE FIELD

Five emergency room social workers were questioned to learn more about their opinions. The five social workers were from a large regional medical center in central Florida, and all were specifically assigned to work in the emergency room. Four of the social workers were Caucasian, one was of Indian descent; these females ranged in age from 35 to 62 years. All had a master's degree in social work. The social workers' experience in the emergency room ranged from 1 to 11 years, with an average of 6 years. The social workers were all experienced in health care, having from 11 to 36 years in the field, with 3 to 13 years of this experience in an acute care setting.

To learn more about the opinions of these emergency room professionals, the following questions were asked:

- What is the role of a social worker in the emergency department?
- What tasks or concrete services do social workers provide in the emergency room?
- What do you see as the most significant need of the clients you serve?
- What client needs have not been reported or referred properly?
- What needs of the clients and their families are not being met in the current system?
- As an emergency room social worker, what would you change to make your work environment better?

INTERVIEWEE COMMENTS

What is the role of a social worker in the emergency department?

All of the social workers believed that the primary role of the social worker was to identify and meet the psychosocial needs of the client being admitted. This often included services such as: discharge planning, case management, advocacy, support, and counseling. The second most important role identified by these social workers was that of someone who makes the staff, doctors, and family aware of the client's needs. Social workers also coordinate services for the client; serve as a liaison between the patient/family and the staff/doctor; provide supportive services such as crisis intervention, bereavement counseling, support counseling, team participation, trauma follow-up, location of next of kin, and appropriate referrals to community resources; and often work on complicated discharge issues. These emergency room social workers also believed it was critical to provide crisis intervention and comfort and support to the families of the clients served.

In terms of referrals, these social workers stated that they often did assessments in the areas of abuse (adult and child), domestic violence, drugs and alcohol, suicide, depression, and mental health. As discharge planners, these social workers needed to know what referrals were available within the community. Three of the social workers reported that flexibility was crucial in this area of social work because often client needs went beyond what most would consider part of necessary medical practice. For example, upon discharge from service the social worker might have to secure emergency housing for a client, or in a situation of domestic violence ensure that the woman and her family have a safe place to go upon discharge. This requires both good assessment skills and being well versed in community services. Having these skills allowed the social worker to design an individualized comprehensive strategy emphasizing client strengths and resources, while striving to achieve measurable outcomes.

What tasks or concrete services do social workers provide in the emergency department?

The primary tasks identified by the social workers were identification of psychosocial issues, needs assessments, counseling, advocacy, referrals, education, linkage, placement, discharge planning, assessment, crisis management, bereavement counseling, adjustment issues, coordination of services needed to meet client psychosocial issues, financial assessment and assistance with indigent clients, location of next of kin, work with law enforcement and trauma patients and their families, and interfacing with staff throughout the hospital. As a source for referrals, these social workers all felt that they often were assigned what they referred to as "complicated" discharge planning cases (i.e., clients were homeless, had no insurance for follow-up). Furthermore, issues related to domestic violence, abuse/neglect cases, and sexual assault cases required the completion of complex assessments that required a great deal of time and creative energy, and when these cases were handled properly, they always required more than a simple referral.

The social workers also commented that although after assessment their official duties were to make referrals for addressing and referring abuse, neglect, or exploitation they were often called on to go beyond the initial problem assessment. Therefore, it was not uncommon to be expected to provide follow-up in these cases, particularly in the areas of sexual assault and child abuse. In addition, all of the social workers expressed a need for more community supports, since for the most part the referral possibilities and services that existed were simply not adequate to meet the needs of the client and his or her family. Additional tasks included helping clients with financial concerns and assisting indigent clients to get medication. These social workers also reported providing a great deal of informal support in terms of identifying and diffusing anxiety-related issues within the emergency department created by other staff members and/or patients and their families.

What do you see as the most significant need of the clients you serve?

All of the social workers had the same responses. The most significant need was for work with adjustment issues, regardless of whether they were related to a crisis situation or a long-term problem. The second most important need was for linkages, referrals, and follow-ups with community resources. These social workers also agreed that although providing psychosocial and supportive counseling was essential to helping these clients, it was the service considered least important by others on the trauma team or other support personnel who were not directly involved in the intervention process. Other services needed by clients included counseling and advocacy, and helping clients and/or families to negotiate the hospital and posthospital health care system. In summary, all of these social workers identified the most significant need for clients and/or their families in the emergency room setting as being of a supportive nature.

What client needs have not been reported or referred properly?

All of the social workers agreed that other team members and emergency room staff often did not identify high-risk situations that required advocacy or appropriate emotional support. In addition, when referrals were made for high-risk cases, it was often so late in the intervention process that issues that might have been simply addressed if presented earlier had magnified into much larger problems. Similarly, many of the referrals to the social worker were not made on admission to the emergency room but rather on discharge or while families were waiting for excessive periods of time. When services were provided on discharge, they were often provided in the waiting room. Several of the social workers stated that at times nurses did not recognize the need for community referrals, and therefore clients were discharged without adequate follow-up or coordination. Overall, these social workers felt that more information was needed to explain what they did and how providing timely referrals could benefit the process for all involved. Four of the five respondents reported that referrals were not always timely or were sometimes perceived as an afterthought. These late referrals set the stage for rushed or inadequate problem resolution.

What needs of clients and their families are not being met in the current system?

All of the social workers reported that a private place was needed regardless of the type of social work intervention, and in the emergency room this was rarely available. These social workers also reported problems with mental health and substance abuse services related to limited community resources. These contributed to the problem of the revolving door. The referral process was also listed as a problem area because often social workers had little or incomplete information on which to act. With the primary focus in the emergency room being on medical problems, the relationship between health and mental health was often ignored. This further complicated overall treatment efficacy. The last area they mentioned was "providing after-care services such as follow-up with phone calls, . . . offering bereavement counseling and assisting with home-based non-medical care." Since this was needed after the client had been discharged from the emergency room, this detail was not given the time and attention that was needed to complete this duty adequately.

As an emergency room social worker, what would you change to make your work environment better?

All of the social workers reported that they would like to see more education and team building to help others in the hospital setting realize what their role was. For the most part there was a desire to have more education for nurses and doctors to reinforce more appropriate referrals, promote the social work service, and reinstate supervisory meetings to make sure all were in sync with each other and with policy. In the words of one social worker, "Through education and support from emergency department management, I would place social workers on the forefront as an active part of the team, rather than being the clean-up batter on the team!"

SUMMARY OF FINDINGS

In summary, most of these social workers defined similar roles and tasks. All of the emergency room social workers agreed that the main services they should provide were risk assessment, supportive counseling and case management, and discharge planning and referrals. Three of the six social workers interviewed said they often provided advocacy services and counseling for their clients and their families in the areas of support and/or bereavement. Two of the respondents listed crisis intervention as the primary role of the emergency room social worker, and one listed education and advocacy as central to each task provided.

All respondents listed case management and community referrals as well as supportive counseling services such as bereavement counseling, as concrete tasks. All five respondents listed counseling, crisis intervention, coordination of services, and handling of abuse cases, as well as services in the emergency department. Two of the social workers stated that they often had to address problems with indigent individuals who did not have insurance. All of the social workers stated they often tried to locate next of kin, and they were very active in helping to address trauma-based services by providing staff support and counseling. Assessments and referrals for domestic violence issues, mental health issues, and substance abuse issues were all common tasks with in the assessment and referral process.

Overall, the responses of these social workers are similar to those in the existing literature. In identifying the roles, tasks, and duties of the emergency room social worker, Bristow and Herrick (2002) also listed psychosocial assessments, substance abuse counseling, crisis intervention, discharge planning, education of patients, bereavement counseling, and advocacy as roles for social workers. What was different about these social workers is the increased emphasis that each of them placed on the team concept, and how as a team member they were invaluable for linking the team to the clients and their families. They also felt that better education for team members and emergency room staff was needed. This increased education and awareness could assist with more timely referrals. Bergman et al. (1993) also advocated that social workers be familiar with high-risk screening and how to educate others on the team to the types of problems these cases generally involve.

Bristow and Herrick (2002) also noted that social workers were often viewed as an information source on medical legal issues, guardianship, and community resources in the emergency department. These social workers said the same; however, they warned that if this recognition and referral occurred at client discharge rather than at admission, there would not be adequate time to address problems. Kerr and

Siu (1993) say, it is important to remember that if important medical and social problems are deferred until discharge they may be inadequately treated or not receive any treatment at all.

Like Keehn et al. (1994), who examined recidivism, these social workers felt that proactive services such as crisis intervention, psychosocial assessment, discharge planning, and consultation with medical staff could indeed reduce recidivism rates. They felt that more research in this area was needed to help them make a databased case that this indeed was true.

One last point these social workers made was that it is important to maintain a sense of humor in such a high-stress environment (Van Wormer & Boes, 1997). Without a sense of humor, the emergency room social worker can easily become overwhelmed and stressed. Humor was believed to provide one means of immediate stress relief for these workers.

CHAPTER SUMMARY AND FUTURE DIRECTIONS

Social work in the emergency department plays an important role in providing for the psychosocial needs of patients in a time of crisis. Although this role is important, emergency room social workers warn that medical staff may overlook social work services because of their focus on the medical needs and not the psychosocial needs of the client being served. Thus, to better utilize the services of social workers in the emergency department, it is vital that the emergency room staff as well as hospital administrators be educated about the role of the social worker in the emergency department. This discussion only surveyed the opinions of five social workers currently working in the field. Therefore, the information in this chapter is not considered generalizable to all emergency rooms across the country. It does, however, provide fertile ground for future thought and activism in this area. More research is needed to demonstrate the role of social workers in the emergency department, and the importance of this role.

The issue of usage and referral to community supports and the relationship this has to cost reduction also needs to be explored (Hughes, 1999). More research is needed into whether or not having these valuable services available can reduce recidivism or readmission rates for hospitals. Until social work services have been researched and their benefits demonstrated from an evidence-based perspective services such as these will be vulnerable to budget cuts in today's behaviorally based managed care system. In the future, social workers involved in emergency department social work should push forward with more innovative evidence-based information to advocate for the availability of these services for their patients.

REFERENCES

Bergman, A. L., Wells, L., Bogo, M., Abbey, S., Chandler, V., Embleton, L., Guirgis, S., Huot, A., McNeill, T., Prentice, L. Stapleton, D., Shekter-Wolfson, L., & Urman, S. (1993). High-risk indicators for family involvement in social work in health care: A review of the literature. *Social Work, 38,* 281–288.

Boes, M. (1998). Battered women in the emergency room: Emerging roles for the ER social worker. In A. R. Roberts (Ed.). *Battered women and their families* (pp. 205–229). New York: Springer Publishing Co.

Boes, M., & McDermott, V. (2002). Helping battered women: A health care perspective. In A. R. Roberts (Ed.), *Handbook of domestic violence intervention strategies: Policies, programs and legal remedies* (pp. 255–277). New York: Oxford University Press.

Boes, M. & Van Wormer, K. (1997). Social work with homeless women in emergency rooms: A strengths-feminist perspective. *Journal of Women and Social Work, 12,* 408–426.

Bristow, D., & Herrick, C. (2002). Emergency department: The roles of the nurse case manager and the social worker. *Continuing Care, 21*(2), 28–29.

Dane, B., & Chanchkes, E. (2001). The cost of caring for patients with illness: Contagion to the social worker. *Social Work in Health Care, 33*(2), 31–51.

Friend, C., & Mills, L.G. (2002). Domestic violence and child protective services: Risk assessments. In A.R. Roberts & G.J. Greene (Eds.), *Social workers' desk reference* (pp. 679–683). New York: Oxford University Press.

Hughes, W. E. (1999). Managed care, meet community support: Ten reasons to include direct support services in every behavioral health plan. *Health and Social Work, 24*(2), 103–111.

Keehn, D., Roglitz, C., & Bowden, M. (1994). Impact of social work on recidivism and non-medical complaints in the emergency department: A cost-benefit analysis of an extended coverage program. *Health and Social Work, 17* (1), 67–74.

Kerr, E. A., & Siu, A. L. (1993). Follow-up after hospital discharge: Does insurance make a difference? *Journal of Health Care for the Poor and Underserved, 4*(3), 133–143.

Ponto, J. M., & Berger, W. (1992). Social work services in the emergency department: A cost benefit analysis of an extended coverage program. *Health and Social Work, 17*(1), 67–75.

Spitzer, W. J., & Kuykendall, R. (1994). Social work delivery of hospital-based financial assistance of services. *Health and Social Work, 19,* 295–298.

Van Wormer, K., & Boes, M. (1997). Humor in the emergency room: A social work perspective. *Health and Social Work, 22*(2), 87–92.

Wells, P. (1993). Preparing for sudden death: Social work in the emergency room. *Social Work, 38,* 339–342.

Zugazaga, C. (2002). *Pathways to homelessness.* Unpublished doctoral dissertation, University of Central Florida.

GLOSSARY

Case management subteam: In some emergency room departments the tasks of case management and discharge planning are now being shared by social workers and nurses, who both serve as case managers. In these situations both professionals are expected to perform the same duties.

QUESTIONS FOR FURTHER STUDY

1. What do you see as the role of the emergency room social worker?
2. What services do you believe social workers in this setting should highlight to project their abilities to others on the interdisciplinary team?
3. This chapter presented the opinions of the social workers working in this area, and all of them stated that they would like to see more evidence- or outcomes-based research to substantiate that emergency room social work could actually reduce recidivism rates. In what ways could this be accomplished?

CHAPTER 13

Case Management and Discharge Planning

Sophia F. Dziegielewski and Alicia Kalinoski

CASE MANAGEMENT AND DISCHARGE PLANNING IN HEALTH CARE SOCIAL WORK

The purpose of this chapter is to explore and identify issues related to professionals working in case management. It is not uncommon for both social workers and nurse case managers to perform this function. Since these two professionals often share the same roles and responsibilities, learning more about how their jobs are perceived is critical. To explore this issue further, four professionals that are working in the area were interviewed about their roles and responsibilities. Topics explored included the role and tasks of the manager and the amount of time involved in direct patient care by each professional.

Case management is a collaboration process that assesses, plans, implements, coordinates, monitors, and evaluates the options and services required to meet an individual's health needs, using communication and available resources to promote quality, cost-effective outcomes (Mullahy, 1998). Case management services seek to ensure that all clients receive the services that they need in a system that sometimes appears fragmented and difficult to navigate (Rothman & Sager, 1998). The tasks in case management can vary; however, for the most part they include the concrete tasks of completing of psychosocial assessments, initiating and implementing advanced directives, assisting in connecting to resources and insurance verification for hospital stays, providing of community resources, and completing referrals for services and durable medical equipment. It also includes more supportive services such as crisis intervention support services, and assisting clients with medication understanding and compliance (Hawkins, Veeder, & Pearce, 1998).

In today's environment of managed behavioral health care social workers are no longer the primary agents providing case management services. Nurses continue to take a more assertive role in what used to be the domain of social work. Generally, nurses working in case management perform tasks similar to social workers; however, more emphasis is placed on performing medical case management tasks such as patient/family education, infection control, quality management, pharmacy inventory, teaching of professional responsibilities, budgeting, and facilitating patient discharges (Bower, 1992; Hawkins et al., 1998; Snow, 2001). In general, nurse case managers focus on the medical condition of the patient, on the patient's insurance, and on ensuring that hospital admissions and lengths of stay remain reasonable (Noetscher & Morreale, 2001). According to Holliman, Dziegielewski and Teare (in press), the duties that are shared are attending meetings, providing documentation, fulfilling outpatient responsibilities, budgeting, and facilitating patient discharges (see Table 13.1).

Although there are similarities in the roles of both the nurse case manager and social worker, there are also differences. One basic difference is in philosophy. Nurses are trained in the medical model, tend to perceive consumers as patients, and focus on concrete services; social workers often assume a more empowering stance and stress self-determination, advocating on behalf of the client. With this different focus it is not uncommon for conflicts to arise between these two disciplines. Some social workers feel that nurses focus too much on the medical needs of the patient, often ignoring the social needs; some nurses may feel that social workers spend too much time on social needs and do not have enough expertise in a client's medical condition to make informed decisions. Therefore, often when the nurse case manager determines that a client is medically ready to leave the hospital plans to initiate this process begin. Some social workers would argue, however, that before this process can begin "person-in-situation" issues need to be explored. For example, what type of support system does the client have? This must be evaluated before concrete plans can be made. It is not uncommon for the social worker to expect to assess the client's environment or situation prior to discharge. When this assessment is

TABLE 13.1 Duties of Case Managers

Tasks of all discharge planners

Task	Percentage (%) who performed the task frequently or almost always
Coordinate services and patient discharge	96.0
Interview caregivers for assessment	95.0
Make contacts for referrals	92.2
Review record prior to contact	91.6
Reassure, support, and reduce anxiety	91.5
Establish rapport	90.4
Documentation	89.9
Review workload to set priorities	86.0
Treatment Team Responsibilities	85.4
Discuss discharge/treatment options with patients/caregivers	85.4

Tasks Exclusive to Social Work and Nursing

Task	Percentage (%) who performed the task frequently or almost always
Performed by Social Workers	
Assess to see if mental health services are needed	63.3
Provide support to unpaid caregivers	63.3
Performed by Nurses	
Review records to ensure standards are met	75.4
Assess treatment plans and quality of care and service effectiveness	64.1
Know current rules/policies	62.3
Gather, enter, and compile data for reports	62.2
Verify eligibility and insurance status	60.4
Educate patients about medical symptoms	60.3

TABLE 13.1   *(continued)*

Comparison of Responsibilities in Addition to Discharge Planning Performed by Social Workers and Nurses

Social Workers	Nurses
Psychosocial Assessments	
Initiate and Implement Advanced Directives	Patient/Family Education
Child/Elder Abuse Screening	Insurance Verification
High Risk Screening	Infection Control
Substance Abuse Intervention	Employee Health
Crisis Intervention	Quality Management
Individual/Family Therapy	Pharmacy Inventory
Group Therapy	Critical Pathways
Grief Therapy	Teaching Professionals
Employee Assistance Programs	Research
Conduct Home visits	

Performed by Both Social Workers and Nurses

Attend Meetings
Documentation
Treatment Team Responsibilities
Conduct Inservice Training for Staff
Supervision
Outpatient Responsibilities
Fundraising
Preparation for Audits
Organ Donation Coordinator
Budgeting

Adapted from Holliman, Dziegielewski & Teare (in press).

not done and limited supports are available, discharges can become complicated.

It is a delicate situation when a client is to be discharged and refuses to go to a nursing home but is unable to handle his or her own activities of daily living (ADL's) or own affairs. The pressure remains great, however, for the case manager to push the patient out the door because there is a lack of coverage or a lack of cooperation from a payer source (Powell, 1996). Every day that the client stays in the hospital under these circumstances costs the hospital money, and pressure for discharge will mount.

The Role of Case Management

In the broadest sense, a case manager is the person who makes the health care system work, influencing both the quality of the outcome and the cost (Mullahy, 1998). Roles are diverse, but perhaps the case manager can facilitate an earlier more supported and stable discharge, negotiate a better fee from a medical equipment supplier, or encourage the family to assume responsibility for assistance with the day-to-day care of the patient. She can be a catalyst for change by seeking solutions that promote improvement or stabilization rather then simply monitoring patient status (Mullahy, 1998). Most professionals agree that for the case manager to be best utilized in a medical setting, there must be well-rounded, broad-based knowledge of all aspects of the hospital (Easterling, Avie, Wesley, & Chimmer, 1995). Overall, it appears that social work case managers have greater contact with patients than do nurse case managers. Social workers see the patients when they are admitted to the hospital and can assess the patients' initial needs. The social worker documents the needs of the patient and follows the patient throughout his or her entire hospital stay, making sure that those needs are being met. The social worker may have to arrange home health care for the patient, arrange for nursing home placement, arrange for medical equipment, arrange for hospice, arrange for transplants, or simply arrange transportation for the patient (Nelson & Powers, 2001). He or she is often able to assess all of the previously stated needs in the short time he or she meets with the patient. The social worker takes into account in the discharge plan the patient's desires, the patient's family's desires, the needs of the patient, the history of the patient, and the potential future of the patient.

The nurse case manager reviews the patient's chart, reviews the social worker's notes, and assesses the patient and his or her medical needs. The nurse's primary focus is business rather then health care (Noetscher & Morreale, 2001). If the patient is medically ready to leave the hospital, the nurse advocates for the hospital, making sure that the patient's length of stay is financially acceptable for the hospital

(Taylor, 2002). In this process the nurse can overlook the social and environmental needs of the patient.

The social work case manager has a broader knowledge of the patient's needs, and the nurse case manager has a broader knowledge of the hospital's needs. At times, instead of working together to facilitate an efficient system, the social worker and nurse are pushing in opposite directions, actually extending the stay of the patient and increasing the cost to the hospital (Hou, Hollenberg, & Charlson, 2001).

Social work case managers are making approximately $32,000–40,000 a year, depending on experience (Hawkins et al., 1998). Nurse case managers are making approximately $36,000–50,000 a year, depending on experience (Hawkins et al., 1998). Social workers' input and services are an effective means of shortening a patient's length of stay, and as a result decreasing the cost to the hospital (Keefler, Duder, & Lechman, 2001). Nurse case managers also lessen the hospital's cost by facilitating a faster move of a patient out of the hospital when medically ready. Social workers and nurses do the same job, but are being paid very different salaries.

OPINIONS OF SOCIAL WORKERS THE FIELD

To better understand the role of the social worker in case management, four professionals were interviewed that all currently work in a medical setting in case management. Each of the four case managers were asked five identical questions. Each interview lasted about 20 minutes and was conducted in the actual work environment. Notes were taken during the interviews by one of the authors. Table 13.2 gives the relevant information on the four case managers.

INTERVIEW QUESTIONS

1. What services do you provide the patient?
2. What do you see as the most significant needs of the patients you serve?
3. What patient needs appear to be met in the current system?
4. What patient needs are not met in the current system?
5. If you could do things differently, what would you change?

TABLE 13.2   Interviewee Information

MSN (A)	Social Worker (B)	Social Worker (C)	Social Worker (D)
48 year old White female	43–year-old White female	45–year-old White female	23-year-old White female
Working with MSN 20 years	Licensed MSW 11 years	Licensed MSW 6 years	BSW
Working in case management 7 years	Working in case management 2 years	Working in case management 15 years	Working in case management 3 months
Working at hospital 7 years	Working at hospital 2 years	Working at hospital 2 years	Working at hospital 3 months
Approx. salary $46,000.00	Approx. salary $40,000.00	Approx. salary $40,000.00	Approx. salary Income not reported

MSN = Master of Science in Nursing, MSW = Master of Social Work, BSW = Bachelor of Social Work.

INTERVIEWEE OPINIONS

Four subjects were interviewed to find out what they saw as their role in providing case management services.

What services do you provide the patient?

- Professional A: I complete chart assessments to determine potential discharge needs for the patient. I do utilization reviews, making sure the patient needs to be hospitalized so there are no unexpected denials by insurance companies.
- Professional B: Discharge planning, community information, assist in connecting to resources, evaluate support system and medical needs, identify gaps, connect to resources to fill gaps, crisis intervention.
- Professional C: Discharge planning, arrange home health care, equipment, outpatient services, skilled nursing facilities, community resources, supportive counseling, and crisis intervention.

- Professional D: Discharge planning, crisis intervention, connecting to community resources, support groups, outpatient services such as home physical therapy, home health nurse, medical equipment, patient support, family support.

What do you see as the most significant needs of the patients you serve?

- Professional A: Arranging for proper placement if patient is unable to return home.
- Professional B: Discharge from acute medical hospital to home, skilled nursing facility, nursing home with no needs, home with home health, home with physical therapy, extended care facility, or rehabilitation.
- Professional C: Financial resources for patients on fixed incomes, some need help with medications, family support is not always given by family members and it is important to connect the patient with a support system in the community.
- Professional D: Discharge plan based on current and past living situation, assisting family support of the patient, connecting the patient to community resources.

What patient needs appear to be met in the current system?

- Professional A: We only meet the immediate health and home care needs of the clients we serve.
- Professional B: At times we have adequate resources and I can help find funds to help supplement insurance coverage or secure private funds.
- Professional C: Medical, acute care, and plan for follow-up care, some limited financial assistance, emotional support, crisis intervention, and limited education.
- Professional D: Discharge plan, connecting to resources, medical, emotional, answering questions and concerns through education.

What patients' needs are not met in the current system?

- Professional A: Cardiac rehabilitation immediately after surgery.
- Professional B: Mental health services are often overlooked with concentration on the client's medical condition, lack of resources.

- Professional C: Financial assistance, patient family education, limited time to provide emotional support, and mental health or psychiatric issues are often not addressed.
- Professional D: Therapy, some medical needs are not met due to lack of insurance, other services lacking include access to medication, education, and support.

If you could do things differently, what would you change?

- Professional A: Add more inpatient cardiac rehabilitation, stronger policies to disallow physician reimbursements for patients that stay in the hospital unnecessarily.
- Professional B: The number of patients that the case manager is expected to cover, this limits service and individualized plans. Need more comprehensive resources for patients.
- Professional C: Be more proactive by intervening with patients earlier in hospitalization to identify needs, and refer to appropriate resources. Be able to do more patient and family education on psychosocial needs by providing families and patients some idea of what to expect.
- Professional D: Ability to address all patients' needs, providing them with a better understanding of the medical procedure that they are going through.

In summary, these interviews are not meant to be representative of any type of formidable research. These professionals were interviewed to help the reader to see exactly what individuals in the field have to say about their area of work. In the future, more research is needed to establish how to join social work and nursing and help social workers and nurses work closer as a team. Enhanced teamwork would allow nurse case managers and social work case managers to use the resources and skills inherent in each profession toward the best interest of the patient. In this small sample, although there is a case management team, each individual reported that he or she often worked in isolation and did not collaborate much with the other. Allowing the nurse and the social worker to collaborate on each patient and his or her needs will allow the team to facilitate an accurate, efficient, and useful discharge plan.

In closing, probably one of the biggest areas of contention with this group was salaries. Currently, nurse case managers are getting paid on average $10,000 a year more than social work case managers for doing basically an identical job (Hawkins et al., 1998). This salary differential alone has created a rift between those working in the same role. More research is needed to see if this is considered the norm, and if it is, social workers need to advocate for at a minimum "equal pay for equal work."

CHAPTER SUMMARY AND FUTURE DIRECTIONS

Case management in the behaviorally based managed care setting is an evolving art. Many new nurses and social workers are coming into case management and are surprised by the differences in job rules and responsibilities. Case management in the medical setting involves discharge planning from the hospital, placement in nursing homes, placement for rehabilitation, placement in a transitional care facility, or placement in a facility that the client was in previously. Case management in a medical setting also involves providing clients with medical equipment, verifying insurance claims, and linking clients to community resources for support groups, educational groups, individual family or group therapy, and community resources to help a client pay for hospital bills and/or medication (Nelson & Powers, 2001).

What seems most unfortunate is that social workers are performing nurse components of the case management job; however, nurses are not performing social work components. This means that many times social workers are given the more difficult and time-consuming cases that require counseling or additional supports. These social workers are well versed in medical terms and procedures as well as in financial information about Medicare and Medicaid. They also need to be aware of community resources and what is needed to qualify for these services. The social worker needs to have background knowledge in mental health, mental illness, domestic violence, child abuse, drug and alcohol abuse, and sexual abuse, and an overall understanding of how people live. All of these components are necessary to be able to help clients.

Furthermore, for case management teams to function more efficiently in the medical setting, the social worker needs to play a crucial role in getting all medical staff more involved in understanding the needs of the clients. The social work case manager can also facilitate helping the client to get his or her needs met as quickly and as accurately as possible. Medical social work is not for all social workers. Some professionals believe it is less "clinical" than traditional social work. Regardless, these social workers help in recognizing what a client needs, in advocating, and in many cases directly providing for those services from an individualized perspective. After all, historically, hasn't that been the clinical core of social work practice?

REFERENCES

Bower, K. (1992). *Case management by nurses*. Washington DC: American Nurses Association.

Easterling, A., Avie, J., Wesley, M., & Chimmer, H. (1995) *The case manager's guide*. New York: American Hospital Publishing.

Hawkins, J., Veeder, N., & Pearce, C. (1998). *Nurse social worker collaboration managed care: A model of community case management*. New York: Springer Publishing Co.

Holliman, D., Dziegielewski, S. F., & Teare, R. (in press). Differences and similarities between social work and nurse discharge planners. Accepted December 18, 2001 in *Health and Social Work*.

Hou, J., Hollenberg, J., & Charlson, M. (2001). Can physicians' admission evaluation of patients' status help to identify patients requiring social work interventions? *Social Work in Health Care*, 33(2), 17–28.

Keefler, J., Duder, S., & Lechman, C. (2001). Predicting length of stay in an acute care hospital: The role of psychosocial problems. *Social Work in Health Care, 33* (2), 1–15.

Mullahy, C. (1998). *The case manager's handbook*. Gaithersburg, MD: Aspen.

Nelson, J., & Powers, P. (2001). Community case management for frail, elderly clients: The nurse case manager's role. *Journal of Nursing Administration, 31*, 444–450.

Noetscher, C., & Morreale, G. (2001). Length of stay reduction: Two innovative hospital approaches. *Journal of Nursing Administration, 16*(1), 1–14.

Powell, S. (1996). *Nursing case management*. Philadelphia: Lippincott-Raven.

Rothman, J., & Sager, J. S. (1998). *Case management: Integrating individual and community practice*. Needham Heights, MA: Allen & Bacon.

Snow, J. (2001). Looking beyond nursing for clues to effective leadership. *Journal of Nursing Administration, 31*, 440–443.

Taylor, C. (2002). Assessing patients' needs: Does the same information guide expert and novice nurses? *International Nursing Review, 49*(1), 11–19.

GLOSSARY

Nurse case managers: Generally, nurse case managers review charts and assess for medical needs. The primary tasks include patient/family education, insurance verification, infection control, employee health, quality management, pharmacy inventory, critical pathways, teaching professionals, and research.

Social work case managers: Generally, social work case managers complete psychosocial assessments, conduct patient/family education, initiate and implement advanced directives, do child/elder abuse screening, do high risk screening, do substance abuse intervention, do crisis intervention, conduct individual/family therapy, lead group therapy, do grief therapy, manage employee assistance programs and conduct home visits.

QUESTIONS FOR FURTHER STUDY

1. Identify what you believe to be the differences and similarities between social work and nurse case managers.
2. What services do you believe social workers in this setting should highlight to project their abilities to others serving as part of an interdisciplinary team?
3. In this chapter all of the social workers stated that they would like to see more evidence- or outcomes-based research to substantiate that the services they provided were important. In what ways can this be accomplished?

CHAPTER 14

Home Care Social Work

Sophia F. Dziegielewski and Dawn Townsend

Home care agencies have been providing high-quality, in-home services to Americans for more than a century and have remained an integral part of the provision of health services since 1905. Health care social workers help patients and their families cope with chronic, acute, or terminal illnesses and handle problems that may stand in the way of recovery or rehabilitation. On October 1, 2000, home care entered a new era of reimbursement when the Medicare Perspective Pay System took effect in all home health agencies. Acknowledging this change from "per visit" to "per episode" is critical because it can affect how social workers are utilized in home care. This chapter introduces the health care social worker to the Perspective Pay System and explains how it impacts the role of the social worker. To further exemplify the changing role of the health care social worker in this area of practice, interviews with home care social workers were conducted. These interviews identify perceptions of social worker effectiveness, roadblocks in performing their job to their satisfaction, ethical dilemmas experienced, and job satisfaction. Strategies are suggested to survive the changes in this area of home care social work.

THE TRANSITION TO HOME CARE SERVICES

Home care refers to health care and the social services that are provided to individuals and families in their home or in communities and other homelike settings. Home care includes a wide array of services, including nursing, rehabilitation, social work, home health aids and other services. This rapidly expanding area of health care social work can be traced back as far as the early nineteenth century (Cowles, 2000; National Association for Home Care, 2000). In 1955, the United States Public Health Services endorsed a physician-oriented organized home health care team designed to provide medical and social services to patients within their home. The team consisted of a physician, nurse, and social worker (R. Goode, 2000). Since that time social workers have continued to provide social services in the home care setting, and this area of health care social work remains a diverse and dynamic service industry.

One reason cited for the increase in demand for home care services is that hospital stays have decreased through the years. Other reasons for the increasing demands for home care services include (1) the aging of the population with a high rate of functional disabilities; (2) the shift from acute infectious diseases to chronic diseases as major health problems; (3) the increase in technology that allows people to be cared for at home in spite of the need for medical equipment such as IVs, catheters, suction machines, portable oxygen, and infusion pumps; (4) the fear of nursing home placement, which prompts people to choose home care instead; (5) the AIDS epidemic; and (6) the increase in medically fragile children (Cowles, 2000).

The majority of home care services are considered third party and are reimbursable by Medicare, Medicaid, private insurance policies, health maintenance organizations (HMOs), and group health plans. These types of payments are determined by several factors, including client diagnosis and the types of services required. Medicare recipients are the largest group of clients needing home health care services.

On October 1, 2000, home care entered a new era of reimbursement when the Medicare Prospective Payment System (PPS) took effect in all home health agencies. Previously, home health agencies received payment from Medicare under a cost-based reimbursement system subject to limits referred to as the Interim Payment System (IPS). This per visit cost allowed as many visits by skilled nurses, therapists, and social workers as were deemed necessary for patient recovery. Payments under the PPS are based on a sixty-day "episode" of care, instead of the "per visit" reimbursement that Medicare had formerly paid. This episodic reimbursement system is based on a national payment rate that is adjusted to reflect the severity of the patient's condition (Moore, 2000; Grimaldi, 2000).

The Health Care Financing Administration (HCFA) developed the Outcome and Assessment Information Set (OASIS), which is a core standard assessment data set for home care. OASIS data are federally mandated assessment questions that must be collected every 60 days. Based on the responses to items on the OASIS assessment, the patient will fall into one of the 80 Home Health Resource Groups (HHRGs). Each HHRG has its own weighted score intended to result in a payment that reflects the intensity of care required (Health Care Financing Administration, 2000; Moore, 2000; Vladeck, 1997).

Each payment is based on the episode experienced by the individual beneficiary. An agency is paid for a 60-day period of care without regard to the amount of services it provides in the 60-day period. Therefore, an agency receives incentive to provide short-term, service-limited care in the most cost-effective way for the agency possible. It is believed that this system has seriously jeopardized patient's access to home health care benefits, especially for social work.

Each agency must manage its utilization of services in order to keep expenses down. As the number of elderly individuals grows, so does the number of individuals who require home care. Since the sheer numbers of elderly individuals are growing so rapidly, this population group is making the greatest demand on home care services. More frequently than not, the services they need often involve social as well as medical supports, making the role of social work crucial in the field of home care. "When psychosocial needs go unmet whether through lack of detection or lack of treatment, elderly patients are at risk of further health problems that can lead to physical deterioration, reduced independence, and eventually to the need for more intensive and expensive services" (Berkman et al., 1999, p. 9).

For many years, NASW has encouraged the HCFA to grant skilled status to social work services. This would require that each social worker provide for each client an evaluation to assess for psychosocial needs. Unfortunately, this advocacy has failed, and now with the new PPS, this seems even less likely to happen (R. Goode, 2000). It is not yet known how the changes in Medicare reimbursement will affect home care social workers. Little research has been done to date that explores how these changes have impacted the role of the home care social worker.

EVIDENCE-BASED PRACTICE IN THE HOME CARE SETTING

Health care social workers help patients and their families cope with chronic, acute, or terminal illnesses and handle problems that may stand in the way of recovery or rehabilitation. Cowles (2000) identifies six categories of home care client problems: "(1) barriers to admission to the service; (2) problems of adjustment to the service; (3) problems of adjustment to the diagnosis, prognosis, or treatment/care plan; (4) lack of information to make informed decisions; (5) lack of needed resources; and (6) barriers to discharge from the service " (p. 176).

Rossi (1999) describes home care social workers' duties as the following: "(1) helping the health care team to understand the social and emotional factors related to the patient's health and care; (2) assessing the social and emotional factors to estimate the caregiver's capacity and potential, including but not limited to coping with the problems of daily living, acceptance of the illness or injury or its impact, role reversal, sexual problems, stress, anger or frustration, and make the necessary referrals to ensure that the patient receives the appropriate treatments; (3) helping the caregiver to secure or utilize other community agencies as needs are identified; and (4) helping the patient or caregiver to submit paperwork for alternative funding" (p. 335).

Although there is little research on the impact of the PPS on social work utilization in home care, there is research that explores the utilization of social work in the field of home care and the ethical dilemmas social workers may encounter.

A research study by C. J. Goode (1995) focused on primary service providers (nurses, physical and occupational therapists, and administrative staff) and their attitudes, beliefs, and perceptions in regards to social work services. C. J. Goode (1995) used unstructured interviews with a sampling of twelve home health agencies that included four for-profit agencies, four nonprofit agencies, and four hospital-based agencies. C. J. Goode's data were gathered from the administrator or director, the director of nursing, and clinical staff. The clinical staff included physical and occupational therapists, RN case managers and home health aides.

According to R. Goode (2000), there were three major obstacles to providing social work services: "lack of knowledge on the part of physicians and the public about the benefits of social workers—reported by five agencies; lack of knowledge among agencies—reported by ten agencies; and no reimbursement for social work visits, which prevented many patients from obtaining services—reported by all twelve agencies" (p. 25). All 12 agencies identified no reimbursement for social work visits as a major obstacle to providing social work services. This is significant in that it could support the possibility that changes in Medicare reimbursement could affect utilization of social workers in home care, since social work visits are no longer reimbursable by Medicare.

Egan and Kadushin (1999) have done extensive research on home care social workers. They believe that "empirically based research on social work practice in home health agencies is essential to help the profession explain its function to other disciplines, to educate practitioners for community based practice and to serve as the basis for the development and measurement of outcomes for social work practice in home health" (p. 44). Initially their focus was to identify types of services provided and agency auspice. Through their research, they were able to "identify a high degree of consensus that the respondents performed functions such as coordination of services, assessment, counseling, interagency collaboration and home visits" (Egan & Kadushin, 1999, p. 46). Additional social work functions included advocating for clients and providing health education. Over 80% of the social workers also spent time educating coworkers about social work.

An interesting finding was that the "auspices of the social workers' agencies were associated with practice activities" (Egan & Kadushin, 1999, p. 51). It appears that social workers in proprietary settings provide more advocacy and health education to patients than those social workers in a nonprofit setting. This can be attributed to reimbursement criteria. This means that social workers in proprietary settings advocated for patients for needed visits. Social workers in proprietary settings also had more opportunity to experience denials for requests for services and identified this barrier to services as an ethical dilemma.

Kadushin and Egan (2001) later expanded on their previous research and targeted the ethical dilemmas experienced by home care social workers. Their survey examined several factors related to the frequency and difficulty of resolving four ethical conflicts in a national sample of 364 home health care social workers (Kadushin & Egan, 2001). Eligible participants rated four ethical conflicts: (1) assessing patients' mental competence, (2) patient self-determination, (3) implementation of advance directives, and (4) patient access to service.

The findings indicated that social workers rated assessing patient's mental competence, patient access to service, and patient self-determination as similarly frequent and difficult to resolve. They rated patient self-determination as moderately frequent. On average, respondents reported rarely having to compromise their ethics. When faced with ethical dilemmas, social workers identified social work colleagues and consulting nurses as being helpful in resolving conflicts (Kadushin & Egan, 2001).

The research also identified reimbursement restrictions as "creating pressures for social workers to restrict services or prematurely terminate care to patients who require a higher intensity of services" (Kadushin & Egan, 2001, p. 15). Social workers are ethically obligated to advocate for their patients, yet this presents an ethical dilemma when trying to stay within the guidelines of the agency's expectations.

It is apparent that research has defined the ongoing need for social work in the home care setting. It is also evident that social workers do encounter ethical dilemmas when working in home care (Barber & Lyness, 2001). What is not known at this time is how the changes in Medicare reimbursement have impacted the utilization of home care social workers. To explore this issue further, individual interviews with social workers in the field were conducted to ask questions about the newly implemented Perspective Pay System.

OPINIONS OF SOCIAL WORKERS IN THE FIELD

To find out opinions of social workers actively working in the field, six home health care social workers were interviewed. Each of the social workers was familiar with the changes created after October 1, 2000. Three of the social workers had been hired less than 6 months before the PPS, and the other three social workers had secured their employment after the PPS was in place.

To find social workers in the field, several agencies were contacted that were listed as licensed home care agencies in the central Florida area, and six social workers agreed to be interviewed. Each of the participants had been employed in a home care agency between 2 and 11 years. Three social workers were licensed clinical social workers, two were bachelor-level social workers, and one was a master-level social worker (who had not gotten her license yet). Interviewees # 5 and # 6 were both bachelor-level social workers and had the longest employment in home care, with 8 and 11 years, respectively. The bachelor-level social workers who were in the setting longer performed most of the entry-level tasks and served as generalist practitioners. These social workers performed roles similar to other generalist social workers, including educator, broker, case manager, mediator, facilitator, and advocate (Kirst-Ashman & Hull, 1999). For the master's-level social workers, the primary roles were similar; however, these more educated social workers were often called upon to do counseling and supportive education when confronting clients with adjustment difficulties and those needing short-term therapy.

The interviews began on February 22, 2002, and ended on March 22, 2002, and each interview lasted 30 minutes. The questions asked were as follows:

- Has your job changed since the introduction of the PPS? If so, in what ways has it changed?
- Have you had any social work staffing changes since the PPS?
- Do you think the PPS has impacted your effectiveness within the agency?
- Are there any ethical dilemmas that have resulted from the changes? Can you tell me about them?
- What would you identify as the biggest roadblock in performing your job to your satisfaction?
- Would you say you are satisfied or dissatisfied with your job in home care?

INTERVIEWEE COMMENTS

Has your job changed since the introduction of the PPS?

Interviewee #1 answered no. Interviewee #2 answered yes. Interviewee #3 answered yes. Interviewee #4 answered yes. Interviewee #5 answered no. Interviewee #6 answered yes.

In what ways has it changed?

Interviewee # 1 reported being a salaried employee who had little restrictions attached to the job and being able to self-define the role of the social worker within the home care agency. Interviewee #2 reported that incoming referrals were reduced. Interviewee #3 reported that there were fewer referrals, fewer numbers of visits to the same patient, and patients were discharged from social services sooner. Interviewee #4 reported that there were fewer visits made and more phone contacts. Interviewee #4 also reported having to provide inservice training about community resources to the nurse case managers. Interviewee #5 reported no changes. Interviewee #6 reported a decrease in the number of referrals and a decrease in the frequency of visits. In the past visits ranged from three to four visits to resolve issues and now visits are limited to one to two for a patient.

Have you had any social work staffing changes since the PPS?

Interviewee #1 reported the elimination of one per diem position. Interviewee #2 reported elimination of one full-time position. Interviewee #3 reported a reduction in staff. Interviewee #4 reported that the full-time social worker was downsized to part time and one full-time position was eliminated. Interviewee #5 reported that their social work staff has increased with the hiring of an additional part-time social worker. Interviewee #6 reported the elimination of one full-time position.

Do you think the PPS has impacted your effectiveness within the agency?

Interviewee #1 answered no. Interviewee #2 answered yes. Interviewee #3 answered yes. Interviewee #4 answered yes. Interviewee #5 answered no. Interviewee #6 answered yes.

Are there any ethical dilemmas that have resulted from the changes?

Interviewee #1 answered no. Interviewee #2 answered yes. Interviewee #3 answered yes. Interviewee #4 answered yes. Interviewee #5 answered no. Interviewee #6 answered yes.

Can you tell me about them?

Interviewee #1 reported no ethical dilemmas. Interviewee #2 reported that using nurses as social workers to identify needs and often to resolve patients' issues was not providing expert services to the patients.

Interviewee #3 reported that there is often pressure from nurses and management to discharge patients sooner from social services. Interviewee #4 reported that there are boundary issues when nurses are attempting to do social work tasks without having the social work skills. Interviewee #4 also reported that having to refer patients out for counseling instead of providing it within the home care system was an ethical dilemma. Another dilemma reported was that sometimes nurses may avoid identifying problems in an effort to contain costs, especially if they think the social worker will not have adequate time to resolve the problem in the one or two visits that may be allowed. Interviewee #5 reported no ethical dilemmas. Interviewee #6 reported that when patients have adjustment problems it takes time to resolve the problem.

What would you identify as the biggest roadblock in performing your job to your satisfaction?

Interviewee #1 reported no roadblocks. Interviewee #2 reported the mixed responsibilities between nurses and social workers, with nurses doing case management. This interviewee also reported that when social workers are considered adjunct services as opposed to main-line services roadblocks to providing services result. Interviewee #3 reported that nurses have the tendency to focus mainly on the physical unmet needs of the patient instead of psychosocial issues. This often leaves some issues that are not addressed that could have benefited from social work intervention. Interviewee #4 reported that trying to accomplish everything that needs to be done for a patient in a "one-time" visit is very difficult. Interviewee #5 reported the lack of funds in the community for things such as medications as being the biggest roadblock. Interviewee #6 reported working with nurses who are case managers and want social work knowledge of systems and community resources but do not want to give the social worker credit for her input.

Would you say you are satisfied or dissatisfied with your job in home care?

Interviewee #1 reported being satisfied. Interviewee #2 reported being dissatisfied. Interviewee #3 reported being dissatisfied. Interviewee #4 reported being dissatisfied. Interviewee #5 reported being satisfied. Interviewee #6 reported being satisfied.

SUMMARY OF FINDINGS

In summary, the majority of the social workers interviewed reported a change in their duties since the introduction of the Perspective Pay System. A decrease in the number of referrals and/or a decrease in the number of visits allowed were identified most frequently. This is supported by the research, which indicates that when social work visits are not reimbursable, social work services are limited (Kadushin & Egan, 2001; Egan & Kadushin, 1999; Goode, 2000). Other changes included more phone contacts and providing inservices and education to non-social work staff.

Five of the six interviewees reported a reduction in social work staff at their agency. Although it is not known why two of the intervivewee's were not impacted by the changes in Medicare reimbursement, as were the others, it is evident that social work services have decreased in the majority of the home care agencies where the interviewees were employed. This decrease could be reason for alarm because clients in home care often require supportive services due to chronic conditions and declining functional and cognitive capacities (Wholey, Burns, & Lavizzo-Mourey, 1998).

The majority of the interviewees reported having experienced ethical dilemmas since the Medicare reimbursement change. Ethical dilemmas included (1) using nurses instead of social workers to identify needs and to resolve patients' issues, (2) pressure from nurses and management to discharge patients sooner from social services, (3) referring weak and ill patients out for counseling instead of providing counseling within the confines of home care services, (4) the often impossible task of meeting patients' needs within a one-time visit, and (5) the knowledge that sometimes a nurse may avoid identifying problems in order to not utilize social work.

The social work profession has a well-developed formal code of ethics that provides the guidelines and boundaries in which the profession operates. Bateman (2000) discusses the importance of always acting in the client's best interest but acknowledges the difficulty when faced with the many pressures to "compromise the vigor of one's advocacy or to work in partnership with the other side" (p. 48). In a multidisciplinary setting, it may be unrealistic to expect that differences among team members in their recommendations of patient care will not create ethical dilemmas. How these dilemmas are addressed by social workers is paramount to being a strong advocate for patients (Rehr, Rosenberg, & Blumenfield, 1998).

The majority of the interviewees identified roadblocks in performing their job to their satisfaction. These roadblocks were similar to the ethical dilemmas that the interviewees experienced. The roadblocks identified were (1) mixed responsibilities between nurses and social workers, (2) having social workers being considered as adjunct services, (3) the nurses' tendency to focus on physical unmet needs instead of the psychosocial issues, (4) the difficulty in trying to meet all the needs of the patient in one visit, (5) lack of funding in the community, and (6) working with nurses who want social workers to share their knowledge of resources, yet do not want to credit the social worker for his or her efforts. The last finding indicated that only half of the interviewees were satisfied with their job in home care.

CHAPTER SUMMARY AND FUTURE DIRECTIONS

There can be much speculation on why social workers may be dissatisfied in the home care setting. Part of this can be related to the roadblocks and ethical dilemmas that the interviewees identified. Frustration from not feeling like a valued professional, and a sense of powerlessness to impact change may also contribute to this dissatisfaction.

Watt and Kallman (1998), when discussing managed care conflicts and dilemmas of professionals, indicated that policy changes and organizational responses could create anxiety, confusion, and dissatisfaction among the professions. Some of this response to change is related to the disruption of comfortable patterns of behavior and insecurity with the unknown changes. "Some of the resistance to the changes may stem from ethical concerns about the nature of the required shifts in practice and the impact on those of the client population" (Watt & Kallman, 1998, p. 2). Furthermore, the subsequent demand for greater clinical accountability with behaviorally based outcomes that are considered essential benchmarks for effective care may also be causing difficulty (Watt, 2001). Regardless of the exact reason, this warrants further research on the direct causes of job dissatisfaction, and how satisfaction could be increased in home care social workers.

A sense of satisfaction is necessary for social workers to decrease the chances of burnout and to enable social workers to want to provide the best services they can for the clients they serve. The opinions of these social workers support the notion that home care social workers are being underutilized since the introduction of the Perspective Pay System. Additional research is needed to explore this topic and to identify the role changes and barriers to job satisfaction.

Armed with a wealth of experiences, varying health conditions, and differing attitudes, behaviors, and levels of functional impairment, elderly clients are possibly the most diverse group of clients with whom social workers will work with. McLeod and Bywaters (2000) validate the need for social workers in health care and report that there is substantial scope for social work involvement through working toward greater equality of access to existing health and social services. Furthermore, social workers need to be active in securing more information and a better understanding of the balancing of responsibility that needs to occur between the federal government and the states in providing adequate funding and reimbursement for home care services (Caro et al., 2002)

Strategies for surviving the changes in the home care system will include social workers realistically assessing their position. This includes careful appraisal of the sources of support for the social worker within the agency. Equally important is to participate in shaping how social workers are viewed to establish their role as knowledgeable, positive, and supportive resources to support staff, coworkers, and administration (Neuman, 2000).

New and different ideas and contributions to increase client empowerment in home care are needed (McWilliam et al., 2001). Ideas such as cross-disciplinary patient case review and consultation ensure that patients receive the benefit of a broad range of expertise, including nursing, therapies (occupational, physical, and speech), and social work (Byrne, 1999). Inservice education programs and ongoing case review with other disciplines give social workers the opportunity to display clinical expertise. Establishing standardized biopsychosocial screening criteria for nurse case managers can be instrumental in incorporating social workers in the care plan (Moore-Greene, 2000). To ensure increased cost effectiveness of the home care services provided, information should always be gathered on incidence of institutionalization, hospitalization, functional impairment, and mortality (Miller & Weissert, 2001), in addition to resource utilization measures such as the number of visits, length of stay, and total direct care time spent with each client (Adams & Michel, 2001).

Social workers are uniquely qualified to provide clinical services in home care. The home care social worker can instruct staff in the intrapsychic, interpersonal, and psychosocial aspects of patients' lives, demonstrate the efficacy of clinical social work interventions, and support staff who are encountering difficulties in providing patient care. By blending their knowledge of environmental and systems assessment and intervention with psychosocial expertise, they can play a fluid role that is frequently demanded as the dynamic needs of the patient shift (Byrne, 1999). Social workers should take advantage of opportunities in this change process by being proactive and creative as the home care social work profession redefines itself.

REFERENCES

Adams, C. E., & Michel, Y. (2001). Correlation between home health resource utilization measures. *Home Health Care Services Quarterly, 20*(3), 45–56.

Barber, C. E., & Lyness, K. P. (2001). Ethical issues in family care of older persons with dementia: Implications for family therapists. *Home Health Care Services Quarterly, 20*(3), 1–26.

Bateman, N. (2000). *Advocacy skills for health and social care professionals.* Philadelphia: Jessica Kingsley.

Berkman, B., Chauncey, S., Holmes, W., Daniels, A., Bonander, E., Sampson, S., & Robinson, M. (1999). Standardized screening of elderly patients' needs for social work assessment in primary care: Use of the SF-36. *Health and Social Work, 24*(1), 9–17.

Byrne, J. (1999). Social work in psychiatric home care: Regulations, roles and realities. *Health and Social Work, 24*(1), 65–72.

Caro, F. G., Porell, F. W., Sullivan, D. M., Safran-Norton, C. E., & Miltiades, H. (2002). Home health and home care in Massachusetts after the Balanced Budget act of 1997: Implications of cost containment pressures for service authorizations. *Home Health Care Services Quarterly, 21*(1), 47–66.

Cowles, L. A., (2000). *Social work in the health field.* Binghamton, NY: Hawthorne.

Egan, M., & Kadushin, G. (1999). The social worker in the emerging field of home care: Professional activities and ethical concerns. *Health and Social Work, 24*(1), 43–55.

Goode, C.J. (1995). Impact of CareMap and case management on patient satisfaction and staff satisfaction, collaboration, and autonomy. *Nursing Economics, 13*, 337–348, 361.

Goode, R. (2000). *Social work practice in home health care.* Binghamton, NY: Hawthorne.

Grimaldi, P. (2000, November). Medicare's new home health prospective payment system explained. *Healthcare Financial Management,* 46–56.

Health Care Financing Administration. (2000, April). Role of physician in the home health perspective payment system. (NCFA Pub. 6OB). *Program Memorandum Carriers,* 1–4.

Kadushin, G., & Egan, M. (2001). Ethical dilemmas in home health care: A social work perspective. *Health and Social Work, 26*(3), 136–161. Retrieved January 4, 2002 from Ehost online database.

Kirst-Ashman, K., & Hull, G. (1999). *Understanding generalist practice.* Chicago: Nelson-Hall.

McLeod, E., & Bywaters, P. (2000). *Social work, health and equality.* New York: Routledge.

McWilliam, C.L., Ward,-Griffin, C., Sweetland, D., Sutherland, C., & O'Halloran, L. (2001). The experience of empowerment in home care services delivery. *Home Health Care Services Quarterly, 20*(4), 49–71.

Miller, E.A., & Weissert, W.G. (2001). Incidence of four adverse outcomes in the elderly population: Implications for home care policy and research. *Home Health Care Quarterly, 20,*(4), 17–47.

Moore, M. (2000). PPS takes effect in home health care. *American Speech-Language-Hearing Association Leader, 5*(19), 1.

Moore-Greene, G. (2000). Standardizing social indicators to enhance medical case management. *Social Work in Health Care, 30*(3), 39–53.

National Association for Home Care (2000). Basic statistics about home care. (pp. 1–25). Retrieved February 11, 2002 from the World Wide Web: *www.nach.org.Consumer/hcstats.html*

Neuman, K. (2000). Understanding organizational reengineering in health care: Strategies for social work's survival. *Social Work in Health Care, 31*(1), 19–32.

Rehr, H., Rosenberg, G., & Blumenfield, S. (Eds.). (1998). *Creative social work in health care.* New York: Springer Publishing Co.

Rossi, P. (1999). *Case management in healthcare.* Philadelphia: W.B. Saunders.

Vladeck, B. (1997). Testimony on Medicare payment for home health agency and skilled nursing facility services (pp. 1–14). *Health Care Financing Administration.* Retrieved February 21, 2002 from the World Wide Web: *www.hhs.gov/asl/testify/t960723a.html*

Watt, H.M. (2001) Community-based case management: A model for outcome-based research for non-institutionalized elderly. *Home Health Care Services Quarterly, 20*(1), 39–65.

Watt, W., & Kallman, G. (1998, July 1). Managing professional obligations under managed care: A social work perspective. In *Family and community health* (pp. 1–10). Retrieved March 6, 2002 from Findarticles.com on-line database.

Wholey, D., Burns, L., & Lavizzo-Mourey, R. (1998). Managed care and the delivery of primary care to the elderly and the chronically ill. *Health Services Research, 33,* 322–354.

GLOSSARY

Home care services: This refers to social services that are provided to individuals and families in their home or in community and other homelike settings. Home care includes a wide array of services, including nursing, rehabilitation, social work, home health aids, and other services.

Home Health Resource Groups (HHRGs): Based on the responses to items on the OASIS assessment, an HHRG consists of a weighted score that is intended to result in a payment that reflects the intensity of care required.

Interim Payment System: This is a system where home health agencies received payment from Medicare under a cost-based reimbursement system where per visit cost is implemented and as many visits as deemed necessary for patient recovery by skilled nurses, therapists, and social workers are allowed.

Outcome and Assessment Information Set (OASIS): This is a core standard assessment data set to be used in home care. It was developed by the Health Care Financing Administration (HCFA). The OASIS is a federally mandated assessment tool that must be completed every 60 days.

Prospective Payment System (PPS): On October 1, 2000, home care entered a new era of reimbursement. Payments under the PPS are based on a 60-day "episode" of care, instead of the "per visit" reimbursement that Medicare had formerly paid. This episodic reimbursement system is based on a national payment rate that is adjusted to reflect the severity of the patient's condition.

QUESTIONS FOR FURTHER STUDY

1. Would you like to be a home care social worker?
2. If you were a home care social worker, in what ways would your job have changed since the introduction of PPS?
3. Find a social worker working in the home care field and ask him or her the following questions:
   - In the area of home care social work, what ways would your job have changed since the introduction of PPS?
   - Do you believe there will be social work staffing changes since PPS?
   - Do you think PPS has impacted your effectiveness within the agency?
   - Are there any ethical dilemmas that have resulted from the changes?
   - Can you tell me about them?
   - What would you identify as the biggest roadblock in performing your job to your satisfaction?
   - Would you say you are satisfied or dissatisfied with your job in home care?

CHAPTER 15

The Roles and Services Provided by the Hospice Social Worker

Sophia F. Dziegielewski and Joanna Kaevats

HOSPICE SOCIAL WORK

This chapter explores the roles of the hospice social worker. Social workers were interviewed to help increase understanding and to help identify their current roles and functions. To facilitate this process, five social workers from a central Florida hospice were interviewed who have 38 years of combined hospice social work experience. The opinions of these social workers actively working in this area of health care are explored. This chapter also discusses additional and/or needed services as perceived by these social workers to better serve clients and their families. The chapter concludes with an emphasis on quicker and timelier referrals to hospice programs. It is also believed that more attention needs to be given to provision of continuous respite care. Additional services that need to be increased include personal care services, education and support in regard to the dying process, homemaking services, and the development of a Hospice House. An argument is also made for additional funding through Medicare to increase patient and family satisfaction with the quality of care and service.

WHAT IS HOSPICE?

Hospice care is a special way of caring for people who are terminally ill and their families. Basically, the goal of a hospice is to care for the patient and the family, with open acknowledgment that no cure is expected for patient's illness. Hospice care includes physical, emotional, social, and spiritual care; usually a public agency or private company that may or not be Medicare approved provides this service. All age groups are serviced, including children, adults, and the elderly during their final stages of life (Facts and Figures, 2001).

The goals of hospice are to provide for the care and needs of the terminally ill; to furnish both inpatient and in-home services; and to make available educational programs to the patient, the families involved, and interested community members. The premise that provides the basis for these programs is the belief that a hospice can create a supportive environment in which a person who has a life-threatening illness is treated with respect. In addition, the individual is prepared for a dignified death that is satisfactory to the person and to those who participate in the person's care (McSkimming, Myrick, & Wasinger, 2000).

The role of the social worker is crucial to the family planning process, and efforts are made to help family members deal with the client's illness and impending death in the most effective way possible. To foster an atmosphere of support and caring, the social worker tries to facilitate open communication between patient and family. It is believed that successful transition and eventual acceptance of the diagnosis and prognosis will allow the grief work to begin. The hospice social worker will be expected to assess levels of stress—especially the ones that affect coping and prognosis. In addition, special attention needs to be given to assessing the spiritual needs of the client and his or her family and helping them continue to adjust and accept. The hospice setting has a strong interdisciplinary focus and uses a team approach to continually assess environmental safety concerns.

One of the first tasks of the social worker is to address grieving with an initial *bereavement risk assessment* for the caregiver, thereby assisting the patient and family to identify strengths that help cope with loss. Families are supported as time is allowed for the patient and family to progress through stages of grieving. Other duties of the hospice social worker involve updating the bereavement care plan after the death of the patient and assessing the type of bereavement program to be initiated upon death of the patient. Also, referrals are provided for bereavement support services. The goal of the service is to provide superior quality, competitive value, and outstanding service in collaboration with the interdisciplinary team. Long-term goals are to provide the medical community and community-at-large with education and outreach. The delivery of services to the patient and family is the one of the most important aspects of the hospice's responsibilities (Johnson, 1998).

PROVISION OF QUALITY HOSPICE CARE

What about quality? While there are no standardized measures of quality for hospice care as advanced in the National Committee of Quality Assurance's Health Plan Employer Data and Information Set 3.0, many hospice providers seek certification from Medicare and the Joint Commission on Accreditation of Healthcare Organizations. Since the outcome is death, there are no specific performance measures (Hunt, Gabel, & Hurst, 1998). The National Hospice Organization suggests that it is important to validate the effectiveness of the program and that every hospice should have a method by which to survey the effectiveness of all services, including social work services (Archer & Boyle, 1999; Kovacs, 2000).

The effectiveness of hospice services needs to be evaluated by all participants involved in the giving and receiving of services (Fontaine & Rositiani, 2000). The impact of hospice care can potentially be evaluated at several different levels, and would be demonstrated in different ways at each level. In day-to-day practice at the individual level, hospice care meets the needs of terminally ill patients and their families by improving clinical status and maintaining or improving quality of life. At this level, the impact of hospice services can be documented through measurement of clinical, psychosocial, needs fulfillment, and quality-of-life outcomes. Outcome measurement is still a relatively new concept in hospice care, but many Hospices are now adding this technique to their quality and performance improvement efforts (Merriman, 1999). The lack of performance and outcome measures is problematic and needs to be addressed in each hospice so that service delivery and patient and family satisfaction are of the highest quality.

One way to measure service delivery and satisfaction in this area is to look directly at the opinions of social workers working in this behaviorally based managed care environment. These social workers have firsthand knowledge from the patient and family and from their own experiences with service delivery, and can thus be an effective voice in how and what services are needed to better serve this client population in the health care setting. It is imperative to identify and address all factors and issues concerning end-of-life care to best achieve quality of life for the patient and his or her family, and who better to ask than the people receiving and delivering hospice social services?

EVIDENCE-BASED PRACTICE IN HOSPICE

Evidenced-based research is limited for assessing the impact of hospice services. Even more disconcerting is the fact that there is very limited information and research available that addresses what additional services are needed to make the hospice experience more effective for the patient and the family. The majority of literature reviewed discusses how to assess patient and family satisfaction through various measurement tools and surveys. It does not address specifically what are the service delivery concerns of the patient, family, or hospice worker. Perhaps the lack of evidence-based practice in hospice care can be attributed to the difficulty of measuring the aspects of hospice that differentiate it from traditional acute medical care. Most of the scales and instruments currently developed to measure a person's quality of life follow the assumption of traditional medicine (Archer & Boyle, 1999). This may make hospice services nonmeasurable from a traditional perspective. Perhaps the most logical solution would be to ask the people responsible for service delivery and the people receiving services what outcomes are related to hospice care and, how these outcomes are different from traditional medical services.

Archer and Boyle (1999) conducted an evaluation of caregiver satisfaction with social services in a large hospice in Atlanta, Georgia. The purpose was to obtain information from the primary caregivers regarding their degree of satisfaction with the services provided by the social work staff. The last question on the survey asked how the social worker could have made the hospice services more beneficial to the family. The majority (84%) of the responses were extremely positive. Other respondents (9%) stated that they would have wanted hospice services sooner, and 7% stated they had experienced some difficulty with coordination and delivery of hospice services.

A large long-term study of families served by hospice found that nearly 95% said that hospice had been helpful (Nolen-Hoeksema, Larson, & Bishop, 2000). Still, about 30% of family members said there was something they wish hospice had done differently. Again, the participants in this study were "overwhelmingly" positive in their views of the hospices. People with some complaints stated they needed (1) more daily or constant care; (2) more "good" information about preparing for the patient's condition and death; and (3) more or less information and support from the hospice staff

Other respondents had a conflict with an individual hospice staff member. Many felt that any deficits in hospice's terms of care were due to lack of adequate funding or resources. Although this study looked at the characteristics of the family members that are associated with their satisfaction, and not the actual satisfaction with services provided, it does support my findings of what the perceived service needs of the family are.

Teno (1999), in her article regarding care for the dying, provides the reader with a brief overview of current problems with measuring satisfaction. Again, the author does not address what the problems with service delivery are as viewed by the patient, family, or caregiver; but she does support the assertion that the patient, caregiver, and family are key factors in improving services for the terminally ill. She believes that individuals that are dying are not the only clients being served; the family in the treatment process is also important.

OPINIONS OF SOCIAL WORKERS: TOWARD A BETTER UNDERSTANDING OF HOSPICE

To facilitate a greater understanding of the role of the hospice social worker, five social workers from a hospice program were queried in Florida in 2002. Each social worker interviewed agreed to participate, and the interviewer explained the reason for the interview and how the information given would be utilized. The 30-minute structured interviews involved answering the six questions outlined. The five female participants are all Caucasian and ranged from 31 to 64 years of age. The combined social work experience of the five participants is approximately 87 years, with 38 of those years being involved with hospice social work. Two participants are licensed clinical social workers, two have attained their master's degree in social work and are eligible to sit for licensure, and one has a bachelor in social work and is pursuing her master's degree.

Based on the in-depth and interrelated responses to the questions, the information gathered is presented for each participant on an individual basis. Each participant was asked to answer six questions:

1. What is the role of the hospice social worker?
2. What services do you provide?
3. What additional services that are already in place need to be changed or enhanced to benefit the patient and family, in your view? In your patients' and/or families' view?
4. What services not already in place need to be provided to benefit the patient and family, in your view? In your patients' and/or families' view?
5. What are the patient's and caregiver's most prevalent concerns about hospice services?
6. What can be done to provide these additional and/or needed services?

Social Worker A: Social worker A reported that she has been a social worker for eight years. Two of those years she has been working at her current hospice agency. She stated that her role as a hospice social worker is to enhance her client's quality of life in several ways, including spiritually, physically, socially, and emotionally. The services she provides are assessment of psychosocial needs, advocating for the patient and family, counseling, completion of advanced directives, and providing referrals to community resources. She stated she felt there is a desperate need in her community for increased respite in the home and the building of a Hospice House. Her patients and families have told her that they need more respite in the home. The reality is that shift work, home health aides, and other services are costly. Since some hospice programs cannot afford gemcitabine, blood transfusions, low-molecular-weight heparin, vancomycin, or parenteral nutrition, or cannot provide one-on-one 8–hour shifts of aide care, the burdens often fall on the family to supplement what can be provided. Unfortunately, extensive care of this nature will exceed the total per diem hospice payment (Lynn, 2001). Social worker A believed that the most prevalent concerns that the patient and family have are with pain management and the death and dying process. To be able to meet the needs of the patient and family, she stated that more funding through Medicare would be helpful.

Social Worker B: Social worker B had been a social worker for seven years, and all of her experience was in the hospice setting. She stated that her role as a hospice social worker is to provide education about death and dying and to support the patient and family. The services she provides involve linking the patient and family to appropriate community resources, education about advanced directives, helping patients through life review, and teaching coping skills to the patient and family. She felt that to benefit the patient and family there should be homemaking services, additional respite, more shift work, and continuous care for imminent death. Her patients and families have verbalized to her the need for homemaking services and additional respite time. She believes that the most prevalent concern for the primary caregiver is how best to assume the responsibility of caregiving for his or her loved one. These individuals need a great deal of support, and this support needs to come from family, friends, hospice, the community, and the church. Nolen-Hoeksema et al., (2000) agree with her perspective, and feel strongly that the most common benefit from hospice that participants mention is emotional support. She also believed that to meet the additional service needs of the clients serviced, an increase in the Medicare benefit is essential.

Social Worker C: Social worker C has a bachelor in social work (BSW) degree and was pursuing her master's degree in social work at the time of the interview. This social worker had been in the field for 13 years, and 12 of those years had been in the area of hospice. She stated that her role was to help keep the terminally ill patient at home until his or her death occurs. She feels strongly about the need for provision of emotional support and for inviting all caregivers involved with the client's care to participate in treatment planning. This requires that the caregiver be involved in either direct or indirect care.

The primary services this health care social worker provided included education in the area of death and dying, teaching and patient and family education, referrals to outside community resources to assist with basic human needs, education and assistance in regard to advanced directives, and end-of-life decision making. She also provided referrals within the agency for spiritual interventions, volunteered support and provided children's services, provided assistance with transportation arrangements, did nursing home placement, and monitored financial status to secure additional care for the patient. Of the services she felt were most needed, additional respite services for caregivers were at the forefront. She stated over and over again that families become very exhausted while trying to assume the role of full-time caregiver. If nurses could spend more time at the bedside of the client, it would assist family members to feel more at ease. She also stated that it would be very convenient to have a van to transport patients to their doctor's appointments and radiation treatments.

Many families have expressed to her that they wish the patient could go "somewhere" with a homelike setting, where he or she could be cared for compassionately until he or she dies. A Hospice House would provide palliative 24–hour care by professionals, and the family would still be very involved, but not the actual full-time caregivers. Social worker C reported that she believed the greatest concerns for a family member was the fear of caregiving. Families often admitted that they felt medically naïve and had no past caregiving experience to cope with this new role. Many of the families were apprehensive because they just did not know how to cope with people who were that ill. Many family members feared they would not take adequate care of their loved one. Another major concern by the families was that of pain management, since many family members did not want their loved one to be in pain. This was especially important if they felt guilty about possibly doing something improperly as the new caregiver (e.g., gave wrong dosage of medicine).

This social worker also believed that many caregivers had employment problems and could not afford to give up their income while trying to take care of their loved one in the home. For families this fear is a real one, since they face not only the intense emotional burden of losing a loved one, but also the expense of end-of-life care. Costs of medications, personal assistance, institutional care, and lost wages are quite substantial and often are not covered by insurance. For hospice patients the benefits do generally cover most medications and some personal assistance.

Social worker C believed the best way to address the needs of the client and family was to provide short-term intervention to address the above-mentioned problems. She explained the role of the hospice social worker as providing compassionate, palliative care and counsel to others involved in the dying process. More services are needed to help with psychosocial problems; with the extra support, caregivers could focus only on the patient and the grieving process. "They wouldn't have to worry about juggling caregivers to care for the patient at home, picking up prescriptions, taking time off from work, and so on."

Social Worker D: Social worker D, a licensed clinical social worker (LCSW) with a master's degree in social work (MSW), had 22 years of experience in the field and had been with hospice for 10 months. She stated that her role as a hospice social worker is to be an empathetic listener, provide information, facilitate admissions with the nurse case manager, and provide concrete services such as billing. She also felt that she filled a supportive role and was supportive toward the patient and family, helping them with coping and grief work. Services provided include assessment of client and family needs, coordination of services such as spiritual help, transportation, and education concerning advanced directives, and death and dying. She believes that more home health aides at lower prices, and more respite care designed to reduce nursing home placement would be beneficial to the patient and family. She states that many of her patients have also suggested the need for a Hospice House, along with longer hours of service for personal care and respite. Her patients' and families' most prevalent concerns are how to deal with misconceptions that hospice hastens death and that the patient will become addicted to morphine or other drugs. Social worker D feels strongly that more Medicare support is needed to help individuals and their families cope with problems and stressors, allowing clients to die with dignity.

Social Worker E: Social worker E also had her master's degree (MSW) and is a licensed clinical social worker (LCSW). She has been a social worker for 39 years and has been with Hospice for 13 years. She stated that her role as a hospice social worker is to help patients and families cope with the dying process. The services she provides are psychosocial assessment and intervention, information about community resources, education about death and dying, and advanced directives. She feels the services that are most needed for the patient and family are housekeeping and more respite. Her patients and families have expressed the need for more respite, night sitting, shift work, more volunteer time, and more home health aide visits per week. Her caregivers expressed concerns about coping with anticipatory grief and loss, the dread of losing the loved one, and how they will get along without him or her. She also has seen many of her patients struggle to express their concerns about the sense of loss that occurs when they have to say good-bye to those they love.

Summary of Findings

In summary, it was interesting that all five of the hospice social workers interviewed identified their roles and tasks in similar ways. In addition, all were in agreement that there is a great need for additional respite in the home to benefit the caregiver. Similar to Lynn (2001), who believed that one third of families of seriously ill, hospitalized, well-insured patients report a major financial change such as loss of most income or having to move because of the costs of illness, these social workers reported similar problems. Three out of the five participants specifically mentioned the need for a Hospice House to be built; and all of them reported the need for more home health aides and/or homemaking services to assist the patient and caregiver. The general consensus of additional services needed and/or more services needed (i.e., respite and homemaking services) associates strongly with the amount of care each patient needs and the toll it takes on the caregiver.

The most prevalent concerns of the patient, caregiver, and family were in regard to pain management, the fear of being a caregiver, and the fear of caring for the patient incorrectly. In addition, the social workers felt that clients needed more supportive information about medications—especially the misconceptions that surround morphine addiction and giving too much pain medication. Many clients requested help with learning how to deal with their condition, as well as the need for outside and family support. In a study done with an Australian palliative home care service, the most compelling predictors of family satisfaction and outcome were family care perceptions (ranked number one), family members' ages, family functioning, and the length of time that clients received the care service (Medigovich, Porock, Kristjanson, & Smith, 1999).

In general, satisfaction surveys regarding hospice care have been found to have a high number of positive responses. To assess the needs of families more effectively, one must be aware of the possible caregiver bias and significant factors that may contribute to that bias (Archer & Boyle, 1999). A factor that may bias the information is the possibility that the person who responded to the survey was caring for a patient who was not as incapacitated, had fewer nursing issues, and died at home.

CHAPTER SUMMARY AND FUTURE DIRECTIONS

The opinions of these social workers can provide valuable information about the current roles and services provided by the hospice social worker. Social workers in the hospice setting provide a valuable service to the client, caregiver, and family, allowing them to better attain quality of life and service. The main areas for continued advocacy appear to be related to respite services provided in the home. When a client stays at home to die, the family can be encumbered with a terrible burden if the family members do not feel supported; therefore, the entire situation must be addressed immediately. This difficulty is linked directly to the amount and intensity of care needed by the patient, the ability of the caregiver to care for the patient, the support system of the patient and caregiver, and the services available to the patient and caregiver. There are other mitigating factors, such as the physical and mental health of the patient and caregiver, the ability of the caregiver to take time off work, and the financial concerns of the patient, caregiver, and family that add to the challenge of caring for the dying patient at home. This is one the most intense and trying circumstances, and it can leave the patient, caregiver, and family very vulnerable.

All of the social workers interviewed agreed that to adequately meet the needs of their clients and families, more funding is needed through an increase in the hospice Medicare benefit and/or the use of fundraisers. One participant felt that a short-term "hospice-type house" would be beneficial, while another expressed concern over funding a Hospice House when there is so much other need now in the agency. Although an increase in the hospice Medicare benefit seems the most logical solution, hospice organizations are still suffering from the Medicare cutbacks imposed by the Balanced Budget Act of 1997. Recent revisions have reduced the rate at which Medicare payments have been cut. The Centers for Medicare and Medicaid Services did provide an increase of 5 percent in the payment rates for hospice care services (effective April 1, 2001); however, reimbursement remains stagnant at a time when the costs of drugs and supplies are rising and hospice organizations face pressure to raise nursing salaries and benefits (Asch-Goodkin, 2000; Facts and Figures, 2001).

The term "MediCaring," as used in Lynn (2001), offers one way to learn how to finance and deliver care for the terminally ill by consciously matching payment coverage with the appropriate service group(s). This would target services for patients who are ill enough to die (instead of using the six-month guideline), build a continuum of care from provider to provider (that is, home, hospital, nursing home), and provide flexibility in financial reimbursement to cutting-edge care providers. Yet, there is the ever present uncertainty about the future of Medicare as a whole, and this in a time when the baby boomers are coming of age and people will live longer with more chronic illness. The challenge now becomes finding an assessment tool or measurement outcome that can be utilized to address the needs of the interdisciplinary team, the patient, the caregiver, and the family.

One way to meet these challenges with respect to documenting impact to outside audiences may be to focus less on measuring the most unique aspects of hospice, which include such difficult concepts to measure as dying with dignity. Merriman (1999) found that it might be more useful to use universally accepted measures of aspects of "dying well" that are based in ethical principles or on consumer research. It is generally accepted that, with few exceptions (so few that they would not skew the data in populations), individuals should not die in pain, alone, or while enduring medical treatments they do not want. These measurements may be fairly easily devised, although other challenges remain in their implementation.

Our health care system is more adaptive to dealing with prevention and efforts to save lives rather than allowing nature to take its natural course; this emphasis on life over death, creates a clear gap between acute care and hospice care. Continuity and comprehensiveness of care for all people are main concerns and key factors to the quality of life that a person can expect. Using national guidelines, two breakthrough collaboratives involving 83 provider organizations generated a list of the promises that a good care system should make to patients who face serious, life-threatening, and eventually fatal illnesses (Lynn, 2001):

- Proven medical treatments
- Treatment that ensures comfort and avoids overwhelming symptoms
- Continuity, coordination, and comprehensiveness

- Advance planning, so that complications are anticipated and optimum treatment is ready to be implemented, rather than emergency efforts
- Customized care reflecting patient preferences
- Thoughtful use of patient and family resources (financial, emotional, and practical)
- Assistance to make the best of every day

Dying and death are universal realities, but these taboo subjects are not often talked about with family members, and even less frequently in mixed company. It is imperative to discuss end-of-life wishes with family or those who may have to make financial and medical decisions for another. is imperative. The best time to discuss views about end-of-life care is before a life-threatening illness has been diagnosed or a crisis happens. This helps reduce the stress a family member may experience in making decisions for a loved one's end-of-life care. The living will, a designated health care surrogate, and a prepared durable power of attorney can help a client to avoid causing a loved one anxiety and doubt. Often loved ones may not know what the client would have wanted done with respect to medical treatment and financial responsibilities. Having such information can also assist the physician in providing the care the person wants and addressing issues surrounding the choices made by that person.

Advanced directives are very important for the client, along with a detailed personal conversation with family and loved ones about the issues surrounding the client's end-of-life care. Hospice social workers can help the client and family approach such difficult subjects, allowing for a plan that honors the client's wishes and desires about end-of-life care.

REFERENCES

Archer, K. C., & Boyle, D. P. (1999). Toward a measure of caregiver satisfaction with hospice social services. *Hospice Journal, 14*(2), 1–15.

Asch-Goodkin, J. (2000). The virtues of hospice. *Patient Care,* 21–34.

Facts and Figures. (2001). *National Hospice and Palliative Care Organization.* Abstract retrieved February 20, 2002, from http://www.nhpco.org/public/articles/factsandfigures121001.pdf.

Fontaine, K., & Rositiani, R. (2000). Cost, quality, and satisfaction with hospice after-hours care. *Hospice Journal, 15*(1), 1–13.

Hunt, K. A., Gabel, J. T., & Hurst, K. M. (1998, September). The truth about hospice. *Business and Health,* 9–12.

Johnson, P. (Ed.). (1998). *Hospice of Health First student orientation* [Brochure]. West Melbourne, Florida: Hospice of Health First, Inc. (Original work published 1992).

Kovacs, P. J. (2000). Participatory action research and hospice: A good fit. *Hospice Journal, 15*(3), 55–62.

Lynn, J. (2001), Serving patients who may die soon and their families—the role of hospice and other services. *Journal of the American Medical Association, 285,* 925–932.

McSkimming, S., Myrick, M., & Wasinger, M. (2000). Supportive care of the dying: A coalition for compassionate care—conducting an organizational assessment. *American Journal of Hospice and Palliative Care, 17,* 245–252.

Medigovich, K., Porock, D., Kristjanson, L. J., & Smith, M. (1999). Predictors of family satisfaction with an Australian palliative home care service: A test of discrepancy theory. *Journal of Palliative Care, 15*(4), 48–56.

Merriman, M. P. (1999). Documenting the impact of hospice. *Hospice Journal, 14,* 177–192.

Nolen-Hoeksema, S., Larson, S., & Bishop, M. (2000). Predictors of family members' satisfaction with hospice. *Hospice Journal, 15*(2), 29–48.

Teno, J. M. (1999). Putting patient and family voice back into measuring quality care for the dying. *Hospice Journal, 14,* 167–176.

GLOSSARY

Bereavement risk assessment: This is an assessment that the hospice social worker completes with the caregiver of the loved one who is receiving the hospice service. The assessment is designed to identify strengths that help cope with loss. Once the risk assessment is completed, it is used to identify where families need the greatest support while progressing through the stages of grieving.

Hospice: Hospice care is a special way of caring for people who are terminally ill and their families. The goal of hospice services is to care for the patient and the family, with open acknowledgment that no cure is expected for patient's illness.

Hospice care: Hospice care includes physical, emotional, social, and spiritual care provided by either a public agency or private company that may or may not be Medicare approved.

Hospice house: A place of care for terminally ill patients that require inpatient hospice care or inpatient care.

QUESTIONS FOR FURTHER STUDY

1. What is the role of the hospice social worker?
2. What services do you provide as a hospice social worker?
3. What services or additional services do you feel need to be provided to benefit your patients and families?
4. What services or additional services need to be provided as expressed to you as a social worker by your patients and families?
5. What are the patients' and families' most prevalent concerns that are expressed to you?
6. How could we meet or provide these needed or additional services?

CHAPTER 16

Social Work in Long-Term Care Facilities

Sophia F. Dziegielewski and Depsy Bredwood

THE LONG-TERM CARE FACILITY

The latest government census shows that the fastest-growing population is adults 65 years and older. These individuals consume the highest medical cost, and most often this is the population group in need of long-term care facility placement. The major funding sources for this type of service are Medicare, a private HMO, or Medicaid. For social workers working in long-term care, it is crucial to be familiar with the OBRA'87 reform act and the way it is used for preadmission screening. In this chapter, consultations with five long-term care social workers were solicited. The questions asked focused on what the social workers knew about long-term care assessment policies, Medicare, HMOs, and Medicaid payment sources in regard to admission, and quality and quantity of care. The opinions of these social workers are utilized to help clarify and provide voices from the field to gain a greater understanding of the role of this health care social worker.

THE SKILLED NURSING FACILITY

As part of the Social Security Act, section 1819, 42.U.S.C. 13951–3, a *skilled nursing facility* is an institution that primarily provides skilled nursing care and related services for residents; it is not primarily for the care and treatment of mental diseases (Senior Care Resources, n. d., p. 1). The *Joint Commission on Accreditation of Healthcare Organizations*

381

(1996) governs all skilled nursing facilities. Its mission statement "is to improve the quality of care provided to the public through the provision of health care accreditation and related services that support performance improvement in health care organizations." Their accreditation covers three forms of services: long-term care, subacute care, and dementia special care. Although the services can vary at each level of care, the purpose of this chapter is to *identify* factors and issues related directly to facilities that deal directly with long-term care. In the provision of long term care resident quality of life must be maintained. Therefore, "the skilled nursing facility must care for the individual in such a manner and in such an environment that promotes enhancement, or maintenance of the quality of life" (Senior Care Resources, n. d., p. 1).

According to Dhooper (1997), there are four basic types of services the skilled nursing facility provides: basic nursing care, which includes giving medicines orally and by injections, tube feeding, and wound care and which may involve physical, occupational, and speech therapy services; personal care services, which include helping residents, with their activities of daily living such as walking, bathing, dressing, and eating; the provision of residential services that provide a safe haven for residents, allowing for adequate assistance and supervision; the facilitation of medical care, providing direct access to physician visits and health care issues involving medications, special diets, and restorative and rehabilitative procedures (p.85).

To ensure that each resident receives the benefit of enhancement and maintenance of the quality of life, a comprehensive quality assessment is completed on each individual upon admission. This reproducible assessment describes the resident's functional capacity. As specified, the standardized Minimum Data Set (MDS) Version 2.0 (2000), form 1721ORNH, must be completed on all residents promptly within 14 days of admission.

The assessor must represent a coordinated effort on the part of all health professionals involved in the resident's care. To insure accuracy, the resident must have had periods of interaction with the assessor/s within the last seven day, as stated in the MDS Version 2.0. This is an extensive evaluation that takes into account both subjective and objective information in regard to cognitive patterns, mood and behavior patterns, and psychological well-being. Once the initial assessment is completed, additional assessments may be required when there is a significant change in physical and mental status, and every 3 months thereafter (Senior Care Resources, n. d.). This makes the evaluator's capacity to interpret, assess, and understand the resident's individualized needs critical. Because of differing assumptions and commitments to resident care, Silberfeld and Checkland (1999) warn that these assessments may not be as objective as most believe.

All professionals directly involved in the resident's care are encouraged to participate. This means that the resident's physician needs to participate not only in the medical care of the client but also in identifying the resident's needs. Conversely, Robinson, Barry, Resnick, Bergen, and Stratos (2001) warn that for physicians this can be a problem because many physicians currently in practice were not exposed to specific topics in geriatric medicine in medical school or during residency training. Therefore, some professionals are concerned that there may not be a lot of interest leading to creative initiatives on the part of these physicians. In an attempt to measure physician's confidence and interest in geriatric topics and assessment; Robinson et al., (2001) surveyed 242 North Carolina community physicians. Only 53% of the physicians in practice claimed that at least half of their caseload was constituted of seniors, although interest in learning more about this population was high. The highest area of interest was in learning more about dementia, urinary incontinence, and completing functional assessments. What is interesting about this study is that the senior physicians in practice showed a higher confidence in geriatric care, in comparison to recent graduates, but less interest in learning more about geriatric topics. To assist physicians to be better prepared to work with geriatric populations, Robinson et al., (2001) discussed the need for continued efforts to improve geriatric education in medical school and residency.

In the long-term care setting, one topic of concern for most professionals is how to best address psychiatric issues and mental health problems. Snowdon (2001) reported the prevalence of residents with psychiatric disorders in skilled nursing homes at 80–91%. The author referred to clinical data that suggested that the most common mental health condition was dementia, at approximately 80%, with 25% to 50% of residents with dementia also displaying psychotic symptoms. Similarly, significant depressive symptoms were reported in 30% to 50% of nursing home patients who could be assessed, and major depression was found in 6% to 25% of those who were not cognitively impaired (Snowdon, 2001). Snowdon (2001) warned, however, that it was highly possible that this summary of prevalence was inadequate because of problems in the assessing process. Snowdon believed that once admitted to a nursing home, there was no encouragement to recognize or treat the patients' psychiatric problem (Snowdon, 2001).

Problems with how to best assess and treat residents that suffer from mental disorders in the long-term care facility are not unique to the United States. For example, in a survey of Canadian nursing homes, administrators reported that there were no psychiatrists available for consultation in the nursing home setting. In addition, 36.8% reported that residents received no psychiatric care, and 88.2% of those who needed psychiatric care were likely to get less than an estimated five hours per month (Meeks, Jones, Tikhtman, & LaTourette, 2000).

In an attempt to address the unavailability of psychiatric services in U.S. nursing homes, the Omnibus Reform Act of 1987 (OBRA), required preadmission screening and annual review of nursing home residents. Unfortunately, some authors believe this reform act was more of a cost-saving measure designed to restrict resident access to nursing homes, and not to solve the existing problem of unmet mental health needs (Snowdon, 2001). This type of cost reduction strategy is not a surprise, since the cost benefit of long-term care for residents in a skilled nursing facility has been the concern of legislators and community residents for several years. If comprehensive mental health services were readily available, the effectiveness of all the services a skilled facility provides would be greatly enhanced. In addition, helping to provide ongoing consultation-liaison services can help nursing home staff to recognize psychiatric problems more readily (Meeks et al., 2000).

In summary, it appears that most residents admitted to the skilled long-term facility require more than just direct medical care. Often the services require multiple and extensive rehabilitative efforts. To fund these services, Medicare or Medicaid remains the main source of payment. Data from the Health Care Financing Review (1995) reported that Medicare charges increased from $4.4 billion in 1990 to $7.0 billion in 1992 for residents within skilled nursing facilities. The increased charges reflect the 24.9% increase in rehabilitative services offered to incoming residents.

In general, rehabilitative services include physical therapy, occupational therapy, and speech therapy, and do not include any types of mental health therapy. This lack of recognition for mental health services in the skilled nursing facility is unfortunate because often the exclusion of mental health therapy may directly affect the client's progression.

OPINIONS OF SOCIAL WORKERS IN THE FIELD

To better understand the opinions of social workers in this area, five social workers were interviewed. These social workers were asked their opinions of the differences between Medicare, HMO, and Medicaid insurance in nursing home assessment and admittance. To facilitate this process, five social workers with either a bachelor's or master's degree in social work were questioned. Each of these social workers had at least one year or more experience with this system and was employed within a skilled nursing facility. Face-to-face interviews were conducted, and individuals were asked to respond to five semistructured questions. All five social workers were females; four were Caucasian, and one was African American. Their ages ranged from 23 to 40 years. Two had master's degrees (MSW), and the other three had bachelor's degrees (BSW). Their years of working as a social worker in this area ranged from one year to ten years. One master's degree participant held the position of admissions director, and the other four were directors of social services at their facility. Salary ranged from $22,000 to $35,000 annually. The interviews were conducted in the office of the social workers for approximately 15 minutes. The five questions were:

- What kind of admission assessment do you complete
- What services are often linked to the completed assessment?
- What are your opinions of the quantity of services reimbursed by private care payments and managed care payments?
- What are the differences, if any, in the quality of care as a reflection of payment method?
- What services do you believe are needed but are not provided?

INTERVIEWW COMMENTS

What kind of admission assessment do you complete?

All social workers reported that each client they admitted was assessed by the standard guidelines set by the governing laws of the state. They all mentioned the fact that when a referral is made for admission from a hospital, home, or mental health center, a required preadmission screening is conducted.

What services are often linked to the completed assessment?

Each attending physician for the client must complete the CF-MED 3008 form with all the pertinent medical and nonmedical information. When question C-4 on the 3008 forms is answered yes, addressing the client mental health, the treating psychiatrist must provide the exact diagnosis and treatment. According to the admission director (MSW), the screening helps to prevent her facility from admitting any client with a mental diagnosis who displays aggression or could present problems with resistance to care. Upon accepted for admission, the facility physician reevaluates the client and the information from the 3008 forms. An exception is made when the attending physician for the client has practicing privileges at the facility.

The OBRA'87 reform act requires each discipline employed at the facility to collaborate on what services are necessary. All participating disciplines must follow the physician's orders for medical, dietary, or rehabilitative care. The role of the social workers is to complete the Minimum Data Set (MDS) form, which is a psychosocial assessment. Other information on the client is also taken from the family when applicable.

What are your opinions of the quantity of services reimbursed by private care payments and managed care payments?

The quantity of care is based on the client's method of insurance. When Medicare Part-A is the payer source, the quantity of care includes rehabilitation, and the time is limited to 100 days. The rates for charges are negotiated by the facility. Managed care (HMO) sets a standard rate of charges per day for care (i.e., $200.00). The charges are based on what is suggested as the difference between the three levels of care for the client. Clients often were expected to use private funds to assist with supplemental care needs.

What are the differences, if any, in the quality of care as a reflection of payment method?

None of the five social workers stated that there was any difference in the quality of care given to the clients. They explained that the staff assigned to administer care remains unaware of the resident's payer source. One BSW social service director stated, "The quality of care is based on the client's diagnosis and should stay consistent, but the quantity of care is based on the needs of the client as it changes." However, it was suggested that if there were a difference in the quality of care as seen by residents and staff, it is more likely that this difference would be based on personality conflicts rather than administrative or funding considerations.

What services do you believe are needed but are not provided?

All five respondents acknowledged several services as lacking that would possibly enhance the client's life. Suggestions for additional services included adequate dental care; having a physician located directly in the facility; and having a licensed social worker available to provide one-to-one counseling and supportive services for the residents and their families. Also, social workers could help to run educational groups to address family and facility misunderstandings.

Other suggestions included more pet or music therapy, ongoing exercise classes for clients who are ambulatory with minimum cognitive impairment, and funding from the government to run these incentive programs. Several social workers noted that because most of the extended care facilities where they were employed were for profit, it was sometimes difficult to convince administration that supportive services could be cost effective.

For the social workers who were directors of their departments, they all said that even though they were directors they were often left out of the administrative decision making. All of the social workers identified their primary roles as conducting ongoing psychosocial assessment on the clients, and most times this information was accumulated from other facility staff and family. A comment was made by one social worker working in the field for ten years: "My role is advocate for the clients, mediate between family members and explain facility policies, and attempt to empower the clients whenever possible to engage in participation with their own plan for care."

In closing, the information reported by this small sample of social workers in the field is similar to that reported by Reinardy (1999), who identified the challenges social workers face and their feelings of ambivalence over autonomy and beneficence. Reinardy (1999) stated that as a result of this ambivalence, "balancing the client need for autonomy and your desire to act beneficently is indeed difficult to reach. 'Everyone is looking out for their best interest, something that never happened when they lived at home.' They feel that everyone's trying to make decisions for them when we feel we're trying to enable them since they live here and we are the professionals" (Reinardy, 1999, p. 72). The social workers saw their role as encouraging resident independence, discouraging the practice of paternalism, and maximizing personal dignity, justice, culture, respect, autonomy, and spiritual values.

For the health care social worker, factors related to declines in health and mental health status can hamper resident self-determination. This makes the role of the family critical in providing continued care. When residents can no longer make decisions for themselves, family and friends may be forced to assume the role of caregivers. In this situation, parent may assume the role of child, and the child now becomes the parent in terms of decision making. Since it is not always clear how relevant former values are to these new situations or how they might apply (Kuczewski, 1999), values and factors such as race, ethnicity, gender, and support systems cannot be underestimated.

FOOD FOR THOUGHT

Race and Ethnicity in Assessing Caregiver Burden

Caregiver burden is the extent to which caregivers perceive their emotional or physical health, social life, and financial status as suffering because of responsibility of care given for a relative.

In terms of the caregiver and caregiving of the elderly, the caregiver's role in this society is not clearly defined, making the client-caregiver cost-benefit relationship a tenuous one. Therefore, understanding culture or ethnicity and race can serve as the cornerstone for understanding the caregiver's role in society.

Ethnic identity is generally defined as a common thread of heritage, customs, and values unique to a group of people (Casas, 1984; Queralt, 1996; Worden, 1999). Although researchers have gathered information on race and culture or ethnicity at the same time, the difference between the two is pronounced. In race the attributes of the individual are partially based on physical characteristics of genetic origin (Helms, 1990); ethnicity, on the other hand, encompasses a much broader range of commonalties such as religion, customs, geography, or historical events. In ethnicity, it is the commonalties between individuals that define and bond members and thereby produce an ethnic backdrop to everyday life. Actually, the ethnicity of the caregiver can influence thinking and feeling and pattern behavior in both obvious and subtle ways. Generally, however, most individuals remain unaware of the influence of ethnicity because it remains natural and consistent with their daily behaviors (e.g., what they eat, how they react).

Regardless of how easily this factor is recognized in developing a sense of caregiving, it is an important assessment factor to be identified by the health care social worker. Ethnicity or culture and race can be related to an increased sense of responsibility on the part of the caregiver (Cain & Wicks, 2000). In assessing and supporting families, gender is also an important consideration. According to Faison, Faria, and Frank (1999), women predominantly were seen in the caregiver role. They also found that mutuality and caregiver burden are inclusive. "Mutuality is a positive quality of the relationship between caregiver and care receiver. When mutuality exists there is a decreased strain because care giving is found to be meaningful" (p.15).

Furthermore, Cain & Wicks (2000) looked directly at the age of the caregiver and the influence age might have on caregiver burden. In their study female spouses made up 86% of the caregivers, with 72% of the caregivers being 55 years and older. Interesting, from the 21 African American caregivers that participated in the study who were all over the age of 55, 65% reported little to no burden. This remains in strike contrast to the remaining 117 Caucasian caregivers, with 44% reporting mild to moderate burden, 15% moderate to severe burden, and 2% severe burden.

Cains & Wicks (2000) support the notion that a sense of responsibility for the caregiver remains an important concept in American culture. With this expectation, the question is, what can and does happen when the family caregiver's burden becomes psychologically damaging?

For the health care social worker, helping a family to make a decision to place a loved one in a long-term care facility is never an easy one. It requires the social worker to take into account many factors, including the cost-benefit ratio and the burden it can place on the family. Factors such as ethnicity, race, gender, and level of disability in the client are only a few of the factors that need to be considered to assist the client and families in the long-term care admission process. Making the decision to place a loved one in a long-term care facility is never easy, and it is important to make sure that the long-term facility is seen as the best option to ensure that quality of care is maintained. This makes the role of the nursing home social worker crucial in identifying the needs of the client, the family and the facility.

CHAPTER SUMMARY AND FUTURE DIRECTIONS

These social workers were working in Florida, and in this county alone there were 19 open skilled nursing facilities with bed capacity ranging from 30 to 180 (Senior Housing Directory, 2002–03). Of the 19 facilities, only 3 of the facilities would actively accept clients with a diagnosed mental health problem. From the remaining 16 facilities, 6 facilities either had a special Alzheimer unit or a general memory care unit for residents.

Looking at the availability of facilities, the interviews conducted help to highlight the degree to which skilled nursing facilities must adhere to strict state and federal regulations and how admission policies designed to protect the clients we serve could actually present covert barriers preventing certain admissions. Ethically, when a patient lacks decision-making capacity or does not fully understand choices, the physician and the skilled facility staff must take steps to safeguard the patient's welfare (Richards, 2000). Review of the literature suggests that the covert barriers can be related to the prescreening of elderly adults that can prohibit needed admissions, and/or neglect of mental health issues that can lead to misdiagnosis or inappropriate failed interventions. Conversely, the main focus of skilled nursing facilities is centered on acute physical and occupational care; yet, this ignores the simple fact that many acute care residents become long term. Furthermore, if all the emphasis is placed on the medical needs of the client, what will happen with the mental health needs that require increased attention? In the long-term setting, these social workers felt that there was a gap in service for those who have mental health disorders, especially when these disorders are severe enough to make their behavior a problem for the facility or endangering to other clients.

Analyzing the role of the social worker in a long-term care setting presents many challenges. During the interview, most respondents asserted that their autonomy was limited based on the policies that govern the facility. Their covert responsibility is to the company, although they are addressing the care needs of the residents. Unfortunately, the role of a social worker in a skilled facility is not to reduce the power imbalance between residents and staff, but to expect them to fit into bureaucratic and professional agendas. These social workers stated that they loved what they did but that any social worker entering the field should never forget the importance of advocating for the residents served, allowing for individuality, and preparing for the complexity of their needs.

REFERENCES

Cain, C. J., & Wicks, N. M., (2000). Caregivers' attributes as correlates of burden in the family caregivers coping with chronic obstructive pulmonary disease [Electronic version]. *Journal of Family Nursing*, 6(1), 46–68.

Casas, J. M. (1984). Policy, training, and research in counseling psychology: The racial/ethnic minority perspective. In S. D. Brown & R. W. Lent (Eds), *Handbook of counseling psychology* (pp. 785–831). New York: Wiley.

Dhooper, S. S. (1997). *Social work in health care in the 21st century*. Belmont, CA: Sage.

Faison, K. J., Faria, S. H., & Frank, D. (1999). Caregivers of chronically ill elderly: Perceived burden [Electronic version]. *Journal of Community Health Nursing*, 16(4), 243–254.

Health Care Financing Review. (1995, February). *Skilled nursing facility: Charges by the type of services: CYS 1990 and 1992*. Retrieved April 5, 2002, from http://ehostvgw.epnet.com/getxml.asp

Helms, J. E. (Ed). (1990). *Black and white racial identity: Theory, research, and practice*. Westport, CN: Praeger.

Joint Commission on Accreditation of Healthcare Organizations. (1996). *Comprehensive accreditation manual for long-term care: CAMLTC/Joint Commission*. Oakbrook Terrace, IL: Joint Commission on Accreditation of Healthcare Organization.

Kuczewski, M. G. (1999). Ethics in long-term care: Are the principles different? *Theoretical Medicine*, 20, 15–29.

Meeks, S., Jones, M. W., Tikhtman, V., & Latourette, T. R. (2000). Mental health services in Kentucky nursing homes: A survey of administrators. *Journal of Clinical Geropsychology, 6,* 223–232.

Minimum Data Set-Version (MDS) 2.0 (2000): *For nursing home resident assessment and care screening: Basic assessment tracking form* (No. 1721ORHH). Des Moines, IA: Briggs.

Queralt, M. (1996). *The social environment and human behavior: A diversity perspective.* Boston: Allyn and Bacon.

Reinardy, J. R. (1999). Autonomy, choices, and decision making: How nursing home social workers view their role. *Social Work in Health Care, 29*(3), 59–77.

Richards, S. (2000). Bridging the divide: Elders and the assessment process. *British Journal of Social Work, 30,* 37–49.

Robinson, B. E., Barry, P. P., Renick, N., Bergen, M. R., & Stratos, G. A. (2001). Physician confidence and interest in learning more about common geriatric topics: A needs assessment. *Journal of the American Geriatrics Society, 49,* 963–967.

Senior Care Resources (FL) Nursing Home Reporter (n.d.). *Requirements for, and assuring quality of care in skilled nursing facilities.* Retrieved February 25, 2002, from http://www.seniorcarehelp.com/resource/title18.htm

Senior Housing Directory. (2002–2003). *Comprehensive housing information for older adults in Central Florida.* [Brochure]. Senior Housing: Author.

Silberfeld, M., & Checkland, D. (1999). Faulty judgment, expert opinion, and decision-making capacity. *Theoretical Medicine and Bioethics, 20,* 377–393.

Snowdon, J. (2001). Psychiatric care in nursing homes: More must be done. *Australasian Psychiatry, 9,* 108–115.

Worden, M. (1999). *Family therapy basics* (2nd ed.). Pacific Grove, CA: Brooks/ Cole.

GLOSSARY

Joint Commission on Accreditation of Healthcare Organizations: This is the governing body for all skilled nursing facilities. The mission statement of this governing body is to improve the quality of care provided to the public through the provision of health care accreditation and related services that support performance improvement in health care organizations. This accreditation body oversees three forms of services: long-term care, subacute care, and dementia special care.

Omnibus Reform Act of 1987 (OBRA): This act addresses psychiatric services in U.S. nursing homes and requires preadmission screening and annual review of nursing home residents.

Skilled nursing facility: This is a facility that primarily provides skilled nursing care and related services for residents; it is not primarily for the care and treatment of mental diseases.

QUESTIONS FOR FURTHER STUDY

1. What do you see as the greatest challenges for the long-term care social worker?
2. Is this an area of practice you would like to consider? Why or why not?

CHAPTER 17

Children with Chronic and Life-Threatening Illness

Sophia F. Dziegielewski and Breanne Anderson

LIFE-THREATENING ILLNESSES AND HEALTH CARE SOCIAL WORK

Every year thousands of children are diagnosed with chronic health conditions. Current research indicates that approximately 18% of the children living in the United States suffer with severe illness and disabilities (Perrin, Lewkowiez, & Young, 2000). Often, the special needs of these children and their families are overlooked or forgotten by health care providers and agencies. According to Morales and Sheafor (2001), "limited access to health insurance and care is largely a function of income; children below the poverty line are more than twice as likely to have poor health status and almost twice as likely to experience a chronic health condition" (p.304). Chronic physical conditions can place extreme psychological and social burdens on the family system. Therefore, the health care social worker needs to have a working knowledge of specific services offered in the client's local community. In addition, practitioners must be cognizant of the issues families face when dealing with chronic illness in order to provide needed assessments and behaviorally based biopsychosocial services. The purpose of this chapter is to make the health care social worker aware of some of the problems that can occur when working with this population group. To exemplify the issues that clients can face in this area, six social workers were interviewed. These social workers' opinions were evaluated, and suggestions for more efficient evidence-based practice are made.

CHRONIC ILLNESS IN CHILDREN

Hoyt (1995) suggested that "it is becoming increasingly important to learn about and meet the special mental health needs of various subpopulations, which involves addressing issues of cultural diversity as well as the problems of elderly members, the chronically distressed, the dually diagnosed, and the medically complicated" (p. 46). According to Perrin et al. (2000), if children are diagnosed with chronic health conditions and also have terminal illnesses, they are 50% more likely to have emotional, developmental, and educational difficulties when compared with healthy children. For example, the Disaster Center (2002) reports that in 1996, approximately 47,000 children and young adults under the age of 24 died: 1,476 died of cardiac related illness; 3,117 deaths were cancer related; 743 HIV-related deaths were recorded; and 1,476 deaths were the result of congenital anomalies. In 1997 the total number of deaths for children and young adults under the age of 19 had risen to approximately 70,000 (Sahler, Frager, Levetown, Cohn, & Lipson, 2000). In 1999, the number had risen even higher to approximately 95,000 (Sahler et al., 2000). In 2001, there were approximately 13,207 children and adolescents under the age of 19 living with AIDS; there were 452,111 reported deaths from AIDS-related causes (Cichocki, 2002). What is most startling is that every year approximately 12,400 children and adolescents under the age of 20 are diagnosed with cancer, and 2,300 die of cancer related causes (EPA, 2002). With these numbers increasing, it is critical that health care social workers recognize the importance of working with children that have long-term childhood diseases.

ASSESSMENT OF NEEDS

Perrin et al. (2000) explored the types of programs and services required to meet the needs of children suffering with chronic health conditions. To accomplish this the perspectives of both parents and primary care physicians were explored. Both parents and physicians agreed that it was crucial for all service providers to adequately address information, treatment, or long-term effects in regard to a child's condition; however, a lack of family support was identified. The parents in the study requested to have more (1) information and advice about the child's behavior and development; (2) involvement and help to coordinate plans for the child's future needs; (3) teamwork involvement and coordination of care; (4) family-centered support and discussion groups;

and, (5) contact with other families going through similar experiences (Perrin et al., 2000). Parents in the study wanted to be active in their child's care and wanted help in anticipating the current and future treatments that might be needed. The primary care physicians also wanted more parental involvement and advocated for parents being given more (1) treatment plan information; (2) counseling services about their child's behavior and development; (3) help with planning for future needs; (4) assistance arranging for the child's school curriculum; and (5) assistance with helping to reinforce treatment information (Perrin et al., 2000). Other areas requested included social and recreational support and camp activities for children facing the psychological aspects of chronic illness. Perrin et al. (2000) voiced concerns that attempts to identify and meet the needs of chronic health conditions in children were sometimes made in an unproductive, disorganized fashion.

A significant issue to consider when dealing with children that suffer from chronic illnesses is the psychological and social burden that is placed on the child and family. This burden can in turn lead to higher rates of mental health problems (Bauman, Drotar, Leventhal, Perrin, & Pless, 1997). Based on a search of the literature from 1997 to 1993, Bauman et al. (1997) found that children suffer psychologically as well as physically from chronic health conditions. From an environmental or situational (mezzo) perspective, the families of the patient were at an increased risk for psychological disturbances. Yet, Bauman et al. (1997) suggested that although mental health problems can develop, only one quarter of the children with a chronic illness that also have a mental health problem received mental health services.

PSYCHOSOCIAL SERVICES

According to the Child Life Council (2000), hospitals have recently begun to expand and/or implement Child Life Programs to help answer patient and family concerns about hospitalization and/or health care issues. Since 1965, Child Life Programs have doubled in number. These programs generally provide information on therapeutic services in the areas of oncology, radiology, dialysis, surgery, and emergency procedures. The Committee on Hospital Care (as cited by Child Life Council, 2000) reported that several states, including Florida, now mandate that child life programs include services for children and families with training of volunteers while providing services geared toward the provision of age-appropriate play and activities. Family care services are also needed so that therapeutic alliances can be developed, information is provided, and reactions to the illness are monitored (Child Life Council, 2000).

Most professionals working in this area agree that in order to set goals for terminally ill children a broad approach is required. Attention must be given to the "psychosocial, emotional, and spiritual needs" of the child (Sahler et al., 2000). Social workers should be trained to help the family explore the finality of their child's illness, while allowing them to maintain hope. The worker must also be able to empower the parents to communicate their feelings with one another and their child. This attention to supportive adjustment is so important because often children have an intuitive knowledge of their condition and death. In these situations palliative care is recommended in hospice programs, where, rather than being a secret fear, the child's impending death is openly acknowledged. This allows practitioners to talk more freely with patients and families about comfort and preparation for death as the clear explicit goal of treatment (Sahler et al., 2000).

Many countries, including the United Kingdom, Australia, and Canada accept and encourage the use of palliative care with pediatric patients; however, children in the United States that suffer from chronic health conditions may have a harder time receiving palliative care. According to Stephenson (2000), although there are approximately 2,500 hospice programs aimed at adults, there are only 247 geared toward children. It would appear that only 1% of the children in the United States are receiving hospice care.

Using a multidisciplinary team approach, Stephenson (2000) examined the pediatric palliative care provided by physicians, nurses, social workers, therapist, clergy, volunteers, and other psychological, social, and spiritual supports given to children and their families. Overall, services were considered limited, with the major concerns being problems with communication, pain and symptom management, caregiver distress, and limited respite. For the health care social worker in this area, provision of individual, family, and group therapy is an important step to helping the child as well as the family feel more comfortable. To provide more macro support, referrals to the National Institute of

Health, American Cancer Society, and the National Cystic Fibrosis Foundation should be considered (Stephenson, 2000).

OPINIONS OF SOCIAL WORKERS: TOWARD A GREATER UNDERSTANDING

To find out the opinions of health care social workers in the field, six practitioners from a large hospital in the Southeast were interviewed. This large southeastern hospital is equipped to service the everyday medical needs of children, with units specializing in HIV & AIDS care, infectious disease, children's heart care, critical care, trauma, neonatal intensive care, oncology/hematology, sexual trauma, and urgent care (About Us, 2002). The six subjects were members of a psychosocial team that worked primarily with children suffering from a chronic life-threatening illness and their families.

The subjects were interviewed and asked about the services they provide to pediatric clients with chronic or life-threatening illnesses and their families. The interviews lasted approximately 30 minutes and were conducted over a two-week time period at the availability of the professional. Each participant agreed to participate and have the interviews recorded for review. The participants ranged in age from 27 to 42. Five participants were female and one was male, four were Caucasian, one was African American, and one was Hispanic. They have been in practice from 2 to 23 years, and in their current positions between 1 and 17 years. One individual worked with infectious disease, one with oncology, one in the cardiology unit, two float throughout the hospital and cover the ICU and special care units, and one works at an outpatient, infectious disease clinic. Five of the participants also spend time working at an outpatient pediatric behavioral and therapeutic clinic provided by the hospital. They were each asked seven questions related to patient services:

- What services are you providing to clients and their families?
- What services are most important to the clients and families you serve?
- What services had the lowest utilization rate?
- What additional services do you feel need to be offered?
- Are the services you provide generally short term or long term?

- Do you believe adequate services are available to children and families?
- How do the clients and families you serve find out about the services that are available to them?

INTERVIEWEE COMMENTS

What services are you providing to clients and their families?

On the first question subjects provided a wide variety of responses, with little consistency on how often these services were provided. See Table 17.1 for a list of services. Overall, the services reported by these social workers remained similar to those reported in the study by Perrin et al. (2000) and were also considered areas of need and benefit for these children and their families.

What services are most important to the clients and families you serve?

Again, the social workers differed on exactly what services were most important. Most agreed that some consistency in reporting back to clients with follow-up information is crucial. They also reported that therapy or counseling sessions, inpatient services, and education services were requested most often by the clients they served. Similar to Perrin et al. (2000), these social workers felt that counseling and education services were the most important services for clients and their families (see Table 17.2)

What services had the lowest utilization rate

In response to this question, five of the six respondents stated that clients do not often seek out the social worker to see what outpatient referrals are available. They also reported that often clients fail to follow through or schedule second appointments. This worried some of the social workers because they felt that even though many clients and families did not seek them out for these services, they were still needed (see Table 17.3).

What additional services do you feel need to be offered?

Palliative or end-of-life care and bereavement support for families and patients were given as the most important services that needed to be

TABLE 17.1   Service Provided

Coping skills
Bereavement
Behavioral adjustment
Community referrals
Assistance with adjustment to diagnosis
Education
DCF liaison
Discharge planning
Patient counseling
Outpatient counseling
Assessment
Crisis counseling
Play therapy
Assistance disclosing diagnosis to child
Groups

TABLE 17.2   Most Important Services

All services are important
Inpatient services
Support Groups
Crisis Counseling
Therapy or counseling services
Education services
Coping skills

TABLE 17.3   Least Utilized Services

Behavioral services
Outpatient referrals
Education
Assistance in disclosing diagnosis to child

offered. The social workers felt that many of the families and friends of these clients needed support to help deal with the loss of friends and loved ones. In addition, as a supportive measure, groups to address the loss issues were suggested for helping family members to adjust to the serious illness or death of their loved one. The emphasis by these social workers on the need for palliative care and bereavement support for children is similar to Stephenson's (2000) findings that seriously ill children in the United States need to be offered help with end-of-life care (see Table 17.4).

Are the services you provide generally short term or long term?

The response to this question was split. Three social workers reported that services were generally provided on a short-term inpatient basis, and the other three stated that services were available on a long-term basis. All of the social workers agreed that they could be provided, but support and time to engage in these activities was what prompted three of the social workers to say that they did not provide these services. In addition, all six social workers agreed that services could be available a lot longer to clients after discharge from the hospital if the client and family follow-up improved. Perrin et al. (2000) and Child Life Council (2000), reported the same need for long-term services and lack of follow-through on referrals. All agreed that although long-term services were available, utilization rates were low.

Do you believe adequate services are available to children and families?

All of the social workers believed that for the most part the services provided were adequate to meet the needs of the clients and their family members. Two social workers reported that services were not available to the families because their workload demands were prohibitive in this area. The primary concern the social workers voiced was that they wished that all services did not have to be tied to the client. For example, a social worker could not assist a family to meet needs that were not related to the client, such as budget problems that were disruptive to the entire family structure (see Table 17.5).

How do the clients and families you serve find out about the services that are available to them?

The social workers stated that there were certain clients they were required to visit and this is how and when services were explained. These clients included all patients in ICU; those who suffer from *failure to*

TABLE 17.4   Additional Services

Bereavement
Long-term mental health
Government program assistance
Specific diagnosis groups
Parent support groups
Sibling support groups
Psychiatrist on staff
Palliative Care

TABLE 17.5   Parent and Siblings Services

Available to siblings as long as it is related to the patient $(n = 1)$
Referrals are provided to family members $(n = 6)$
Family therapy sessions are provided $(n = 2)$
Counseling services are available to all members of the child's family $(n = 4)$
Services are not available to family members $(n = 2)$

thrive; those who have been in the hospital for more than 6 days; those that are younger than 3 months of age; or any child that has experienced severe trauma or abuse as designated by the hospital on returned visits. The most common reason to see clients was that a physician referred them; five of the six social workers listed that as their primary reason. It is during these visits that clients and their families were informed about the services that the social worker could offer (see Table 17.6).

CHAPTER SUMMARY AND FUTURE DIRECTIONS

It is hoped that presenting the opinions of social workers actually working in the field will give the reader a greater understanding of what is happening in behaviorally based managed care environments. One of the subjective comments that these social workers acknowledged was that there was a desperate need for supportive services with this population. Yet all six reported that there were not enough available

TABLE 17.6   Knowledge of Services

Required visits
Referrals provided by doctors
Make contact if they see signs of needing assistance
Open door policy
Services are offered at patient discharge

resources to address the problems that these clients and their families encounter from a micro, mezzo, or macro level. To add to this discontent, the social workers acknowledged that they often found difficulties in providing services, as well as clients and family reluctance for utilization or follow-through on services provided. It is recommended that further research and study be done to investigate both the needs of these clients and the benefits from services currently provided. It remains unclear why families are not keeping second appointments or utilizing referrals as given. To address this issue more research in the area is needed. In turn, more information is needed as to what can be done to better educate psychosocial providers in the best methods for serving this rapidly growing population. It appears that the number of clients suffering from chronic conditions and life-threatening illnesses is continuing to grow. This unprecedented growth makes it absolutely necessary that an effective system of providing the needed mental health services and additional needed support services be developed.

REFERENCES

About Us. (2002). *Arnold palmer hospital for women and children.* Retrieved on October 9, 2002, from http://www.arnoldpalmerhospital.org.

Bauman, L., Drotar, D., Leventhal, J., Perrin, E., & Pless, I. (1997). A review of psychosocial interventions for children with chronic health. *Pediatrics, 100,* 244–251.

Child Life Council, Inc. (2000). Child life services. *Pediatrics, 106,* 1156–1159.

Cichocki, M. (2002). Basic statistics-cumulative AIDS cases. *What You Need to Know About.* Retrieved on April 1, 2003, from http://aids.about.com/blbasicstats.htm

The Disaster Center. (2002). Death rates for the leading causes of death for people 1–24 years, all causes: United States, preliminary 1996. Retrieved on October 9, 2002, from http://www.disastercenter.com.

Environmental Protection Agency. (2002). *Childhood cancer.* Retrieved on October 9, 2002, from *http://www.epa.gov/children/cancer.htm.*

Hoyt, M. F. (1995). *Brief therapy and managed care: Readings for contemporary practice.* San Francisco: Jossey-Bass.

Morales, A. T., & Sheafor, B. W. (2001). *Social work: A profession of many faces.* Needham Heights, MA: Pearson Education.

Perrin, E. C., Lewkowiez, C., & Young, M. H. (2000, January). Shared vision: Concordance among fathers, mothers, and pediatricians about unmet needs of children with chronic health conditions. *Pediatrics,* 105 (1), 277–285.

Sahler, O., Frager, G., Levetown, M., Cohn, F., & Lipson, M. (2000). Medical education about end-of-life care in the pediatric setting: Principles, challenges, and opportunities. *Pediatrics, 105* (3), 575–584.

Stephenson, J. (2000, November). Palliative and hospice care needed for children with life threatening conditions, *Journal of the American Medical Association, 284* (19), 2437–2441.

GLOSSARY

Failure to thrive: When infants appear to develop normally but for some reason that is usually unexplained they do not grow and gain weight as would be expected for an infant of similar age and size.

QUESTIONS FOR FURTHER STUDY

1. In terms of working with children who suffer from chronic illness, what do you believe are the most important factors for the social worker to be aware of in the assessment process?
2. What types of educational efforts would best serve clients suffering from these types of illnesses?
3. What types of educational efforts would best assist the parents and/or guardians who have a child who has a chronic illness?

CHAPTER 18

Shaken Baby Syndrome

Sophia F. Dziegielewski, Kelly Richards, and Sherri Diebolt

UNDERSTANDING AND RECOGNIZING SHAKEN BABY SYNDROME

A social worker in the health care setting must be aware of early warning signs indicating shaken baby syndrome (SBS). This sometimes brutal and often undetected form of child abuse can be deadly. It was not until 1972 that SBS was first described in medical literature. Physicians used to think that injuries resulting from SBS were accidental, but as child abuse was studied more diligently, more cases of this syndrome were properly diagnosed (Caffey, 1972, 1974). In fact, nearly 50,000 children in the United States are forcefully shaken by their caretakers every year (Ramirez, 1996), and the consequences are dire.

Although approximately one third of victims exhibit little or no adverse effects, another one third suffers significant injury, and the final third die. Of those who are comatose on initial presentation, 60% will die. Those who do survive their initial comas often suffer profound mental retardation, spastic quadriplegia, severe motor dysfunction, blindness, varying degrees of paralysis, cerebral palsy, or other grave consequences. Shaken baby syndrome is a frequent cause of permanent brain damage and intellectual impairment (Sinal & Ball, 1987).

This chapter will examine SBS, overall statistics, and problems encountered by health care social workers; it will end with suggestions for education and prevention in this area. To illustrate these points, case studies and previous research in this area are presented. In conclusion, recommendations are made to help health care social workers in addressing and preventing this problem.

Understanding Shaken Baby Syndrome

The Encyclopedia and Dictionary of Medicine, Nursing, & Allied Health (Brown, 1992, p. 1621) defines SBS as a constellation of injuries to the brain and eye that may occur when a child who is fewer than 3 years old (usually less than 1 year old) is shaken vigorously while being supported. This causes stretching and tearing of the cerebral vessels and brain substance, commonly leading to subdural hematomas and retinal hemorrhages, and these injuries are generally associated with cerebral contusion (an internal bruising of the brain). These injuries may result in paralysis, blindness and other visual disturbances, convulsions, and death.

An estimated 50,000 cases occur each year in the United States (Ramirez, 1996). According to a 5–year-old study (Poissaint & Linn, 1997), one shaken baby in four dies as a result of this abuse, while others have the death incidence as high as one in three. Head trauma is the most frequent cause of permanent damage or death among abused infants and children, and shaking accounts for a significant number of those cases (Showers, 1992a). The victims of Shaken Baby Syndrome range in age from a few days to 5 years, with an average age of 6 to 8 months (Showers, 1997). When this type of abuse is suspected, the law mandates that the health care social worker must report the incident immediately to the State's Department of Children and Families.

Thirty years ago, SBS was not even considered a classification. It now accounts for more than 15,000 infant deaths per year, and that number again of severe injuries (Ramirez, 1996). Unfortunately, SBS is becoming much more common for today's social worker.

Recognition, Identification, and Family Issues

The anatomy of infants renders them more susceptible to shaking than older children or adults. The head of the infant comprises 10% of his or her body weight, compared with just 2% in the adult. Neck muscles have not developed strength compared with later in life, and consequently the neck cannot absorb the energy generated during a whiplash event such as shaking. Infants lack head control, so they cannot resist or minimize the forces of injury (Fulton, 2000).

Unfortunately, the pathophysiology that occurs in SBS starts the moment that the baby is first shaken. Therefore, the severity of cerebral injury will be directly related to the severity of the shaking and the time elapsed during the event. The perpetrator must be aware that the vigorous back-and-forth motion causes intense problems within the baby's skull, resulting in serious bruising to the brain as it hits the skull. It is this shaking that leads to the bruising, which in turn causes the subdural bleeding. These factors contribute to cerebral edema and shearing of the blood vessels. As well as causing increased edema, constriction of the thorax can also lead to retinal hemorrhages, a classic finding in SBS (Fulton, 2000).

Damage also occurs within the eyes of the baby where retinal hemorrhages associated with SBS are attributable to rapid movement of the vitreous body and sudden increased intraocular pressure. This damage is so pronounced because a sudden rise in intracranial pressure is transmitted to the eyes via the optic nerve sheath. This mechanism causes the increased intraocular pressure that could cause permanent visual impairment (Levin, 1990). Based on this finding, it is not uncommon for 30% to 80% of children who have suffered from concomitant intracranial and retinal injury to also have significant visual problems. Therefore, SBS should be a consideration in all children under 4 years of age who present with retinal hemorrhages (Fulton, 2000).

Victims of SBS are infants or children ranging in age from a few days old to 5 years, with the average being 6 to 8 months old (Showers, 1994). Boys are most at risk, and until recently more often white children than black (Brenner, Fischer, & Mann-Gray, 1989). The reasons that boys are more often victims were explored in a 1992 study. The study found that parents believe that boys can withstand rougher handling than girls, or there may be cultural expectations that boys should cry less often (Showers, 1992b).

SBS is characterized as much by what is obscure or subtle as by what is immediately clinically identifiable (Coody et al., 1994). The infant who has been a victim of SBS can present in many ways. In less severe cases, some of the symptoms include:

- History of poor feeding, sucking, or swallowing
- Vomiting
- Lethargy or irritability
- Hypothermia

- Failure to thrive
- Increased sleeping and difficulty arousing
- Failure to smile or vocalize

Because of the vagueness of the symptoms, SBS may remain unidentified (Wehrwein, 1998). These types of symptoms can occur frequently in other infectious processes common to infants and children. Subtle symptoms may occur intermittently for days or weeks preceding the first contact with a health care facility. The caretaker may put the child to bed hoping for natural resolution of symptoms. Instead, the condition of the infant frequently deteriorates (Fulton, 2000).

In more severe cases of SBS, the symptoms are acute and often life-threatening. Irreversible damage may already be present. Some of the more severe symptoms include:

- Decreased level of consciousness
- Seizures
- Coma
- Bulging fontanel (indicative of increased intracranial pressure)
- Periods of apnea
- Bradycardia
- Complete cardiovascular collapse

Even when SBS symptoms are life-threatening, they may go unrecognized. The presentation of such extreme symptoms may lead to misdiagnosis such as traumatic accident, meningitis, sepsis, or unusual neurologic disorders. The characteristic presentation of SBS is the lack of external trauma in the presence of intracranial and intraocular hemorrhage (Fulton, 2000). Suspicion of child abuse may not be a consideration because of the absence of surface trauma.

Again, diagnosis is not easy and computerized tomography (CT) and/or magnetic resonance imaging (MRI) would need to be performed for a complete and accurate diagnosis (Sato et al., 1989). CT has become the first-line technique in imaging evaluation of the patient with brain injury. CT is generally the method of choice for diagnosing subarachnoid hemorrhage, mass effect, and large extra-axial hemorrhages (Sato et al., 1989). The most common CT finding in the shaken baby is subdural hematoma. It is also the most common cause of death in shaken babies when the death is classified as a homicide. MRI is of great value as an adjunct to CT. It offers better contrast sensitivity and clearer evidence of injury and is useful in determining the age of an injury (Chiocca, 1998).

An ophthalmology exam is one of the simplest and cheapest ways of determining closed injury traumas, especially SBS (D'Lugoff & Baker, 1998). Retinal hemorrhages occur in about 75% of victims of SBS, indicating that an ophthalmology consultation is paramount on all patients with suspicious histories, including children with unexplained lethargy or seizures (D'Lugoff & Baker, 1998). Except in the first month of age, the presence of retinal hemorrhage in children younger than 4 years of age should serve as a red flag for SBS (Fishman, Dasher, & Lambert, 1998).

Once the child with a head injury is stable, a skeletal survey may rule out or confirm other injuries. Most abuse is not a single event; therefore, evidence of old injuries may be present. On examination, long bones, skull, spine, and ribs should be x-rayed (Meservy, Towbin, McLaurin, Myers, & Ball, 1987). Old injuries and injuries in various stages of healing are consistent with abuse. Old and new fractures of the midshaft and metaphysics are present in 25% of victims of SBS (Gilliland & Folber, 1996).

According to Showers (1994), the perpetrators are profiled as mostly male (75%), with an average age of 22 years (ranging from 14 to 46 years of age) and related to the victim or to the victim's mother (44% were fathers, 23% were boyfriends of the mother, 2% were stepparents, and 6% were unrelated male baby-sitters). Furthermore, Starling, Holden, and Jenny (1995) concluded that out of 127 cases of head trauma recognized in their study, 65.5% of the perpetrators were male and 31.5% female. An astonishing feature in the study that distinguishes SBS from other forms of child abuse is that the mother is the least likely perpetrator.

SBS is a complex disorder with implications beyond the undeniable need for identification and protection for child victims. Social workers in a hospital setting, office practice, and public health and community practice play a major role in prevention, diagnosis, and treatment of the individual and family affected by SBS.

PREVALENCE OF SHAKEN BABY SYNDROME

There are many risk factors associated with SBS. Frequently, new parents are unaware of a child's normal development or an infant's basic needs. This lack of knowledge can create unrealistic expectations of the infant and/or child. Other parents may have a need for nurturing themselves and look, illogically, to the infant or child to fulfill that need. When these expectations are unsatisfied, a parent's stress and frustration increase. Young parents and single parents fall within the parental risk group. Their lack of life experience and immaturity may create unmanageable frustration when faced with an inconsolable infant. A crying infant, combined with poor impulse control in the parent and not knowing how to console their baby, places the child at high risk for SBS.

Another major risk factor contributing to SBS is substance abuse by the parent (Starling et al., 1995). In general, perpetrators under the influence of drugs, alcohol, or both commit large proportions of violent crimes. SBS is an unquestionable act of violence. Most individuals under the influence of mind-altering substances lose inhibition and impulse control. Consequently, they may do things that they would never do in an unimpaired state.

Infants born to drug-addicted mothers are at extreme risk for SBS (Starling et al., 1995). Addicted themselves, these infants cry for extended periods and are inconsolable and irritable. To compound the situation, the mother under the influence has altered perception. She will frequently perceive the infant as always crying. Her frustration and altered mental status place that infant at high risk for SBS, neglect, and other forms of abuse.

Another factor increasing the risk of SBS is the overall environment. Numerous factors, such as financial, social, and physical burdens, that have changed negatively with the birth of a child contribute to increased levels of stress. Any external factor that places stress on the parent puts an infant at risk for SBS.

Among these factors, lack of financial resources is a major stressor. The infant is at even greater risk if there was a significant effect on the family financial situation with the birth of the baby. Compounding that financial burden is the fact that the presence of a child often decreases the earning potential in a dual-income couple if adequate child care resources are not available.

In the case of new parents or single parents, the responsibility of an infant often creates social isolation. They no longer have the freedom to pursue individual interests. Things previously taken for granted no longer exist or are difficult to attain. These changes can result in resentment toward the infant. As time goes by, the parent may experience a decreased tolerance for the numerous needs of an infant.

In addition, physical elements of the surroundings, parent, or child may be risk factors. A parent with a physical disability may experience increased difficulty caring for an infant, which leads to feelings of inadequacy. A child with a physical or mental disability places additional demands on the parent.

Ironically, infants themselves have intrinsic behavior patterns that place them at risk for SBS. The behavior that most often precedes an episode of shaking is crying. Infants spend about 20% of their time crying even in optimal situations (Butler, 1995). Some parents perceive the crying as constant and unrelenting. It becomes even more frustrating when the infant is inconsolable. For example, infants with colic cry even more and often are inconsolable. An inconsolable infant can make the parent feel helpless and increasingly frustrated.

Previously unrecognized as a potential perpetrator of SBS, the family baby-sitter is emerging as a frequent abuser. Very often the baby-sitter is an adolescent, and this group is considered risky because of immaturity and lack of life experience. When a caretaker from outside of the family is the perpetrator of SBS, there is often a failure to report the onset of symptoms to the parents (Starling et al., 1995). This lack of information makes it difficult to determine the time of injury (Nashelsky & Dix, 1995). Frequently, caregivers claim that the infant was fine when put to bed and then was unresponsive when later checked (Starling et al., 1995). A delay in recognizing and seeking early treatment for symptoms associated with SBS increases mortality and morbidity of injuries sustained. Given the number of families who rely on outside child care, it is essential to target this group for education regarding the danger of SBS.

There have been episodes of SBS that are nonintentional. These "accidents" are linked to lack of understanding of the etiology of SBS. Rough horseplay such as swinging or tossing an infant can cause severe injuries. "Calda de Mollera" is a form of Hispanic folk medicine (Perinatal Education Association, 1999–2000). The purpose of the practice is to raise the sunken fontanel in an infant. The practitioner holds the infant upside down over a pan of hot water. The heels of the infant are then slapped while the infant is simultaneously shaken in an up-and-down motion. The obvious solution to these inadvertent causes of SBS is to educate those who care for infants about the dangers of such practices.

CASE EXEMPLARS

In the emergency room of a local hospital, a 2-month-old baby boy's case was given to the social worker on the unit for assessment. The physician was concerned when the parents were unable to adequately explain what had happened to their baby boy. The baby presented as listless and unresponsive.

When the social worker met the family, she recalled having seen them before. The couple had sought medical attention for another child in the past, when the sister had been treated for several broken ribs and a broken arm that was explained by the parents as a result of a fall from the crib. At that time the social worker reported the case to the Department of Children and Families (DCF). Generally, in cases like this the reporting social worker is not made aware of the disposition, and it was unclear what happened after the referral of this case was made.

In another case, D'Lugoff and Baker (1998) highlighted the difficulties that medical personal can have in diagnosing SBS as well as the problems parents can experience when trying to determine if seeking medical consultation is appropriate. D'Lugoff and Baker (1998) studied a case where a 3–month-old African American boy was brought into the emergency room by his parents. In the initial assessment, the baby appeared lifeless and was believed to be in septic shock. The mother stated for the previous 24 hours her child would not eat, was having trouble breathing, was crossing his eyes, and was having what appeared to be seizures. The parents reported the baby had recently received his immunization shots and the mother noted to staff that his symptoms resembled what his doctor had warned might occur as a reaction to the shots.

During the health assessment, the mother claimed that the baby had fallen off the bed while his father was caring for him 2 weeks earlier. The mother reported she had contacted her doctor but was informed by the nurse that since the baby did not lose consciousness he would not need medical attention. On this occasion, the child was observed in the emergency room for 3 hours without a diagnosis being rendered. No one suspected SBS. Consequently, no referral was made to a health care social worker. It was not until later, when the child was placed in a tertiary care facility, that a report of suspected child abuse was filed. Upon further examination, the baby was found to have a fractured skull, internal bleeding, five fractured ribs, and both wrists fractured. The child's right eye was bruised and his big toe appeared to be smashed.

The father was arrested and charged with child abuse, assault, battery, reckless endangerment, and attempt to murder. He was found guilty and sentenced to a minimum of 15 years in prison. The mother was arrested and charged with failure to seek urgent medical treatment for her son and served 6 months.

It was the opinion of D'Lugoff and Baker (1998) that the mother was not guilty of neglect, nor did she willfully delay getting the child treatment. Furthermore, in reviewing the dynamics that surround this case, it would appear that the child's mother also became a victim. According to D'Lugoff and Baker (1998), the mother did try to help her child by reporting the child's toe to the pediatrician during a checkup, and the doctor gave the child medication. The mother called the pediatrician's office when the child fell from the bed and was informed not to bring the child in. The mother was also informed that after the child was immunized he might have side effects similar to the symptoms he displayed after being shaken by the father. The mother tried to get help for her child but may have been unaware of the extent of his injuries; or she may have not realized what serious injuries the baby could sustain from shaking. The baby was permanently damaged by his injuries and was placed into a foster home (D'Lugoff & Baker, 1998).

Unfortunately, cases like this are becoming more common. In a recent study of 53 infants who died as a result of a nonaccidental head trauma, 37 of them died because they stopped breathing (Trifiletti, 2001). The actual cause of death was damage to the cranio-cervical junction, which is the point of the brain that meets the spinal cord. This joint is very fragile in young babies because of their weak necks and can easily be damaged when shaken or rocked (Coghlan & Page, 2001).

PREVENTIVE EDUCATION

Working with children and families in a health care setting is the social worker's opportunity to listen to parents and to pick up on cues that may lead to the discovery of families at risk and in need of support before SBS occurs. Without preventive interventions, such families may respond to the pressures in the family dynamics with inappropriate parenting behavior (Patrini, 2002). The end result of such behavior may culminate in a shaken baby.

For the health care social worker, it is important to realize how challenging parenting can be for some parents, and not knowing or understanding why a baby is crying can be very frustrating for all involved. For parents, new or additional parental responsibilities often mean juggling with competing priorities to balance work and home life. This juggling is further complicated by simply trying to understand how best to meet children's needs at all stages of their development. Parents themselves require and deserve support. There are some families who are not capable or self-aware enough to be able to recognize their need for help. This is why health care social workers need to be trained to recognize the symptoms of such family pressure, identify needs, and provide or assist in accessing support mechanisms (Patrini, 2002).

According to Poissaint and Linn (1997), helping parents and caregivers to better understand infant behavior can help prevent SBS. Teaching parenting skills and concrete skills to help caregivers manage their frustrations could significantly reduce the occurrence of SBS and other types of abuse. Sometimes parents may shake a child, perceiving it a less violent way than other means to enforce discipline.

The focus of education should be on child care givers and potential child care givers. New parents can be informed through prenatal care, community education, and their primary care provider. In the hospital on the postpartum unit, information about the dangers of shaking an infant should be part of the standard discharge teaching (Chiocca, 1995). Incorporating education about SBS through health education within the school system will reach young potential child care givers. Decreasing mortality and morbidity associated with SBS is achievable through early preventive education.

A health care social worker, as a part of preventive management, should ask about caretaker stress, discipline practices, substance abuse, and responses to the crying infant. Home visitation programs are proven helpful in preventing interfamilial physical abuse. The United States Advisory Board on Child Abuse and Neglect (1991, 1995) has repeatedly recommended nationwide home visitation programs.

There is increasing recognition nationwide that SBS is not a rare phenomenon and that a public education campaign is needed. More and more, agencies have begun to distribute printed material describing the problem. The number of public service announcements and billboard ads has also risen. The most comprehensive campaign to date has been a "Don't Shake the Baby" program begun in Ohio (Showers, 1992a). The "Don't Shake the Baby" approach to education includes a print packet for parents of newborns, a multimedia package consisting of television and radio public service announcements, and reproducible black and white print ads (Showers, 1992a).

Child care providers, another concerning risk group, need to have mandated child abuse training that includes SBS education before they begin caring for children. Funding and monitoring high-quality child care is also important so that parents leave their children with safe caregivers.

Physicians, social workers, educators, attorneys, families, and others should collaborate to educate the public about preventing SBS. In addition to public education, strategies to reduce the problem should include identifying families at high risk for abuse and providing supports to reduce stress.

The Early Childhood Development Parent Education Program (Calming a Crying Baby, 2002) identifies the following information to help prevent SBS:

- Try to stay calm. This isn't easy! NEVER SHAKE YOUR BABY! This can damage your baby's brain.
- If you are upset, it is okay to put your baby in a crib and take a break for up to 15 minutes.
- If you are still feeling upset after this break, you may need to find another adult to care for your baby while you take a longer break.
- If your frustration is high and you are still upset, or feel you may lose control, leave the room and call or contact another adult to watch your child while you calm down. All parents need help and support sometimes. Caring for children can be very stressful.
- If you are upset or angry and think you might hurt your baby...GET HELP!! Call a neighbor, a friend, a church, a health department, a parent assistance center, or a social worker.
- Getting help is a sign of strength. It is the best thing you can do for you and your baby.
- Have hot line information readily available.

CHILD ABUSE SUPPORT LINES

CHILD HELP (800-4-ACHILD)
National Child Abuse Hot line (800-422-4458).

THE SOCIAL WORKER'S ROLE

Shaken baby syndrome is an extremely difficult diagnosis to recognize in the absence of obvious signs of physical abuse. If true for medical personnel, it is at least equally difficult for a layperson. From a health care social worker's point of view, a biopychosocial assessment could contribute information regarding the health and safety of the home. A review of relevant history of behaviors, values, attitudes, and fears is important to understand what might contribute to the parent's delay in seeking medical help.

Furthermore, community health social workers are apt to encounter the barriers that the underprivileged experience through lack of telephones, timely transportation, inaccessible health care, and language and class disparities with caregivers. They are more likely to recognize community-wide illiteracy or compromised educational functioning and can educate and enlighten judges and prosecutors of these problems that are not likely to be present in the life experience of upper-middle-class professionals. Likewise, they can share research evidence of the difficulty that families have in identifying drug use in a family member who wishes to conceal it.

Funding for prevention continues to be limited, although the benefit of prevention can far outweigh the cost of care for a surviving SBS child over his or her lifetime. It has been estimated that just the initial hospitalization for a SBS child is $75,000-$95,000 (Showers, 1996). This does not include continuing rehabilitation or medical expenses incurred after the child goes home. Most of these costs are absorbed by society through insurance, government assistance, and increased special education costs (Showers, 1996).

For the health care social worker there is a need to advocate for agency programs that will facilitate prevention, education, and intervention in regards to SBS. The practitioner must be cognizant of signs and symptoms of SBS when working with clients. Workers must be prepared to train and educate parents and caregivers on how a normal infant will develop and grow, what to expect and how to meet a child's needs, and how to handle frustration when stress does occur.

Health care social workers must be vigilant for the signs of SBS so that appropriate interventions and protection of the child can take place. Risk factors must also be recognized before the occurrence of injury. Intervention before an episode of shaking may save the life of an infant. There is no greater reward than saving a life. The following are important questions for health care social workers to address:

- How can we best be helpful to children and families?
- How do we as health care social workers determine the presence and extent of risk factors for a child to become a victim of SBS?
- How do we best teach parents how to teach, guide, and discipline their children?

CHAPTER SUMMARY AND FUTURE DIRECTIONS

Parenting is a difficult challenge. Under the best of circumstances, the stress of a new baby (particularly to new parents) is intense, not only because of the demands of an infant but also because of the changes that take place in the new parent's life—increased responsibility, financial pressure, a decreased independence. Mix in less than ideal circumstances, poor or no support from family and friends, substance abuse or a combination of other stressors, and the temptation to take out these troubles on an unsuspecting child is sometimes too great. A baby that cries a lot is another target. Frustration can boil over, and picking up a baby and shaking him to stop the crying is sometimes an impulsive action.

No matter why it occurs, the results are devastating (Uscinski, 2002). Thousands of serious injuries and deaths occur each year. The best way for the health care social worker to assist with this problem is by taking a proactive approach of education and prevention: reaching out to caregivers at a young age with more emphasis on SBS in schools; education about SBS as an integral part of prenatal and postpartum care; and diligence among social workers to identify and assess and address potential problems before they occur. A combination of the above could result in many fewer cases of this deadly, brutal, and heartbreaking syndrome.

SPECIFIC RECOMMENDATIONS FOR THE HEALTH CARE SOCIAL WORKER

1. Become educated about the recognition, diagnosis, treatment, and outcome of shaken baby injuries in infants and children.
2. Be aware of and exercise responsibility to report these injuries to appropriate authorities.
3. Provide pertinent medical information to other members of multidisciplinary teams investigating these injuries.
4. Support home visitation programs and any other child abuse prevention efforts that prove effective.
5. Provide or have appropriate referrals to resources to educate parents about healthy coping strategies when dealing with their child.

REFERENCES

Brenner, S. L., Fischer, H., & Mann-Gray, S. (1989). Race and the shaken baby syndrome: Experience at one hospital. *Journal of National Medical Association, 35,* 183–184.

Brown, M. J. (Ed.). (1992). *Miller-Keane encyclopedia and dictionary of medicine, nursing, and allied health* (5th ed.) Philadelphia, PA: W. B. Saunders. (Original work published 1972)

Butler, G. (1995). Shaken baby syndrome. *Journal of Psychosocial Nursing, 33*(9), 47–50.

Caffey, J. (1972). On the theory and practice of shaking infants, its potential residual effects of permanent brain damage and mental retardation. *American Journal of Disabled Children, 124,* 161–169.

Caffey, J. (1974). The whiplash shaken baby syndrome: Manual shaking by the extremities and whiplash induced intracranial and intraocular bleeding linked with residual permanent brain damage and mental retardation. *Pediatrics, 54,* 396–403.

Calming a Crying Baby. (n.d.) Retrieved October 23, 2002 from *http:// www.health.state.ok.us,* MCH Early Childhood Development and Parent Education Program

Chiocca, E. (1995). Shaken baby syndrome: a nursing perspective. *Pediatric Nursing, 21*(1), 33–38.

Chiocca, E. (1998). Action stat! Shaken baby syndrome. *Nursing, 28*(5), 33.

Coghlan, A., & Page, M. L. (2001). Gently does it: Shaken baby syndrome. *New Scientist, 170,* 2295.

Coody, C., Brown, M., Montgomery, D., Flynn, A., & Yetman, R. (1994). Shaken baby syndrome: Identification and prevention for nurse practitioners. *Journal of Pediatric Health Care*, *8*(2), 50–56.

D'Lugoff, M. I., & Baker, D. J. (1998). Case study: Shaken baby syndrome—one disorder with two victims. *Public Health Nursing*, *15*, 243–249.

Fishman, C., Dasher, W., & Lambert, S. (1998). Electroretinographic findings in infants with shaken baby syndrome. *Journal of Pediatric Ophthamology Strabismus*, *35*, 22–26.

Fulton, D. R. (2000). Shaken baby syndrome. *Critical Care Nursing Quarterly*, *23*, 43–50.

Gilliland, M., & Folber, R. (1996). Shaken babies: Some have no impact injuries. *Journal of Forensic Sciences*, *41*(1), 114–116.

Levin, A. V. (1990). Ocular manifestations of child abuse. *Ophthalmological Clinics North America*, *3*, 249–264.

Meservy, C. J., Towbin, R., McLaurin, R. L., Myers, P. A., & Ball, W. (1987). Radiographic characteristics of skull fractures resulting from child abuse. *American Journal of Roentgenology*, *149*, 173–175.

Nashelsky, M., & Dix, J. (1995). The time interval between lethal infant shaking and the onset of symptoms. *Journal of Forensic Medical Pathology*, *16*, 154–157.

Patrini, S. A. (2002). A window of opportunity: Preventing Shaken Baby Syndrome in A&E. *Pediatric Nursing*, *14*(7), 32–35.

Perinatal Education Association. (1999–2000). *Cultural diversity in the perinatal education setting: Hispanic or Mexican American*. (1999–2000). Retrieved October 23, 2002 from *http://www.birthsource.com/proarticlefile/proarticle10.html*.

Poissaint, A., & Linn, S. (1997, Spring 33). Fragile: Handle with care [Special Edition]. *Newsweek*.

Ramirez, D. (1996, November 19). Beware of the dangers of shaking infants. *Forth Worth, Texas: Star-Telegram*.

Sato, Y., Yuh, W. T., Smith, W. L., Alexander, R. C., Kao, S. C., & Ellerbroek, C. J. (1989). Head injury in child abuse: Evaluation with MR imaging. *Radiology*, *173*, 653–657.

Showers, J. (1992a). Shaken baby syndrome. *Children Today*, *21*(2), 34–38.

Showers, J. (1992b). "Don't shake the baby": The effectiveness of a prevention program. *Child Abuse and Neglect*, *16*, 11–18.

Showers, J. (1994). Shaken baby syndrome: What have we learned about victims and perpetrators? *'Don't Shake the Baby" Campaign News*, *8*(2), 1–2

Showers, J. (1995). SBS prevention in America: An update. *Campaign News*, *5*(1), 1.

Showers, J. (1996). A medical, legal, and prevention challenge, executive summary. In *The National Conference on Shaken Baby Syndrome*, Alexandria, VA: National Association of Children's Hospitals and Related Institutions.

Showers, J. (1997). A medical, legal, and prevention challenge, executive summary. In *The National Conference on Shaken Baby Syndrome,* Alexandria, VA: National Association of Children's Hospitals and Related Institutions.

Sinal, S. H., & Ball, M. R. (1987). Head trauma due to child abuse; serial computerized tomography in diagnosis and management. *Southern Medical Journal, 80,* 1505–1512.

Starling, S., Holden, J., & Jenny, C. (1995). Abusive head trauma: The relationship of perpetrators to their victims. *Pediatrics, 95,* 259–262.

Trifiletti, R. (2001). Non-accidental head injury in children: New clues from neuropathology. *Neurology Alert, 20(3),* 19.

U.S. Advisory Board on Child Abuse and Neglect (1991). *Creating caring communities: Blueprint for an effective federal policy on child abuse and neglect* (pp. 141–146). Washington, DC: U.S. Department of Health and Human Services.

U.S. Advisory Board on Child Abuse and Neglect. (1995). *A nation's shame: Fatal child abuse and neglect in the United States.* Washington, DC: US Department of Health and Human Services; 1995. Report No. 5.

Uscinski, R. (2002). Shaken baby syndrome: Fundamental questions. *British Journal of Neurosurgery, 16(3),* 217–219.

Wehrwein, P. (1998). Scientific review on shaken-baby syndrome undermines legal defense. *Lancet, 351,* 1935–1935.

GLOSSARY

Bradycardia: Slowness of the heart beat, as evidenced by slowing of the pulse rate to less than 60 per minute.

Cerebral contusion: Contusion of the brain following a head injury.

Cerebral edema: Fluid collecting in the brain, causing tissue to swell.

Fontanel: A soft spot; one of the membrane-covered spaces remaining at the junction of the sutures in the incompletely ossified skull of the fetus or infant. Though these "soft spots" may appear very vulnerable, they may be touched gently without harm. Care should be exercised that they be protected from strong pressure or direct injury.

Hematoma: A localized accumulation of blood in tissues as a result of hemorrhaging.

Hemorrhage: A condition of bleeding, usually severe.

Intracranial: Within the cranium.

Intraocular: Within the eye.

Retinal hemorrhage: Bleeding of the retina, a key structure in vision located at the back of the eyes.

Shaken baby syndrome: A severe form of head injury that occurs when a baby is shaken forcibly enough to cause the baby's brain to bounce against his or her skull. This jarring can cause bruising, swelling, and bleeding of the brain resulting in permanent, severe brain damage or even death

Subarachnoid hemorrhage or subdural hematoma: A localized accumulation of blood, sometimes mixed with spinal fluid, in the space of the brain beneath the membrane covering called the dura mater.

QUESTIONS FOR FURTHER STUDY

1. What are the risk factors that could facilitate the early risk assessment of shaken baby syndrome?
2. What are the most important points for health care social workers to identify in order to help educate new parents and young babysitters on the danger of shaking a baby?
3. What types of parents are at greatest risk of shaken baby syndrome, and why?

CHAPTER 19

Complementary Therapies: Tips and Techniques for Health Care Social Workers

Sophia Dziegielewski and Patricia Sherman

THE TREND TOWARD ALTERNATIVE APPROACHES TO HEALTH CARE

For many health care social workers, there has been a pronounced movement toward helping clients to take charge of their own mental and medical health. In accepting this responsibility the underlining premise is that good health needs to involve the promotion of health and maintaining wellness. For many individuals this involves exploring nontraditional types of treatment and intervention, such as alternative and complementary or integrative approaches to achieving health and wellness. These can include medications, herbs, vitamins, minerals, and the new so-called functional foods to enhance and support an individual's well-being. Knowledge of these products has become a practice reality because clients use these interventions and preparations as a means to gain greater control over their health and well-being. Effective, efficient, and comprehensive helping relationships require that social workers keep abreast of all types of intervention. The purpose of this chapter is to provide a brief overview of some of these modalities and thereby help the health care social worker become aware of these interventions and some of the problems and benefits that can arise.

THE EXPLOSION OF HEALTH AND WELLNESS EFFORTS

For many health care social workers, there has been a pronounced movement toward helping clients to take charge of their own mental and medical health. Many clients are seeking alternatives or supplements to traditional medical care. Whether out of dissatisfaction with the increasingly impersonal treatment from health care providers or a desire to exercise more control over their own care, clients are using herbs, acupuncture, massage, homeopathic remedies, and a host of other nonallopathic treatments. There are also some clients who desire to utilize remedies traditionally employed within their cultures, such as herbals, amulets, or exorcisms. It is becoming increasingly essential for social workers to have adequate knowledge of these alternatives, since many of them may interfere with or intensify the actions of traditional medications and treatments.

PRACTICE STRATEGY

Medical treatments in this country remain varied and can range from home remedies shared among family and friends to medications that are prescribed by a physician. Basically, there are three primary approaches to the delivery of medical care: traditional mainstream medicine, alternative medicine, and complementary or integrative medicine. Historically, in this country the most traditional and widely used form of medicine involves standard drug therapies and surgical interventions. This type of *traditional mainstream medicine* and the practices that reflect this type of intervention strategy clearly require the skill of a trained professional and are generally referred to as mainstream American medical practice.

Today, the majority of physicians in this country share this philosophical approach to medicine and have been trained primarily in this area. The awareness and belief that physicians are trained in this way may pose a problem, since clients using alternative therapies may be reluctant to tell the physician. Many times they may fear that the physician will be opposed to the treatment, so they do not mention it. Further, they may feel that the physician won't know enough in the area and is not an expert on the client's individual needs. Heart disease, for example, has been conventionally treated through surgery that entails an extensive risk, such as stroke or heart attack that could occur during the operation itself. Many individuals today are electing not to have this invasive procedure at all and choosing to utilize an alternative treatment consisting of a low-fat vegetarian diet, stress management, moderate exercise, and group counseling (McCall, 1998). For some of these clients, it does appear that this less invasive method is working effectively and providing a reasonable alternative to the more invasive surgical procedure that was usually performed.

Those professionals who practice medicine, regardless of whether they specialize in traditional approaches or newer, holistic methods, often agree that when traditionally based medical interventions have been proven to work, it is best to use them (Stehlin, 1995). For example, in childhood leukemia conventional therapies can yield an 80% cure rate; therefore, it would seem unreasonable to switch to something that was not considered to have as reasonable a chance of success. Generally, however, this is not the type of client who will leave traditional medicine. Rather, it is the person who suffers from a complicated or chronic condition, or one for whom allopathic remedies have not been effective enough—the individual who is tired of receiving minimal relief and wants a new and different "get and stay well" approach. For so many individuals whose symptoms cannot be relieved or controlled by conventional medicine, the idea pain-free or symptom-free relief is so seductive that they will quickly drop the more conventional therapies in favor of alternative ones.

A second approach to medical care that has recently gained in popularity is *alternative medicine*. According to Stehlin (1995), most alternative approaches are often described as any medical practice or intervention that is utilized instead of conventional treatment, lacks sufficient documentation in regard to its safety and effectiveness against certain diseases and conditions, is generally not taught in United States medical schools, and is generally not reimbursable by health insurance providers (p. 10). The National Institutes of Health defines alternative medicine as "medical systems, therapies, and techniques that mainstream Western (conventional) medicine does not commonly use, accept, study, understand, or make available" (NIH, 2000, p. 6). These approaches are varied but often involve such techniques as touch therapy and massage (e.g., acupressure), chiropractic, magnets, herbals, and naturopathic remedies. Further techniques that allow for mind and body control, such as herbal preparations and spiritual healing, are also used. See Table 19.1, for a summary and quick reference for some of the different alternative approaches. When clients express interest in this type of therapy, it is important for social workers to encourage them to utilize the services of alternative practitioners who are licensed or certified.

A third type of medicine practiced in this country is referred to as *complementary or integrative medicine.* In this approach to medical care, clients generally receive traditional approaches to therapy such as prescription medications, augmented or supplemented by alternative approaches. In this method a combination approach is explored.

CONSIDERATIONS AND CONCERNS

In 1997, 42% of Americans used an alternative therapy, spending over $27 billion (Eisenberg et al., 1998). Borken et al. (1994) reported a study that showed that more than 60% of doctors from a wide range of specialties recommended alternative therapies to their patients at least once. In addition, 47% of the doctors in this study reported using alternative therapies themselves. Physicians might recommend folic acid to prevent birth defects, Vitamin E to promote a healthy heart, or Vitamin C to boost the patient's immune system. Many United States medical schools are now offering elective courses in complementary or alternative medicine (Wetzel, Eisenberg, & Kaptchuk, 1998). On the other hand, Kroll (1997) found that 60% of retail pharmacists interviewed in a University of Mississippi study learned about herbal medicines from their own patients, and only 25% said they had learned about them during their professional education.

So much interest has been generated in alternative therapies that the National Institutes of Health established the Office of Alternative Medicine (OAM) in 1992, with a budget of $2 million. In 1998, Congress established the National Center for Complementary and Alternative Medicine (NCCAM) as a replacement for OAM to stimulate, develop, and support research on CAM. It now supports both basic and applied research and had a budget of $68.7 million in FY 2000.

Probably the biggest concern for the health care social worker in accepting and supporting clients who utilize alternative remedies is the assumption that because they are natural, they must be safe (Dziegielewski, 2002). Unfortunately, this is not necessarily so. Herbal

TABLE 19.1 Alternative Therapies

Alternative Medicine Systems

Traditional Chinese Medicine (TCM)—uses herbs, acupuncture, accupressure (shiatsu, tsabu, jin shin, jujitsu), and physical exercise like t'ai chi chian or qigong

Ayurveda—uses pranayama (alternate nostril breathing), abhyanga (rubbing skin with oil, usually sesame), rasayana (herbs and mantras during meditation), yoga, panchakarma (intense cleansing therapy including diaphoretics, diuretics, cathartics, and emetics), and herbal remedies

Naturopathy—holistic approach using homeopathy, vitamin and mineral supplements, physiotherapy, TCM, stress management, and herbs

Homeopathy—uses homeopathic (minute doses of herb, mineral or animal products) remedies as catalysts to aid body's inherent healing mechanism. Correct remedy treats the physical, emotional, and mental symptoms

Osteopathy—uses diagnostic and treatment techniques similar to medical practitioners, but also treats the musculoskeletal system with adjustive maneuvers

Chiropractic—diagnoses and treats illnesses that affect the nerves, muscles, bones and joints by relieving pressure through manipulation

Environmental Medicine—focuses on the effect of chemicals, such as pesticides, food preservatives, car exhaust fumes, and formaldehyde, on the immune system. Uses nutritional supplements, immunotherapy, and desensitization

---

Mind/Body Therapies

Hypnotherapy—technique of focused attention; especially helpful for pain management, addictions, and phobias

Biofeedback—relaxation technique to enable people to gain control over autonomic responses, such as heart rate, blood pressure, and voluntary muscle contractions

Relaxation Techniques—autogenic training, progressive muscle relaxation, meditation

---

Bodywork

Massage—lymphatic massage, neuromuscular (deep tissue) massage, rolfing (facial manipulation)

TABLE 19.1 *(continued)*

Postural/Energy Therapies—focuses on relationship between the musculoskeletal system and body movement. Alexander Technique (corrects muscle and joint coordination, balance and ease of movement), Feldenkreis (improves coordination and increases awareness of bodily functions involved with movement), and Therapeutic Touch

---

Dietary Supplements

Nutritional Supplements—deficiencies are determined through blood, stool, urine and hair analyses. Adverse reactions between medications and supplements can occur

Orthomolecular Medicine—uses mega doses of supplements; found useful for hypercholesterolemia and AIDS

Botanical Medicine—herbs are prescribed for specific symptoms (Information obtained from Integrative Medicine Communications, 1998)

---

medications are derived primarily from natural substances and therefore many individuals assume that they are safe. What most people do not realize is that many prescription medications are created similarly and utilize many of the same ingredients. Therefore, it is not uncommon for some of the pharmaceutical drugs used today to be derived from herbs and freely utilize these ingredients in their composition (Dziegielewski & Leon, 2001). For example, aspirin, a commonly used pain reliever, is derived from the bark of the white willow tree. In addition to this, one cancer treatment medication known as Taxol comes directly from the Pacific yew tree.

The implications of this "natural is safe" mentality requires further exploration and study because clients may be unaware that they are taking preparations that could create problems when combined with prescription drugs or with other natural supplements or herbs. It is important to note, however, that mixing herbal remedies and prescription medicine does not always have a negative outcome. For some mixtures the results could be quite positive because the herbal remedies may complement the other medications being taken. The worse case scenario that can result from combining herbal remedies and prescription medicines deserves some attention, though, since it can have serious toxic results that could present severe health risks for clients. For example, drinking the juice of grapefruits seems safe enough, but when a client is undergoing dialysis, drinking grapefruit juice can inhibit or prevent the absorption of medications used in dialysis Goeddeke-Merickel, 1998 a,b,c,). When dealing with any type of medication at all (herbal and natural included), it is essential to remember that any remedy which is powerful enough to affect the body beneficially is also powerful enough to create unwanted side effects (Dziegielewski & Leon, 2001).

Since herbal medications have received an upsurge of interest in the 1990s, they have clearly gotten the attention of the FDA. It may not be long until herbal preparations, similar to their prescription counterparts, are regulated to ensure efficiency and effectiveness for the claims they purport to address. In the United States the importance of the need for more controlled studies has been recognized and will continue to increase (Bender, 1996).

Today, the herbal industry is thriving, with few, if any, requirements placed on them by the government. Generally, most of the herbal products are exempt from federal regulation because they are not considered medications. Rather, to get around regulation, many of the herbal remedies are referred to as dietary supplements. Unfortunately, however, this lack of government regulation can lead to confusion and open misinformation. Further, since the DSHEA makes no requirements for product standardization of the active products it utilizes, does nothing in terms of bioavialability and efficacy, and does not require any testing in terms of combination issues with OTC and prescription drugs, it is incumbent upon the user to exercise caution. Additionally, this lack of regulation can lead to lower quality of the product that is supplied. It has been documented in several case studies (LaPuma, 1999) and reported by the FDA that some of the imported herbal products in the past have been known to have by-products, trace metals or chemicals in them that could indeed prove harmful to those that ingest them. Ingesting lead, for example, could clearly lead to lead poisoning or toxic reactions that might not be easily traced to the herbal product that introduced it. In monitoring this at minimal levels, the FDA has already made harmful links to products such as ephedra, comfrey, chaparral, licorice, pennyroyal, sassafras, and senna.

MEDICINAL HERBS

For the most part *herbal medicines* are derived from plants, leaves, roots, flowers, and fungi by alcoholic extraction or decoction and are used to prevent and treat diseases (Linde et al., 2001). To date, there are well over 600 medicinal herbs available to the consumer (*PDR for Herbal Medications,* 2000) without much regulated and standardized testing to clearly establish their effectiveness (see Table 19.2). In the United States the Dietary Supplement Health and Education Act (DSHEA) of 1994 allows herbs to be sold legally so long as they make no claims for disease treatment on the label (Kroll, 1997). For example, a very popular product used primarily for the treatment of mild depression known as St. John's wort states in ambiguous terms that it is used "for mental well-being" or "to improve mental health.

Probably the single largest concern for social workers who see clients taking these preparations is the lack of formal regulation. Currently, many of the herbal products are limited in the testing that has been performed and therefore cannot clearly link safety to efficacy. To avoid legal penalties it is common for these herbal and natural product manufacturers to use vague terminology such as to "support body function" or "safely balances emotions." The lack of regulation can also lead to limited standardization in terms of harvesting, processing, and packaging. Having active ingredients is essential and ensuring that they stay active is just as important. Without regulation there is no need to guarantee that a product is not old or that the packaging is sufficient enough to keep the active ingredients active (Kroll, 1997). This could be a particular problem if substances are brought in bulk or remain in stores for an extended period of time. Additionally, this lack of regulation can lead to contamination of the product that is supplied. It has been documented in several case studies (LaPuma, 1999) and reported by the FDA that some of the imported herbal products in the past have been known to have by-products in them or trace metals that could prove harmful to those that ingest them. Ingesting lead, for example, could clearly lead to lead poisoning or toxic reactions that might not be easily traced to the herbal product that introduced it. Prices also may vary dramatically and are no indication of quality. A particular challenge is determining which herbal remedies may be efficacious. A meta-analysis of systematic reviews of clinical trials of

2 Popular Herbal Medicines

	Clinical applications	Contraindications	Side effects	Herb–drug interactions
sh	PMS, menopause, arthritis, high blood pressure	First two trimesters of pregnancy	G.I. symptoms	May intensify side effects of syntheti estrogen
	Peptic ulcers, skin irritations, colic, insomnia, nausea	Ragweed allergy	Highly concentrated tea may be emetic	May interfere with anticoagulant thera
	Viral and bacterial illness, immune system booster	Autoimmune diseases, immunosuppressant therapy	G.I. symptoms	Do not use with immunosuppressai therapy
il	Bruises, asthma, chronic fatigue syndrome, congestive heart failure, metabolic disorders, PMS, menopause	May trigger latent temporal lobe epilepsy, particularly in people with schizophrenia	G.I. symptoms	Increases risk of temporal lobe epil when used with epileptogenic drug schizophrenia
	Migraine, allergies, rheumatic diseases	Pregnancy, lactation, children under 2 years	Nervousness G.I. symptoms	May interact with thrombotic drugs s as aspirin and war

Arteriosclerosis, respiratory infections, mouth and pharynx inflammation, cancer preventative	Slow blood clotting pregnancy, lactation	G.I. symptoms, burn-like skin lesions with topical preparation	Increases action o anticoagulant drug
Colic, menstrual symptoms, motion sickness, reduces some chemotherapy side effects	Gallstones, pregnancy	Mild heartburn	In doses exceeding dietary intake, ma interfere with car anticoagulant, or a diabetic medicatio
Allergies, dementia, Alzheimer's, cochlear deafness, macular degeneration, depression, stroke	Ingesting the seed can cause severe adverse effects; the fruit should not be handled or ingested	G.I. symptoms	May interfere with MAO inhibitors
Ulcers, edema, cancer, infertility, fatigue, viral illness, red blood cell depletion	Acute illness, cardiovascular disease, diabetes or blood pressure disorders, pregnancy	None known	May increase the effect of phenelzine (Nar other antipsychoti blood pressure, ant diabetic, or steroid medications

Clinical applications	Contraindications	Side effects	Herb-drug interactions
Gastric inflammation, colds, flu, externally for lacerations, skin eruptions	Pregnancy, hypertension; long-term use of large amounts may lower B vitamin absorption and utilization	Large doses may cause convulsions, long-term use may cause elevated white blood cell counts	None known
Stomach ailments, chemotherapy, dental caries prevention, cancer, obesity	Sensitive stomach, cardiovascular complications, kidney disorders, overactive thyroid	Large amounts can cause restlessness, tremor, heightened reflex excitability	Tea beverages may delay the reabsorp of alkaline medica
Coronary artery disease, congestive heart failure, essential hypertension	Pregnancy, lactation; those using drug therapies for blood pressure disorders and other heart failure medications should be closely monitored	G.I. symptoms, headache	May increase effec of digitalis

2 *(continued)*

Anxiety, stress, insomnia	Pregnancy, lactation, may cause liver damage	Skin rash, G.I. symptoms	May potentiate eff of barbiturates or alcohol
e	Chronic hepatitis B, C, D, E, liver disorders, gallstones, skin problems	Alcohol-based extracts are not recommended for severe liver problems	Mild laxative effect	None known
-)	Depression, osteoarthritis, alcoholic liver disease	None known	May trigger manic episode	May potentiate antidepressant medication
	Stage I and II benign prostatic hypertrophy, female androgen excess disorders	Pregnancy, lactation	G.I. symptoms, headache	May interfere with hormonal therapie
	Mild depression, anxiety, anorexia; topically, promotes wound healing	Pregnancy, lactation	G.I. symptoms, photosensitivity	May interact with L-dopa, MAO inhib

.2 *(continued)*

Clinical applications	Contraindications	Side effects	Herb-drug interactions
Sleep disorders, anxiety, migraine	None known	May have paradoxical effect	May interfere with anxiolytics, hypno analgesics, and anti-epileptics; ma enhance effects of and other herbs

obtained from Integrative Medicine Communications (2000) and Linde et al. (2001).

herbal medicines undertaken by Linde et al. (2001) showed that many herbs, including ginkgo, garlic, St. John's wort, echinacea, and saw palmetto were promising, but that methodological problems, including lack of standardization of the tested compounds, compromised the findings. They report that there is no way to know whether "different products, extracts, or even different lots of the same extract are comparable and equivalent" (Linde, 2001, p. 4). A recent study (Hypericum Depression Trial Study Group, 2002) showed that St. John's wort was no more effective than placebo for patients with major depression of moderate severity. Interestingly enough, this study also compared Zoloft to placebo and found little difference.

CHAPTER SUMMARY AND FUTURE DIRECTIONS

The health care social worker needs to be aware of this growing movement to integrate wellness concepts through alternative and conventional care. This integration can serve to help bridge the gap between the two very different approaches to health care. In the meantime, however, it is extremely important that people share with their physicians what they are taking. A study of breast cancer patients by Adler & Fosket (1999) showed that only 54% of the patients who were using complementary therapy informed their physician. Combining herbs and other supplements and prescription drugs can have unpleasant and even hazardous consequences. If physicians and other health care providers are not informed about what their clients are taking, the professional will be unable to use his or her professional expertise to help the clients determine if this is the best remedy for them. The health care social worker can encourage clients to inform health care providers of all natural remedies they are taking so that the health care professional can also become familiar with the effects these natural remedies are having on the clients that they serve. This requires a type of *educative counseling* that helps clients learn the benefits and risks of such treatments. It is essential that the social worker perform within the bounds of the National Association of Social Workers' Code of Ethics (NASW, 1996) dealing with competence.

In particular, health care social workers should ensure that the host agency will support the client's exploration of complementary treatments. Social workers should encourage clients to make informed decisions in terms of what is best for them. Clients do not have to accept and automatically commit to a traditional approach to medical care (Seligson, 1998), and, with the current trends toward wellness, if clients are forced to accept these traditional approaches they most likely will refuse. All health care social workers need to realize that this trend exists and to assist clients by encouraging them to seek the information that allows them to make informed choices. If a health care provider seems resistant to a method of intervention, encourage clients to ask them why they feel as they do. By understanding that there may be a reluctance to discuss the use of natural remedies with the mainstream medical community, social workers can help clients to prepare for such discussions. Effective, efficient, and comprehensive helping relationships require that social workers recognize other forms of treatments that could potentially be more useful for our clients. Complementary forms of intervention can also serve as a preventative measure, helping to ensure client well-being. Health care social workers need to be aware of these practices and remedies that can be incorporated into conventional therapies. Keeping abreast of all forms of treatment is important to provide the best possible care for our clients, while discouraging the use of either medications and herbal preparations as being the only form of intervention when a complementary approach may prove to be just as or even more effective.

REFERENCES

Adler, S. R., & Fosket, J. R. (1999). Disclosing complementary and alternative medicine use in the medical encounter: A qualitative study in women with breast cancer. *Journal of Family Practice, 48,* 453–458.

Bender, K. J. (October, 1996). St. John's Wort evaluated as a herbal antidepressant. *Psychiatric Times.* Retrieved July 6, 1999 from http://www.mhsource.com/edu/psytimes/p964058.html

Borken, J., Neher, J. O., & Anson, O., Smoker, B. (1994). Referrals for alternative therapies. *Journal of Family Practice, 39,* 545–550.

Dziegielewski, S. F. (2002). *DSM-IV-TR™ in action.* New York: Wiley.

Dziegielewski, S. F., & Leon, A. M. (2001). *Psychopharmacology and social work practice.* New York: Springer Publishing Co.

Eisenberg, D. M., David, R. B., Ettner, S. L., Appel, S., Wilkey, S., Van Rompay, M., & Kessler, R. C. (1998). Trends in alternative medicine use in the United States, 1990–2001: Results of a follow-up national survey. *Journal of the American Medical Association, 280,* 1569–1575.

Goeddeke-Merickel, C. M. (1998a). Alternative medicine and dialysis patients; Part II. *For Patients Only,* May/June, 19–20.

Goeddeke-Merickel, C. M. (1998b). Alternative medicine and dialysis patients: Part III. *For Patients Only,* July/August, 22, 30.

Goeddeke-Merickel, C. M. (1998c). Herbal medicine: Some do's and don'ts for dialysis patients. *For Patients Only,* March/April, 22–23.

Hypericum Depression Trial Study Group (2002). Effect of hypericum perforatum (St.John's Wort) in major depressive disorder: A randomized, controlled trial. *Journal of the American Medical Association, 287,* 1807–1814.

Integrative Medicine Communications. (1998). *An integrative medicine primer.* Newton, MA: Author.

Integrative Medicine Communications. (2000). *A physician's reference to botanical medicines.* Newton, MA: Author.

Kroll, D. J. (1997, September). St John's Wort: An example of the problems with herbal medicine regulation in the United States. *Medical Sciences Bulletin, 240,* 1–5.

LaPuma, J. (1999). Danger of Asian patent medicines. In *Alternative medicine alert: A clinician's guide to alternative therapies, 2,* 6, 71.

Linde, K., Reit, G., Hondras, M., Vickers, A., Saller, R., & Milchart, D. (2001). Systematic reviews of complementary therapies—an annotated bibliography. Part 2: Herbal medicine. *BMC Complement Alternative Medicine, 1*(5). Retrieved 2/10/02 from http://www.biomedcentral.com/1472-6882/1/5.

McCall, M. D. (1998). Alternative medicine: Is it for you? *Orlando Sentinel,* May 12, 1998, Orlando, FL.

National Association of Social Workers (NASW). (1996). *Code of ethics.* Washington, DC: Author.

National Institutes of Health. (2000). Hepatitis C: Treatment alternatives. Retrieved 11/7/02 from http://nccam.nih.gov/health/hepatitisc/index.htm.

PDR for Herbal Medications (2nd ed.). (2000). Montrale, NJ: Medical Economics.

Seligson, S.V. (1998). Melding medicines. *Health,* May/June 1998, 64–70.

Stehlin, I. B. (1995). An FDA guide to choosing medical treatments. *FDA Consumer, 29,* 10–14.

Wetzel, M. S., Eisenberg, D. M., & Kaptchuk, T. J. (1998). Courses involving complementary and alternative medicine at U.S. medical schools. *Journal of the American Medical Association, 280,* 784–787.

GLOSSARY

Alternative medicine. This is often described as any medical practice or intervention that is utilized instead of conventional treatment, lacks sufficient documentation in regard to its safety and effectiveness against certain diseases and conditions, is generally not taught in United States medical schools, and is generally not reimbursable by health insurance providers.

Complementary or integrative medicine. In this approach to medical care a combination approach is utilized whereas clients generally receive traditional approaches to therapy such as prescription medications augmented or supplemented by alternative approaches.

Educative counseling: This is a loosely defined approach to practice that focuses on helping the client to become an "educated consumer" and through this information to better be able to address his or her own needs.

Herbal medicines: These are medicines or preparations used for medicinal purposes that are derived from plants, leaves, roots, flowers, and fungi.

Traditional mainstream medicine: This type of medical practice is most reflective of the application of the general medical model and is generally referred to as mainstream American medical practice.

QUESTIONS FOR FURTHER STUDY

1. What do you see as the role of the health care social worker in this area?
2. What can health care social workers do to assist clients that utilize these types of treatments?

PART V

Conclusion

This page intentionally left blank

CHAPTER 20

Health Care Social Work: A Product of Political and Cultural Times

---

MANAGED BEHAVIORAL HEALTH CARE AND SOCIAL WORK PRACTICE

Managed behavioral health care, first introduced in the 1990s, presents a type of health care delivery never before experienced. Social workers must now show that the time-limited brief services they provide are necessary and effective. If they do not, they may be replaced with other professionals that perform similar functions that do. Today, the managed care has a broad-based emphasis; however, it is important to note that effectiveness goes beyond just helping the client (Dziegielewski & Holliman, 2001). Effectiveness must also involve validation that the greatest concrete and identifiable therapeutic gain was achieved, in the quickest amount of time, and with the least amount of financial and professional support. This means that not only must the interventions that social workers provide be socially acknowledged as necessary, but they must also be therapeutically effective (Franklin, 2002), specific and individualized to guide all further intervention efforts (Maruish, 2002). In addition, these services must be professionally competitive with other disciplines that claim similar treatment strategies and techniques. This has led to the rebirth of all efforts for client betterment to be evidence-based in order to be acknowledged as effective (Donald, 2002). This makes outcomes-based behavioral health care an approach in which disease management and health care risk prevention follow a very specific format (see Figure 20.1).

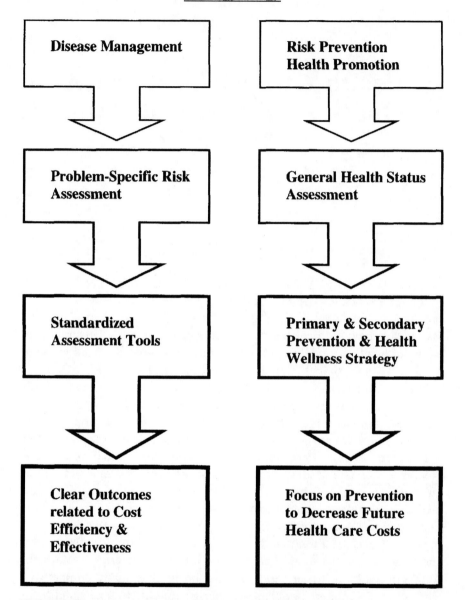

FIGURE 20.1 Outcomes-based behavioral health care.

Evolution of Health Care Social Work

The practice of health care social work has changed dramatically over the years. Traditionally the health care social worker served the poor and the disfranchised. Clarity of a definition of what the health care social worker does has been further complicated by basic changes in the health care environment that include scope of practice, the roles served, and the expectations within the client-practitioner relationship. Furthermore, this definition, along with the focus of care, is shifting. There is less emphasis on inpatient acute, tertiary, and specialty/subspecialty care and more emphasis on ambulatory and community-based care, the role of the physician's office, and group practice and health maintenance organizations (Rock, 2002). These changes require social workers to constantly battle "quality-of-care" versus "cost-containment" measures for clients, all the while securing a firm place as a professional provider in the health care environment.

Today, the health care social worker can be viewed as the professional "bridge" that links the client, the multidisciplinary or interdisciplinary team, and the environment. For future marketability and competition, it is believed that social workers need to move beyond the traditional definition and role of the health care social worker (Dziegielewski, 2002). In the area of clinical practice, new or refined methods of service delivery need to be established and used. Social workers are encouraged to assume positions such as managers, owners of companies, employees, administrators, supervisors, clinical directors, and managed care case managers where they can help influence specific agency policy, services, and procedure.

Managed Care Principles and the Health Care Environment

Many events have occurred over the last 15 years that have truly transformed health care delivery and social work practice. For survival in this environment, several steps are suggested: (a) social workers need to continue to market the services they provide and link them to cost-benefit measurement; (b) social workers need to present themselves as essential team members on the health care interdisciplinary and multidisciplinary teams; (c) health care social workers should never forget the importance of anticipating the environment and the role that political and social influences can have on service delivery; and

(d) social workers need to look beyond the traditional expectations and assumptions historically noted as clinical professional practice in the health care field. New and innovative ideas and methods of service delivery are needed, from rethinking foundations issues in terms of human growth and development (Farley, Smith, Boyle, & Ronnau, 2002), to application of these concepts in an evidenced-based framework (Wodarski & Dziegielewski, 2001). New and revitalized models to guide practice are needed to compete in today's health care environment. Health care remains a changing environment that requires a resilient social work professional.

ROLES AND STANDARDS FOR HEALTH CARE PRACTICE

All social workers, whether in the role of clinical practitioner, supervisor, administrator, or community organizer, have been challenged to anticipate our current health care system and the effects this propensity will have on current and future practice. Incremental changes involve compromising and implementing service agreements that are based on the needs or wishes of various political forces. Integrated services and systems must occur under behaviorally based managed care principles that make teamwork and an awareness of corporate and administrative policies and procedures essential ingredients for success. This type of integrated care requires that adequate links be made between the corporate governance structure and the modes and/or agencies that deliver the services. Furthermore, linkages need to be made between health maintenance organizations, acute care facilities and services, long-term care services and facilities, transitional or home-based services, mental health and substance abuse services, wellness and prevention services, the standard care that may be received in the physician's office (see Figure 20.2). Coordination through referrals, discharge planning, and case management have long since been the responsibility of social work, and never before has this role been more important to ensure the continuity of care for each client served. For each health care social worker engaging in practice, the control of rising health care costs will ultimately be considered his or her responsibility.

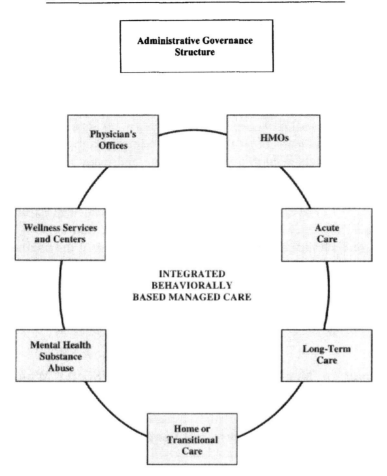

FIGURE 20.2 Administrative governance structure.

Responsibility for quality service delivery in this cost-containment climate has increased the need for greater emphasis on macro practice. This means that health care social workers must take an active role in ethical practice while advocating for social action and social change (Strom-Gottfried & Dunlap, 1999; Strom-Gottfried & Corcoran, 1998). Social workers must work actively to help society to understand its responsibility to control and regulate the health care industry. Health care social workers, no matter what setting they work in, must help to develop and present a format for approaching problems in the current system and establishing means for addressing them.

FIELDS OF HEALTH CARE SOCIAL WORK PRACTICE

Staff reductions and changes continue to happen throughout the field of health care social work. Yet, health care social workers is not the only profession being targeted for reduction; it is happening across all disciplines as a means of cost reduction. To remain competitive, health care professionals need to be flexible, open, and ready to embrace the future. However, we should never lose sight of the ethical and moral judgment that is needed to steer the profession and ourselves for the betterment of the clients we serve. Social workers need to participate in conducting research that can support the work that is being completed on a clinical as well as a research level. Most of the chapters in the special topic section of this book look at issues germane to the field through the eyes of those working in the field. These health care social workers can offer valuable insight into the problems that they confront in everyday practice and how they believe some of these problems can be overcome.

SHORTAGE OF NURSES: AN OPPORTUNITY FOR SOCIAL WORK GROWTH

Officially, after years of speculation, it has been confirmed that there is a nursing shortage. By all reports this shortage will reach crisis proportions by 2015, when the United States will experience a 20% shortage of available nurses (HSRA, 2002). In response to this pending crisis, federal and state agencies, legislatures, professional nursing organizations, the health care industry, labor organizations, and private philanthropies have all responded with analysis, recommendations, and in some cases resources (Buerhaus, Needleman, Mattke, & Stewart, 2002). This marshaling of forces has produced a myriad suggested responses. But the question remains, what does this shortage mean for the role of the nurse as case manager? This role has always traditionally been filled with social workers. Furthermore, nurses in general, report that salary earnings have decreased as well under managed care principles (Bauer, 2001a, 2001b; Buerhaus & Staiger, 1996). Meanwhile, nurses are leaving the profession in record numbers. Research from the University of Pennsylvania suggests that nursing graduates are leaving the profession within the first 4 years at increasing rates (Sochalski, 2002).

In the past, nurse managers would have responded to such a shortage in a fairly typical manner. Retention efforts would have been intensified through improved compensation packages and creative scheduling options until aggressive recruitment efforts by educational programs could increase the supply of available nurses (Tanner & Bellack, 2001). However, by all accounts, for nursing professional this is a shortage unlike any other (Kimball, O'Neil & Health Workforce Solutions, 2002). Managed care has contributed to a significant increase in the acuity of hospitalized patients (Buerhaus et al., 2002), and the aging population is causing an increased demand for patient care services (Quinless & Elliot, 2000).

This shortage of nurses, who have traditionally been considered essential personnel in the health care field, needs to be openly acknowledged by social workers, since many times in today's health care environment nurses continue to assume many of the responsibilities that were traditionally in the domain of social work. For example, this includes services in the area of case management and discharge planning. As discussed in this text, many nurses continue to assume the roles of the social worker and complete similar if not identical duties at a much higher rate of pay. Therefore, this nursing shortage can be of pivotal importance to health care social workers and serve as a means to take back or increase their role in activities that were previously their domain. This, however, can only be accomplished by (1) establishing through evidenced-based practice the importance of what they do in helping the client; (2) responding to social, political, and clinical demands to continue to identify outcomes-based service criteria; and (3) clearly identifying the critical importance of the service they provide in terms of promoting overall health and wellness. Special importance needs to be placed on the increasing numbers of readmissions and recidivism and how social work services, often neglected in today's system, can enhance service provision and decrease recidivism.

CONCEPTS ESSENTIAL TO HEALTH CARE PRACTICE

In social work health care practice, the behaviorally based biopsychosocial approach continues to be the model of choice to integrate the biomedical and the psychosocial approaches to practice. In this approach, social workers are considered leaders regarding their understanding and interpreting of the "behavioral," "psycho," and "social" factors in a client's condition. Teamwork and collaborative efforts are now required in health care service delivery (Abramson, 2002).

Within the interdisciplinary team, it is not uncommon for blurred definitions and diffuse boundary distinctions to occur between professionals. These problems can result in difficulty defining tasks and obligations. Furthermore, these blurred and overlapping functions among professionals can complicate the tasks that need to be performed. After all, this tightly knit group of professionals is expected to always act as a team (Dziegielewski, 1996). To social work professionals, this situation can be viewed as a way to expand their role and the services they provide as part of the team. To exemplify this concept, the social worker is encouraged to become a leading professional in the quality review process. It is also recommended that health care social workers highlight the issues related to informed consent, which requires that health care providers reveal to clients the nature of the medical treatments to be given and the related benefits, risks, and alternatives (Strom-Gottfried & Corcoran, 1998). Health care social workers can make excellent team leaders and can guide this process while ensuring that quality care services are provided.

PRACTICE STRATEGY

Today, the concept of behaviorally based managed care services is creating a practice revolution in which the provision of social work services can remain an integral component. Interest in time-limited brief interventions has greatly increased and will most probably continue to increase over the years (Bolter, Levenson, & Alverez, 1990; Dziegielewski, 1997a). This is especially true in the area of home-based programs or community support services (Hughes, 1999). Long-term care continues to be an area where more attention and health care reform are needed (Wiener, Estes, Goldenson, & Goldberg, 2001). This makes preparing for our elderly population a critical task (Sorenson & Pinquart, 2001), as well as assisting those caregivers that will make up the sandwich generation (Spillman & Pezzin, 2000).

Today, practice strategy in the health care environment is often intermittent; each session stands alone and is conducted as if it is the

only client contact that will occur (Dziegielewski, 2002). Health maintenance organizations and employee assistance programs generally favor
highly structured brief forms of intervention, and as they continue to
grow, so will usage of the time-limited models they support (Wells,
1994). It is suggested that social workers continue to learn and use
education in achieving behavioral outcomes. Use of a health and wellness strategy, as described in this book, is steadily becoming a practice
reality. The goal of insight-oriented intervention and cure-focused therapy seems to have have taken second place to the acquisition of outcomes-based behavioral change, which is considered more realistic and
practical. Health care social workers (similar to physicians) generally
do not cure the problems clients suffer from—nor are they expected to.
What is expected, however, is that they help clients realize and use
their own strengths to diminish or alleviate symptoms or states of
being that cause discomfort. Emphasis on evidenced-based practice
and outcomes-based behavioral changes are not only expected but are
required for "state-of-the-art" practice.

The need for time-limited practice strategies has been clearly established. Models and methods of service delivery, such as those presented in this book, only begin to open the door to what is left to come.
Health care social workers are being forced by an environment of
managed health care policies, fee for reimbursement, capitation, and
so on to continue to demonstrate effectiveness and cost containment
in the intervention methods they employ (Gibelman, 2002). It is important for social workers to realize, whether they like it or not, that
professional survival dictates change. Managed health care has introduced a new practice revolution that social workers need to embrace
with confidence (Dziegielewski, 2002).

In general, no matter what setting the health care social worker
engages, he or she needs to embrace a more eclectic approach to
practice—in which allegiance to one particular model or method is
discouraged (Colby & Dziegielewski, 2001). In selecting a clinical practice method for today's managed health care environment, the following considerations are suggested: (a) it should be a time-limited
intervention approach; (b) it should always stress mutually negotiated
goals and objectives; (c) all practice should include efforts to make it
evidenced-based and objectives should be behaviorally linked, outcomes
based, and measurable; (d) there should always be an emphasis on
client strengths and self-development; (e) the focus of intervention

should always be concrete, realistic, and obtainable; and (f) it should be changeable, based on the needs and desires of the client being served, not the preference of the social worker. By adapting this flexible perspective, the social worker will be better able to prepare to deliver the services expected while maintaining the highest degree of marketability possible.

COST–BENEFIT ANALYSIS

The growth of the over-age-65 population, the rising cost of health care, and numerous other societal events have stimulated attention and subsequently rocked the delicate balance between cost containment and quality of care. In the resultant health care practice environment, cost reduction is considered the primary maintenance issue. This means that health care social workers must now recognize at each stage of the intervention encounter the resultant bottom-line dollar expenditures that are generated or saved by the service provided. Like other professionals in the health care field, to compete successfully social workers must also show that the services they provide can be related to initial dollar savings. An example of this can be viewed in discharge planning from the hospital to home health care services. The social worker must first compute the rate of a general inpatient stay in the medical facility. Generally, most social workers can simply call hospital admissions and ask them for the daily rate for room and board. If a social worker is able to facilitate a discharge home in a timely manner, you can simply compute this amount in relation to the cost of an additional in-house stay. Discharge planning services are important cost-saving strategies for health care facilities. That is why they often receive so much attention. Clients who feel as though they are experiencing a lack of support can also cause numerous readmissions, thus, contributing to high recidivism rates. Direct dollar savings have always been difficult for social workers to calculate because formerly little emphasis was placed on actual prevention of costs. Times, however, are changing. Social workers need to realize the importance of cost-benefit ratios and attach this measurement to every service they provide. Recording and justifying of these costs can help social workers to establish the importance of their service from a dollar-driven administrative perspective.

INCLUSION OF PRIVATE PRACTICE

As changes occur in the modes of health care service delivery, they are also occurring in the field of social work. Today, serving in an independent private practice or within a physician's office remains one of the fastest-growing sectors of social work practice. As social workers become eligible to receive third-party payments for the provision of intervention, the area of private practice becomes more inviting (Dziegielewski, 2002; Schram & Mandell, 1997). Private practice can serve to develop an expanded area of marketability for health care social workers, particularly those with an interest in providing direct therapeutic intervention to clients.

In the field of social work, the disagreement regarding an increasing market for private-practice services continues to rage. Many professionals disagree with the movement toward private practice because they believe it is abandoning social work's original call to serve the poor and underserved. It is further believed that the more social workers enter into private practice, the more spaces will be left open in public-sector jobs that were previously filled by social workers. Because of this withdrawal of professional social workers, these positions are now being filled by other related disciplines (Schram & Mandell, 1997). However, in the area of health care social work, this argument is not nearly as relevant. Health care social workers have generally been employed in many areas of social work and continue to serve in hospital social work, AIDS counseling and education, public health, hospice/counseling and management, home health care, case management, discharge planning, maternal and child health, physical rehabilitation, chemical dependency, and disease prevention and health promotion; employers of health care social workers continue to be health maintenance organizations, nursing homes, hospitals, clinics, hospice programs, and group homes (NASW, 1993). For future growth, particularly in those services affiliated with physicians' offices or HMOs, entering into private-practice arrangements can assist health care social workers to expand their practice arena and, therefore, their marketability. This is particularly true in the area of behavioral health and wellness counseling.

Today, to engage in private practice successfully, the health care social worker must compete for preferred provider status, a position that was virtually unheard of 10 years ago. Membership as providers in these managed care agencies is essential for health care social workers because it will allow the social worker to accept clients from a particular managed care network and get reimbursed for the services he or she provides. Davis and Meier (2001) warn that although many of the practices of managed care organizations will continue, these practices are not always in the best interest of the client. All social workers need to be aware and adapt to this type of thinking which is business or corporate focused. Social workers interested in private practice or contracting for services must be aware of the requirements and subsequent limitations that to-day's PPO, HMO, EAP, and managed care may invoke. For health care social workers who wish to engage in private practice, managed care partnerships will remain a critical necessity. Unfortunately, there is no way around them unless the health care social worker is capable of gen-erating only self-pay clients or limits practice to consultation. For more information on managing and creating private practice partnerships with managed care agencies, the reader is referred to Davis & Meier's (2001) book, *The Elements of Managed Care: A Guide for Helping Professionals.*

CLINICAL LICENSURE

Generally, this area of expansion in medical social work will be offered at the master's of social work (MSW) level, since a graduate level of education is usually required for reimbursement. To date, many states now require that social workers be licensed to qualify as providers. The purpose of licensure is to ensure that clients can receive compe-tent, ethical, and moral services. Licensure ensures that social work practitioners have a minimum level of competence necessary to per-form professional functions. Health care social workers can benefit from licensure, as can all social workers. Whether an individual social worker is practicing under the auspices of an agency or not, more emphasis will be placed on licensure to receive third-party reimburse-ment. Licensure can help health care social workers to maintain cur-rent levels of marketability as well as anticipate of future trends. Thus for health care social workers, licensure at the bachelor's of social work (BSW) or the MSW level is highly encouraged.

AWARENESS OF MEDICATIONS AND ALTERNATIVE TREATMENTS

In this era of managed care, the field of social work, like many other disciplines, has been forced to reexamine its intervention methods and modalities. To compete successfully, or more simply stated, to survive in the health care arena, it has become clear that social workers must provide effective and accountable practice (Thyer, 2002). This type of practice must incorporate health care concepts familiar to social work, particularly for those who work in mental health. The techniques medical social workers are expected to know encompass knowledge regarding diagnostic criteria as well as usage and side effect profiles of the medications so often used in treatment (Dziegielewski, 2002; Dziegielewski & Leon, 2001). Social workers are often called on to give advice for medical treatment or to recommend what medications would best serve as adjunct to the current intervention being provided. And, with the current shortage of nurses, this trend is expected to increase.

Therefore, social workers need to be familiar with current diagnostic guidelines and the medications that are often used. Unfortunately, social work professionals have not readily addressed the clinical application of diagnostic psychotherapeutic treatments. This has resulted in most of the current resources available being written by non–social work professionals. These other disciplines often do not relate this information directly back to a social work treatment regimen. Social workers are therefore expected to incorporate the fields' own practice base and ethical and moral issues into the practice guidelines suggested. Since it is beyond the scope of this text to cover all the basics that are needed in terms of medication knowledge and application, the health care social worker is referred to Dziegielewski and Leon's (2001) text *Psychopharmacology and Social Work Practice.*

Although all accredited social work programs generally offer at least one graduate-level course in psychopathology or clinical diagnosis, few offer separate courses in understanding medication or herbal preparation usage. Considering that most social workers did not receive training in medications and herbal preparations in their social work program, information in this area is essential for those in this area of clinical practice.

Knowledge of alternative treatments is also essential. Health care social workers must consider the various types of alternative treatments in which clients are engaging. Having a knowledge of medications, herbal remedies, and alternative practices is a practice reality for today's health care social worker (Dziegielewski & Leon, 2001). Whether the more radical stance is taken actually to acquire enough education to have limited prescription privileges as suggested by Dziegielewski (1997a), or to take the more conservative role suggested by Bentley (1997), it is clear that social workers must have, at a minimum, a general knowledge of medications and their usage. Health care social workers must be familiar with side effect profiles, dosage routines, and so on to assist clients to obtain and maintain the most therapeutically productive treatment possible. They must be able to recognize potential problem areas to refer the client for adequate or revised treatment. Social workers must stay updated with new trends in the field and how these new medications can affect the client and the counseling relationship.

LINKING EVIDENCE-BASED PRACTICE WITH INTERVENTION EFFORTS

For the social worker in health care practice, the process of recording needs to go beyond the traditional bonds of documentation. Documentation to support and justify evidence-based practice is pivotal. Mixing research and practice yields the type of record keeping employed in the medical setting. This mix must consider the need to achieve both quality of service and cost-effectiveness. Although this union may, at times, be an awkward one, the combination is essential to ensure delivery of efficient and effective services.

In health care, a connection between research and practice is critical, and questions to guide the scientific inquiry process include the following: What does the social worker want and need to know about the problem? For example, if there is interest in studying discharge patterns of elderly, is there already a significant amount of information in this area? Is the health care social worker the one that needs to conduct the research? Are other disciplines more suited to completing the study, and if so, what role can the social worker play in this process? For example, if we want to monitor our clients and the effects of medications in the home, we may need some assistance from the interdisciplinary team to accomplish this.

A second important factor is what to do once the information has been gathered—how to determine how it can be used. For example, can the information gathered be used to facilitate the implementation of teen education groups, AIDS prevention programs, and health and wellness education? Unfortunately, identifying the problem may constitute only a small step toward the solution of the problem—particularly when interest in addressing the problem is not supported in the immediate environment. Many times, the administration may not see the problem as a crucial one to be studied. Administrative nonsupport can leave the health care social worker unaware of the problems and obstacles a nonsupportive environment can create. Administrative interest and investment can be essential in creating an open climate.

The health care social worker must assess if there are any logistical obstacles present. If so, would measurement be an insurmountable problem? Can the necessary data be obtained? Once the information is gathered, where will the social worker put it? Many times, case records are interdisciplinary in nature and there simply is no room for this type of information. These are just some of the questions that health care social workers must face when they engage in evidenced-based practice. Today the pressure to act on this evidenced-based means of practice has never been more intense. There is one addition, however, that must be added to this discussion—and that is the concept of cost-effectiveness. In today's health care environment, it is openly proclaimed that there must be a balance between quality of care and cost-effectiveness; however, few professionals would argue which one appears to carry the most weight (Dziegielewski, 1996, 1997b, 2002). In addition to proving that social work practice is efficient and effective, it also must be established that practice can also be completed with as little effort and expense as possible.

The health care environment is changing rapidly, and with the tremendous increase in allied health professionals (Flood, Shortell, & Scott, 1994), it is believed that "only the strongest will survive." Not only is this survival important for the profession of health care social work, but it is also essential for the clients who are served. Each day and with every task the health care social worker completes, the client's lifestyle and expectations are influenced. Health care social workers help to make their clients better able to relate to their environments. To continue to address the client-in-environment match in the health care setting adequately, there is no choice—practice and research must be one. When practice and research combine, evidenced-based practice results (Wodarski & Dziegielewski, 2001). It is this type of evidenced-based practice that will be best suited to stand the rigor and instability of the managed care practice environment.

This book is written to provide a basis for the integration of basic clinical evidence-based practice strategy with direct linkage to cost containment in the health care practice area. To complete this, changes in both research and practice strategy will be required (Rosen & Proctor, 2002). Research suggestions and compromises are suggested to address scientific vigor and facilitate practicality. In clinical practice, social work practitioners are urged to learn methods of practice that stress measurement and cost containment and incorporate these methods into the delivery of services. The strengths and limitations of these types of methods for service delivery are not well known, and the future task of the health care social worker is to explore this problem further.

In evidenced-based practice, health care social workers must mix practice, research, and cost-containment strategy and document all these accordingly. Intervention plans must show and report success in these areas to justify third-party reimbursement, capitation, and fee for service; yet, this must be done in a limited and often restricted setting. Health care social workers must be able to understand the integration of evidenced-based methods and not fear suggesting new and improved methods of documentation that make justification reflective of the professionally therapeutic and economic reality that has been created through the service implemented. If health care social workers engage in an evidenced-based practice strategy that follows the scientific method, this can also help ensure that clients are not harmed by practice fallacies that do not involve sound critical thinking (Gibbs, 2002).

DEALING WITH STRESS AND PREVENTING BURNOUT

Any book in the area of health care social work would be deficient if it did not recognize the high-stress environment in which most social workers function, as well as the importance of dealing with stress and recognizing potential signs and symptoms that could relate to burnout. To help anticipate this problem, Roembke (1995), Heaman (1995), and Godbey and Courage (1994) stress that seminars and training on stress management and prevention of burnout need to be considered. It is believed that participation in these seminars can be effective in increasing understanding of stress and strategies for dealing with stress, thereby allowing professionals to better cope with stressful situations (Deckro et al., 2002).

Health care social workers need to (1) be able to identify stressful situations; and (2) have an awareness of how to develop and implement strategies to reduce stress. According to Roembke (1995), simply learning about stress and how to identify it can be considered a preventative measure. Furthermore, Godbey and Courage (1994) encouraged applying psychoeducation regarding stress to personal reaction patterns. Therefore, teaching strategies to reduce stress and prevent burnout have also been an integral part of Roembke's (1995), Heaman's (1995), and Godbey and Courage's (1994) studies. Determining which strategies and exactly how they are best taught provides fertile ground for future research.

The type of work that health care social workers perform is considered very stressful because of the nature of the problems they deal with (Pottage & Huxley, 1996). Therefore, training in stress management and prevention of burnout are critical to help better prepare the social work professional (Resnick & Dziegielewski, 1996). Since these social workers will face continued stress throughout their professional careers and these levels of stress will most probably continue in their professional work settings, receiving preventative training on how to handle stress and prevent burnout is essential. Since burnout is prevalent in the helping professions, especially among new professionals, training of this nature can help in the transition between academic and professional life (Roembke, 1995). Training health care social workers and other professionals in the health field on how to better cope with stress and burnout and how to apply this information in their academic and professional lives is without a doubt an important area for further exploration.

FUTURE TRENDS: EXPANDING THE ROLE OF THE HEALTH CARE SOCIAL WORKER

In this book, the basic concepts related to the delivery of social work services in the health care arena have been presented. Health care social work has been influenced greatly by the principles of behaviorally based managed care. This development has changed the role of health care professionals, thus requiring social workers also to question the traditional bounds of service and to change the services they provide to prove that what they do is necessary, effective, and cost-containing. In today's health care environment, effectiveness must go beyond just helping the client. Effectiveness must also involve validation that the greatest concrete and identifiable therapeutic gain was achieved with the least amount of financial and professional support

(Donald, 2002). This means that not only must the intervention that social workers provide be therapeutically effective—it must show cost benefits as well. Health care social workers need to portray themselves as powerful contenders who are professionally competitive with other disciplines that claim similar intervention strategies and techniques. The battle in the health care arena of "more with less" continues to rage. Health care social workers continue to have one strong weapon to bring to the table that should not be underestimated in today's climate of fiscal restraint. Throughout history, social workers have provided similar interventions for less money. In social work, the NASW Code of Ethics clearly advises social workers to provide reasonable fees and base service charges on an ability to pay. This makes the fees social work professionals charge competitive when compared with those of psychiatrists, psychologists, family therapists, psychiatric nurses, and mental health counselors, who profess they can provide similar services. This cost-containment factor can provide enticement to managed care agencies to contract with social workers instead of other professionals to provide services of a health and wellness nature. In this era of managed health care, this strength should not be underestimated, and with the right marketing, it can help social workers gain additional ground, adding to their employment desirability in this era of managed care.

In general, social workers need to understand the philosophy of the current health care environment; based on this philosophy, they must be willing and able to use evidenced-based social work practice strategy with an emphasis on cost containment and outcomes measures to assist individuals, groups, and families (Frager, 2000; Rudolph, 2000).

In closing, it is important to remember that the cultural and political environment in which health care delivery finds itself today is changing (Meenaghan, 2001); however, it is not necessarily the downfall of clinical health care social work practice as we have known it. Although crisis can be intimidating, it is also a catalyst to change. Changes that could never have been made in the previous system may now become possible. Health care social workers need to acknowledge and accept this challenge swiftly and eagerly. New frontiers that can increase marketability need to be explored and pursued. Challenge, opportunity, and subsequent risk remain part of the health care social worker's future. Today, this era of managed health care is creating a whole new practice revolution for which the provision of social work services must remain an integral component. As health care social workers struggle for survival, they are not alone. The other professional specialties are scared of these practice changes, too.

The traditional view of health care social work, with its perspective of "treating the total person" and "the person-environment stance," fits beautifully into the current demand for holistic practice intervention that focuses on wellness and prevention. The task for health care social workers remains clear.

The revolution in health care delivery is well under way. Now social workers must decide whether we want to take an active part in this fight or whether we just want to sit at the "gate" and make sure the other medical specialties get through. If we decide that the role of the health care social worker is essential to the delivery of competent, effective, and efficient health care services, we will have to fight for it. By engaging in this fight, I believe we will benefit our clients and ourselves as a profession. If we decide not to advocate for ourselves and assume a position of hesitance and apathy for too long, the importance and strength of the social worker as a crucial member of the health care delivery team will go untold, and the other more assertive professions will be free to claim what once was our "turf."

REFERENCES

Abramson, J. S. (2002).Interdisciplinary team practice. In A. R. Roberts & G. J. Greene (Eds.) *Social workers' desk reference* (pp.44–50). New York: Oxford.

Bauer, J. (2001a). The other half of the picture. *RN, 64*(11), 38–45.

Bauer, J. (2001b). Higher earnings, longer hours: 2001 earnings survey. *RN, 64*(10), 56–63.

Bentley, K. J. (1997). Should clinical social workers seek psychotropic medication prescription privileges? No. In B. A. Thyer (Ed.), *Controversial issues in social work practice* (pp. 152–165). Boston: Allyn & Bacon.

Bolter, K., Levenson, H., & Alverez, W. (1990). Differences in values between short-term and long-term therapists. *Professional Psychology, 21,* 285–290.

Buerhaus, P. I., Needleman, J., Mattke, S. & Stewart, M. (2002). Strengthening hospital nursing. *Health Affairs, 21*(5), 123–132.

Buerhaus, P. I., & Staiger, D. O. (1996). Managed care and the nurse workforce. *Journal of the American Medical Association, 276,* 1487–1493.

Colby, I., & Dziegielewski, S. F. (2001). *Social work: The people's profession.* Chicago: Lyceum.

Davis, S. R., & Meier, S. T. (2001). *The elements of managed care: A guide for helping professionals.* Belmont, CA: Brooks/Cole.

Deckro, G. R., Ballinger, K. M., Hoyt, M., Wilcher, M., Dusek, J., Myers, P., et al. (2002). The evaluation of a mind/body intervention to reduce psychological distress and perceived stress in college students. *Journal of American College Health, 50* (6), 1–14. Retrieved June 20, 2002, from http://ehostvgwll.epnet.com/ehost.asp.

Donald, A. (2002). Evidenced-based medicine: Key concepts. *Medscape Psychiatry and Mental Health Journal, 7*(2) 1–5. Retrieved from *http://www.medscape.com/viewarticle/430709.*

Dziegielewski, S. F. (1996). Managed care principles: The need for social work in the health care environment. *Crisis Intervention and Time-Limited Treatment, 3,* 97–110.

Dziegielewski, S. F. (1997a). Should clinical social workers seek psychotropic medication prescription privileges? Yes. In B. A. Thyer (Ed.), *Controversial issues in social work practice* (pp. 152–165). Boston: Allyn & Bacon.

Dziegielewski, S. F. (1997b). Time–limited brief therapy: The state of practice. *Crisis Intervention and Time Limited Treatment, 3,* 217–228.

Dziegielewski, S. F. (2002). *DSM-IV-TR™ in action.* New York: Wiley.

Dziegielewski, S. F., & Holliman, D. (2001). Managed care and social work: Practice implications in an era of change. *Journal of Sociology and Social Welfare, 28*(2), 125–138.

Dziegielewski, S. F., & Leon, A. M. (2001). *Psychopharmacology and social work practice.* New York: Springer Publishing Co.

Farley, O. W., Smith, L. L., Boyle, S. W., & Ronnau, J. (2002). A review of foundation MSW human behavior courses. *Journal of Human Behavior and the Social Environment, 6*(2), 1–12.

Flood, A. B., Shortell, S. M., & Scott, W. R. (1994). Organizational performance: Managing for efficiency and effectiveness. In S. M. Shortell & A. D. Kaluzny (Eds.), *Health care management: Organizational behavior and design* (3rd ed., pp. 316–351). Albany: Delmar.

Frager, S. (2000). *Managing managed care.* New York: Wiley.

Franklin, C. (2002). Developing effective practice competencies in managed behavioral health care. In A. R. Roberts & G. J. Greene (Eds.), *Social workers' desk reference* (pp. 1–9). New York: Oxford.

Gibbs, L. (2002). How social workers can do more good than harm: Clinical thinking, evidenced-based clinical reasoning, and avoiding fallacies. In A. R. Roberts & G. J. Greene (Eds.), *Social workers' desk reference.* (pp. 752–756). New York: Oxford.

Gibelman, M. (2002). Social work in an era of managed care. In A. R. Roberts & G. J. Greene (Eds.), *Social workers' desk reference.* (pp. 16–22). New York: Oxford.

Godbey, K. L., & Courage, M. M. (1994). Stress-management program: Intervention in nursing student performance anxiety. *Archives of Psychiatric Nursing* 8, 190–199.

Heaman, D. (1995). The Quieting Response (QR): A modality for reduction of psychophysiologic stress in nursing students. *Journal of Nursing Education, 34* (1), 5–10.

HSRA: Health and Human Services. (2002, June 4). *HHS Awards $30 Million to Address Emerging Nursing Shortage* [Press Release]. Retrieved 11/8/02 from http://www.hhs.gov/news/press/2002pres/20020604.html.

Hughes, W. C. (1999). Managed care meet community support: Ten reasons to include direct support services in every behavioral health plan. *Health and Social Work, 24,* 103–111.

Kimball, B., O'Neil, E., & Health Workforce Solutions. (2002, April). *Health Care's Human Crisis: The American Nursing Shortage* [For The Robert Wood Johnson Foundation]. Retrieved 11/8/02 from http://www.rwjf.org/publications/publicationsPdfs/nursing_report.pdf.

Maruish, M. E. (2002). *Essentials of treatment planning.* New York: Wiley.

Meenaghan, T. M. (2001). Exploring possible relations among social sciences, social work and health interventions. In G. Rosenberg & A. Weissman (Eds.), *Behavioral and social sciences in 21st century health care* (pp.43–50). New York: Haworth Social Work Practice Press.

National Association of Social Workers. (1993). *Choices: Careers in social work.* Washington, DC: National Association of Social Workers.

Pottage, D., & Huxley, P. (1996). Stress and mental health social work: A developmental perspective. *International Journal of Social Psychiatry, 42*(2), 124–131.

Quinless, F. W., & Elliot, N. L. (2000). The future in health care delivery. *Nursing and Health Care Perspectives, 21*(2), 84.

Resnick, C. A., & Dziegielewski, S. F. (1996). The relationship between therapeutic termination and job satisfaction among medical social workers. *Social Work in Health Care, 23* (3), 17–34.

Rock, B. (2002). Social work in health care in the 21st century. In A. R. Roberts & G. J. Greene (Eds.), *Social workers' desk reference.* (pp. 10–16). New York: Oxford.

Roembke, J. E., Jr. (1995). Prevention of burnout among graduate students and new professionals in mental health (Doctoral dissertation, Rosemead School of Psychology, Biola University, 1995). *Dissertation Abstracts International, 56* (6-A), 2177.

Rosen, A., & Proctor, E. K. (2002). Standards for evidenced-based social work practice: The role of replicable and appropriate interventions, outcomes and practice guidelines. In A. R. Roberts & G. J. Greene (Eds.), *Social workers' desk reference* (pp. 743–747). New York: Oxford

Rudolph, C. S. (2000). Educational challenges facing health care social workers in the twenty-first century. *Professional Development, 3*(1), 31–41.

Schram, B., & Mandell, B. R. (1997). *Human services: Policy and practice* (3rd ed.). Boston: Allyn & Bacon.

Sochalski, J. (2002). Nursing shortage redux: Turning the corner on an enduring problem. *Health Affairs, 21*(5), 157–164.

Sorenson, S., & Pinquart, M. (2001). Developing a measure of older adults' preparation for future care needs. *International Journal of Aging and Human Development, 53*, 137–165.

Spillman, B. C., & Pezzin, L. E. (2000). Potential and active family caregivers: Changing networks and the "sandwich generation." *Milbank Quaterly, 78*, 347–374, 339.

Strom-Gottfried, K., & Corcoran, K. (1998). Confronting ethical dilemmas in managed care: Guidelines for students and faculty. *Journal of Social Work Education, 34*(1), 109–119.

Strom-Gottfried, K., & Dunlap, K. M. (1999). Unraveling ethical dilemmas. *New Social Worker, 6*(2), 8–12.

Tanner, C., & Bellack, J. P. (2001). Resolving the nursing shortage: replacement plus one!. *Journal of Nursing Education, 40*(3), 99–100.

Thyer, B. A. (2002). Principles of evidenced-based practice and treatment development. In A. R. Roberts & G. J. Greene (Eds.), *Social workers' desk reference* (pp. 739–742). New York: Oxford.

Wells, R. A. (1994). *Planned short-term treatment* (2nd ed.). New York: Free Press.

Wiener, J. M., Estes, C. L., Goldenson, S. M., & Goldberg, S. C. (2001). What happened to long-term care in the health reform debate of 1993–1994?. *Milbank Quarterly, 79*, 207–252.

Wodarski, J., & Dziegielewski, S. F. (2001). Human behavior and the social environment: Integrating theory and evidenced-based practice. New York: Springer Publishing Co.

QUESTIONS FOR FURTHER STUDY

1. What do you see as the current role of the health care social worker?
2. What changes in the delivery of health care services should social workers be prepared to face?
3. What changes do social workers in this field need to be aware of? Once identified, what are some of the ways that these changes can be incorporated into the practice environment?

WEBSITES

AMSO Managed Care Forum
Home page for the American Medical Specialty Organization Managed Care Forum

The Brown School of Social Work at Washington University
University site with articles and information on health care and reform issues.
http://www.gwbweb.wustl.edu/websites.html

Health Care and Social Work
Accesses online articles from the above journal.
http://www.naswpress.org/publications/journals/journals.html

Health Care and Social Work Jobs
Job openings in the field.
http://www.quintcareers.com/healthcare_jobs.html

Home Page
A forum for debate on social work and health care research.
http://www.elsc.org.uk/

Journal of Social Work Practice
Contents and abstracts of articles in past issues.
http://www.tandf.co.uk/journals/carfax/02650533.html

National Council for Community Behavioral Healthcare
Advocates in Washington to advance the interests of members and consumers.
http://www.nccbh.org/

The New Social Worker's Online Career Center
Employment opportunities and job-seeking tips.
http://www.socialworker.com/career.htm

World Federation of Mental Health
An international nonprofit advocacy organization. Consultant to the UN and of public education programs such as World Mental Health Day.

http://www.wfmh.com
and other related health care issues. Forum to read and submit ideas
and information.
http://www.amso.com/

MEGASITES WITH LINKS TO HUNDREDS OF OTHER SITES

Health Finder
Selected online publications, databases, websites, government agencies, and not-for-profit organizations information.
http://www.healthfinder.org/

Social Work Search .Com
Provides over 500 different Internet links and related services
devoted solely to the social work profession.
http://www.socialworksearch.com/html/about.shtml

SWAN
The Social Work Access Network is sponsored by the University of
South Carolina College of Social Work; hundreds of links to social
work resources.
http://www.sc.edu/swan

World Wide Web Resources for Social Workers
Developed by New York University, this website contains hundreds
of links to social work resources in a wide range of topics.
http://www.nyu.edu/socialwork/wwwrsw/

Index